Phenolic Compounds: Extraction, Optimization, Identification and Applications in Food Industry

Editors

Ibrahim M. Abu-Reidah
Amani Taamalli

MDPI • Basel • Beijing • Wuhan • Barcelona • Belgrade • Manchester • Tokyo • Cluj • Tianjin

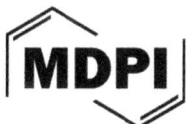

Editors
Ibrahim M. Abu-Reidah
Memorial University of Newfoundland
Canada

Amani Taamalli
University of Hafr Al Batin
Saudi Arabia

Editorial Office
MDPI
St. Alban-Anlage 66
4052 Basel, Switzerland

This is a reprint of articles from the Special Issue published online in the open access journal *Processes* (ISSN 2227-9717) (available at: https://www.mdpi.com/journal/processes/special_issues/Phenolic_Compounds_Industry).

For citation purposes, cite each article independently as indicated on the article page online and as indicated below:

LastName, A.A.; LastName, B.B.; LastName, C.C. Article Title. *Journal Name* **Year**, *Volume Number*, Page Range.

ISBN 978-3-0365-4175-4 (Hbk)
ISBN 978-3-0365-4176-1 (PDF)

© 2022 by the authors. Articles in this book are Open Access and distributed under the Creative Commons Attribution (CC BY) license, which allows users to download, copy and build upon published articles, as long as the author and publisher are properly credited, which ensures maximum dissemination and a wider impact of our publications.

The book as a whole is distributed by MDPI under the terms and conditions of the Creative Commons license CC BY-NC-ND.

Contents

About the Editors vii

Ibrahim M. Abu-Reidah and Amani Taamalli
Special Issue on "Phenolic Compounds: Extraction, Optimization, Identification and Applications in Food Industry"
Reprinted from: *Processes* **2022**, *10*, 128, doi:10.3390/pr10010128 1

Maria G. Campos, Christian Frigerio, Otilia Bobiş, Adriana C. Urcan and Nelson G. M. Gomes
Infrared Irradiation Drying Impact on Bee Pollen: Case Study on the Phenolic Composition of *Eucalyptus globulus* Labill and *Salix atrocinerea* Brot. Pollens
Reprinted from: *Processes* **2021**, *9*, 890, doi:10.3390/pr9050890 7

Colin M. Potter and David L. Jones
Polyphenolic Profiling of Green Waste Determined by UPLC-HDMS[E]
Reprinted from: *Processes* **2021**, *9*, 824, doi:10.3390/pr9050824 21

Josipa Vukoja, Ivana Buljeta, Anita Pichler, Josip Šimunović and Mirela Kopjar
Formulation and Stability of Cellulose-Based Delivery Systems of Raspberry Phenolics
Reprinted from: *Processes* **2021**, *9*, 90, doi:10.3390/pr9010090 35

Ivana Ivić, Mirela Kopjar, Lidija Jakobek, Vladimir Jukić, Suzana Korbar, Barbara Marić, Josip Mesić and Anita Pichler
Influence of Processing Parameters on Phenolic Compounds and Color of Cabernet Sauvignon Red Wine Concentrates Obtained by Reverse Osmosis and Nanofiltration
Reprinted from: *Processes* **2021**, *9*, 89, doi:10.3390/pr9010089 47

Shusheng Wang, Amy Hui-Mei Lin, Qingyou Han and Qin Xu
Evaluation of Direct Ultrasound-Assisted Extraction of Phenolic Compounds from Potato Peels
Reprinted from: *Processes* **2020**, *8*, 1665, doi:10.3390/pr8121665 63

Andreea Puşcaş, Andruţa Mureşan, Floricuţa Ranga, Florinela Fetea, Sevastiţa Muste, Carmen Socaciu and Vlad Mureşan
Phenolics Dynamics and Infrared Fingerprints during the Storage of Pumpkin Seed Oil and Thereof Oleogel
Reprinted from: *Processes* **2020**, *8*, 1412, doi:10.3390/pr8111412 77

Colin M. Potter and David L. Jones
Polyphenolic Profiling of Forestry Waste by UPLC-HDMS[E]
Reprinted from: *Processes* **2020**, *8*, 1411, doi:10.3390/pr8111411 93

Florin Banica, Simona Bungau, Delia Mirela Tit, Tapan Behl, Pavel Otrisal, Aurelia Cristina Nechifor, Daniela Gitea, Flavia-Maria Pavel and Sebastian Nemeth
Determination of the Total Polyphenols Content and Antioxidant Activity of *Echinacea Purpurea* Extracts Using Newly Manufactured Glassy Carbon Electrodes Modified with Carbon Nanotubes
Reprinted from: *Processes* **2020**, *8*, 833, doi:10.3390/pr8070833 105

Cecilia Castro-López, Catarina Gonçalves, Janeth M. Ventura-Sobrevilla, Lorenzo M. Pastrana, Cristóbal N. Aguilar-González and Guillermo C. G. Martínez-Ávila
Moringa oleifera—Storage Stability, *In Vitro*-Simulated Digestion and Cytotoxicity Assessment of Microencapsulated Extract
Reprinted from: *Processes* **2020**, *8*, 770, doi:10.3390/pr8070770 123

Cristian Hernández-Hernández, Cristóbal Noé Aguilar, Adriana Carolina Flores-Gallegos, Leonardo Sepúlveda, Raúl Rodríguez-Herrera, Jesús Morlett-Chávez, Mayela Govea-Salas and Juan Ascacio-Valdés
Preliminary Testing of Ultrasound/Microwave-Assisted Extraction (U/M-AE) for the Isolation of Geraniin from *Nephelium lappaceum* L. (Mexican Variety) Peel
Reprinted from: *Processes* **2020**, *8*, 572, doi:10.3390/pr8050572 137

Haifa Jebabli, Houda Nsir, Amani Taamalli, Ibrahim Abu-Reidah, Francisco Javier Álvarez-Martínez, Maria Losada-Echeberria, Enrique Barrajón Catalán and Ridha Mhamdi
Industrial-Scale Study of the Chemical Composition of Olive Oil Process-Derived Matrices
Reprinted from: *Processes* **2020**, *8*, 701, doi:10.3390/pr8060701 147

Thi Thuy Nguyen, Lan Phuong Doan, Thu Huong Trinh Thi, Hong Ha Tran, Quoc Long Pham, Hai Ha Pham Thi, Long Giang Bach, Bertrand Matthäus and Quoc Toan Tran
Fatty Acids, Tocopherols, and Phytosterol Composition of Seed Oil and Phenolic Compounds and Antioxidant Activity of Fresh Seeds from Three *Dalbergia* Species Grown in Vietnam
Reprinted from: *Processes* **2020**, *8*, 542, doi:10.3390/pr8050542 161

Mohamad Nasser, Hoda Cheikh-Ali, Akram Hijazi, Othmane Merah, Abd El-Ameer N. Al-Rekaby and Rana Awada
Phytochemical Profile, Antioxidant and Antitumor Activities of Green Grape Juice
Reprinted from: *Processes* **2020**, *8*, 507, doi:10.3390/pr8050507 173

Dongdong Wang, Jiansheng Huang, Andy Wai Kan Yeung, Nikolay T. Tzvetkov, Jarosław O. Horbańczuk, Harald Willschke, Zhibo Gai and Atanas G. Atanasov
The Significance of Natural Product Derivatives and Traditional Medicine for COVID-19
Reprinted from: *Processes* **2020**, *8*, 937, doi:10.3390/pr8080937 185

Mónica L. Chávez-González, Leonardo Sepúlveda, Deepak Kumar Verma, Hugo A. Luna-García, Luis V. Rodríguez-Durán, Anna Ilina and Cristobal N. Aguilar
Conventional and Emerging Extraction Processes of Flavonoids
Reprinted from: *Processes* **2020**, *8*, 434, doi:10.3390/pr8040434 211

About the Editors

Ibrahim M. Abu-Reidah has a Ph.D. in natural products and food chemistry and works at The Memorial University as a researcher. He manages several projects with the aim of developing new plant-based functional foods enriched with functional and active ingredients. His research approach involves multidisciplinary research themes from the industry and academia in the areas of agriculture, food science, analytical chemistry, biostatistics, and nutritional biochemistry; to assess the roles of phytochemicals in agriculture production, food, and human health outcomes. He has analytical expertise in pressurized solvent extraction, mass spectrometry, chromatography, and phytochemical identification. His research interests include functional foods production, bioactive phytochemical identification and separation, biological activities, R&D, safety, and preservationas well as to increase the yield, nutritional and value-added production in control systems agriculture.

Amani Taamalli has a PhD in Chemistry and works as an assistant professor. Her research interests focus on the extraction, analysis, and valorization of bioactive natural compounds. She is a reviewer and guest-editor in several ISI scientific journals, and is the author of 53 papers published on international peer-reviewed journals and scientific books. She was project coordinator and member in international scientific projects.

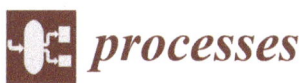

Editorial

Special Issue on "Phenolic Compounds: Extraction, Optimization, Identification and Applications in Food Industry"

Ibrahim M. Abu-Reidah [1,*] and Amani Taamalli [2]

1. School of Science and Environment, Memorial University of Newfoundland, St. John's, NL A1B 3X5, Canada
2. Department of Chemistry, University of Hafr Al Batin, P.O. Box 1803, Hafr Al Batin 31991, Saudi Arabia; amani.taamalli@cbbc.rnrt.tn
* Correspondence: iabureidah@grenfell.mun.ca

Interest has grown regarding natural plant extracts in food and beverage applications, their vital role in food quality and technology, and their therapeutic use in inhibiting several diseases. The protective properties of healthy diets rich in fruits, vegetables, and whole grains are due not only to fiber, vitamins, and minerals, but also to a variety of plant secondary metabolites, particularly phenolic compounds, which are considered among the most important classes originating in plant-derived secondary metabolites. Phenolic compounds or phenolics are well-renowned for their possession of a wide array of remarkable biochemical and pharmacological properties, namely, antioxidant, antiviral, anticancer, and anti-inflammatory activities, etc. Therefore, these compounds can be functional in the prevention of many diseases and in health maintenance, in addition to phenolic-varied applications in the food, nutraceutical, and pharmaceutical industries, and due to their importance in the pharma- and nutraceutical arenas. This Special Issue (SI) aims to gather the most recent contributions concerning their chemistry, extraction methods, and analytical techniques, along with their biological activities. The interpretation of phenolic bioactivities on a molecular basis by means of both well-established and advanced bio-analytical techniques is also covered in this SI.

This Special Issue of *Processes*, entitled "Phenolic Compounds: Extraction, Optimization, Identification and Applications in Food Industry" (https://www.mdpi.com/journal/processes/special_issues/Phenolic_Compounds_Industry, accessed on 23 December 2021), gathers the recent work of leading researchers in a single collection, and the content covers a variety of theoretical studies and experimental applications, focusing on the phenolic compounds extraction, identification, and applications in industry. We think that the advances described by the contributors in this SI have significantly helped accomplish this target. Aside from the research articles, the Special Issue features two reviews, covering a range of topics, which highlight the versatility of the area.

The topics covered in this SI include: advanced analytical methodologies for the isolation, purification, and analysis of phenolics from food, food wastes, and medicinal plants; phenolic compounds and metabolites in plants, food, and biological samples; biological activities and mechanisms of action; health benefits, in vivo evaluation; development of novel antioxidants and phenolics-based nutraceuticals and functional ingredients.

For instance, Campos et al., [1] discuss the drying impact on the phenolic composition of pollens of *Eucalyptus globulus* and *Salix atrocinerea* plant models by using infrared irradiation technology. This technique is used to determine the moisture content in pollens. Moreover, the influence of the IR radiation over the phenolic and flavonoid profiles has also been examined by HPLC/DAD profiling and radical scavenging ability by the DPPH assay. The IR-based method shows good reproducibility and, furthermore, it reduces drying time and energy consumption, thus having a low environmental impact, and it is suitable for

---

Citation: Abu-Reidah, I.M.; Taamalli, A. Special Issue on "Phenolic Compounds: Extraction, Optimization, Identification and Applications in Food Industry". *Processes* **2022**, *10*, 128. https://doi.org/10.3390/pr10010128

Received: 23 December 2021
Accepted: 24 December 2021
Published: 9 January 2022

Publisher's Note: MDPI stays neutral with regard to jurisdictional claims in published maps and institutional affiliations.

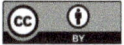

Copyright: © 2022 by the authors. Licensee MDPI, Basel, Switzerland. This article is an open access article distributed under the terms and conditions of the Creative Commons Attribution (CC BY) license (https://creativecommons.org/licenses/by/4.0/).

industrial scaling-up once no more degradation is found to occur during the radiation process.

Potter and Jones [2] studied the (poly)phenolic profiles of green waste determined by UPLC-HDMSE separation and detection techniques to identify the main phenolics present in four contrasting green waste feedstocks, viz. *Smyrnium olusatrum*, *Ulex europaeus*, *Allium ursinum*, and *Urtica dioica*. In this work, over 70 phenolic compounds with reported benefits to human health were identified, where *U. europaeus* was the most abundant in these compounds. Important components identified include among others procyanidins, naringenin, (−)-epigallocatechin, eriodictyol, naringenin, eriodictyol, iso-liquiritigenin and eriodictyol, plus several phytoestrogens, which highlights the importance of food waste through the formation of nutritional supplements.

Vukojaet al. [3] formulated raspberry juice phenolics and freeze-dried cellulose/ raspberry encapsulates by using cellulose as carrier and studied the influence of cellulose amount and time on the complexation of cellulose and raspberry juice. An increase in the amount of cellulose during formulation resulted in the decrease in the content of total phenolics and anthocyanins. Encapsulates with 2.5% of cellulose had the highest and those with 10% of cellulose the lowest capability for inhibition of α-amylase. They concluded that cellulose in low proportions could be used as a good encapsulation material for delivering bioactives as well as for the formulation of encapsulates.

Ivić et al. [4] studied the influence of processing parameters on phenolics and color of red wine concentrates attained by reverse osmosis and nanofiltration under different pressures and membrane conditions, in order to obtain highly enriched concentrates of phenolics. It was shown that the higher the pressure applied, the greater was the drop in retentates' temperature, as a favorable technique for higher phenolics retention. Several factors can affect the retention of individual compounds such as the operating conditions, membrane properties, chemical structure, and membrane fouling. Out of the two membrane types used, the highest concentrations of phenolics were detected in retentates obtained at around 50 bars, involving a cooling process.

The work of Wang et al. [5] involved the evaluation of phenolic compounds from potato peels and by-products by using direct ultrasound-assisted extraction system. In their study, they estimated the efficiency of various ultrasound-assisted extraction techniques, namely, direct ultrasound-assisted extraction (DUAE), indirect ultrasound-assisted extraction (IUAE), and conventional shaking extraction (CSE) in recovering antioxidants from potato peels. It was found that DUAE was more effective in extracting phenolic compounds than IUAE and CSE. Temperature, time, acoustic power, ratio of solvent to solids, and size of PPs particles were found to affect the yield of total phenolic compounds (TPC) in DUAE. DUAE was found with a higher yield TP comparable to commercial synthetic antioxidants, and the extraction rate was faster than IUAE and CSE. Furthermore, TPC yield was strongly correlated to the temperature of the mixture of the potato peels suspension. The study concluded that DUAE has the potential to transform potato peels from agricultural waste to functional ingredients.

In the work of Pușcaș et al. [6], phenolics dynamics and infrared fingerprints during the storage of pumpkin seed oil, and oleogel thereof, have been established. The work aimed to assess individual phenolics' dynamics and infrared fingerprints during the ambient storage of pumpkin seed oil, and oleogel thereof. Several phenolics including isolariciresinol, vanillin, caffeic and syringic acids were quantified. The main changes were determined for isolariciresinol, which decreased in liquid pumpkin seed oil samples from 0.77 to 0.13 mg/100 g, whereas for oleogel samples, it decreased from 0.64 to 0.12 mg/100 g. However, during the storage at room temperature, it was concluded that the oleogelation technique might display potential protection of specific phenolic compounds such as syringic acid and vanillin after 8 months of storage. For isolariciresinol, higher amounts are registered in the oleogel than in the oil after 5 months of ambient temperature storage, which may be due oxidation processes occurred after 5 months storage for both oil and oleogel samples.

Profiling of polyphenolics of several agro-forestry by-products by using UPLC-HDMSE was reported by Potter and Jones [7]. They used UPLC-HDMSE tool to profile ethanol extracts of three common tree barks (*Pinus contorta*, *Pinus sylvestris*, *Quercus robur*). About 35 high scoring components with reported significance to health were tentatively characterized across the three bark extracts. Scots Pine showed generally higher compound abundances than the other two extracts. Although Oak bark extract had the lowest abundances, it exhibited higher amounts of naringenin and 3-O-methylrosmarinic acid. The study concluded that forestry bark waste can provide a rich source of extractable polyphenols suitable for use in food supplements.

In their study, Banica et al. [8] used a newly sensitive invented glassy carbon sensitive electrodes with carbon nanotubes to assess the total polyphenols content and antioxidant activity of *Echinacea purpurea* extracts. In this investigation, three glassy carbon electrodes (GCE) were used; three different pharmaceutical forms (capsules, tablets, and tincture) were assessed, which contain aerial or root parts of *E. pururea* extracts. The modified [1 mg/mL CNTs/CS 5%/GCE] electrode has superior properties compared with the other two (the unmodified and (20 mg/mL CNTs/CS 0.5%/GCE-modified)) electrodes used in the study. Echinacea tincture had the highest antioxidant capacity and total amount of polyphenols, whereas capsules and tablets had the lowest antioxidant capacity and the lowest total amount of polyphenols. Pulse-differential cyclic voltammetry represents a rapid, simple, and sensitive technique to establish the entire polyphenolic amount and the antioxidant activity of the *E. purpurea* extracts.

The storage stability of microencapsulated extract of *Moringa oleifera* was studied by Castro-López et al. [9], by assessing its in vitro-simulated digestion and cytotoxicity assessment. The extract was processed by spray-drying technique using tragacanth gum (MorTG) to improve its stability. The results of the study showed that TPC was as follows—oral (9.7%), gastric (35.2%), and intestinal (57.6%). The in vitro antioxidant activity in digestion was 300% higher than the initial value. Moreover, microencapsulated moringa extract presented a half-life up to 45 days of storage, where the noticeable change was observed at 35 °C and 52.9% relative humidity. Caco-2 cells' viability demonstrated non-cytotoxicity, which supports the safety of the proposed formulation and potential use within the food field.

A preliminary testing of ultrasound/microwave-assisted extraction (u/m-ae) for the isolation of geraniin from *Nephelium lappaceum* l. peel was reported by Hernández-Hernández et al. [10]. Five extractions were performed using different (mass/volume) and ethanol/water ratios. Condition 1:16-0 was defined as the best extraction condition (only water). The major compound isolated in the two separations was geraniin, according to HPLC/ESI/MS analysis.

Jebabli et al. [11] designed an industrial-scale study of the chemical composition of olive oil process-derived matrices to investigate the effect of the industrial process and collecting period on produced olive oil and by-products was evaluated. The obtained results showed significant variations for most quality indices before and after vertical centrifugation between all samples from the three collecting periods. All the tested samples were enriched in monounsaturated fatty acid: Oleic acid (C18:1) with a maximum of 69.95%. The total polyphenols and individual phenolic compounds varied significantly through the extraction process, with a significant variation between olive oil and by-products. Remarkably, the percentage of secoiridoids and their derivatives was significant in paste and olive oil, emphasizing the activity of many enzymes released during the different extraction steps. Regarding antioxidant capacity, the most remarkable result was detected in olive oil and olive mill wastewater samples.

Nguyen et al. [12] investigated Vietnamese Dalbergia species for their fresh seeds and oil composition of fatty acids, tocopherols, and phytosterol, phenolic compounds and antioxidant activity. Among the examined samples, *D. tonkinensis* seed oils showed high contents of linoleic acid, whereas in *D. mammosa*, oleic acid was predominant. Moreover, α- and γ-tocopherol and β-sitosterol were major ingredients in the seed oils, whereas ferulic acid and rosmarinic acid are usually predominant in the seeds of these species. Concerning sterol composition, the *D. entadoides* seed oil figured for remarkably high content of Δ7-stigmastenol and Δ5,23-stigmastadienol. Moreover, extracts with methanol/water of seeds displayed significant in vitro antioxidant activity which was determined by DPPH free radical scavenging assay.

In his study, Nasser et al. [13] explored the phytochemical profile, biological properties of green grape verjuice. Antioxidant and antitumor activities have been assessed and various conventional methods were used to quantify the alkaloids and tannins. Results show that the verjuice extract contains alkaloids, tannins, and a high quantity of total flavonoids and total phenols. Aside from its antioxidant activity, verjuice significantly repressed human pulmonary adenocarcinoma (A549) cells' viability in both time- and dose-dependent manners. Furthermore, verjuice extract significantly enhanced the anticancer potential of cisplatin. This study suggests a potential use of verjuice as a natural antitumor therapy.

The review of Wang et al. [14] reported an overview of natural products and their derivatives, the traditional medicine products, already described in the literature with potential to inhibit and manage SARS-CoV-2 in vitro, in vivo, or in clinical reports or trials. The study proposed that randomized, double-blind, and placebo-controlled large clinical trials are necessary to deliver solid evidence for the potential effective treatment. In addition, they suggested that carefully combined cocktails need to be assessed for preventing the COVID-19 pandemic and the resulting global health concerns thereof.

The review of Chávez-González et al. [15] entailed a comparison between the conventional and emerging extraction processes of flavonoids, which are found in plant-based foods and beverages as anon-energetic components. In this study, they examine, analyze, and discuss recent methodologies for biotechnological recovery/extraction of flavonoids from agro-industrial residues, describing the challenges and advances in the topic.

We would thank all the contributors and the Editor-in-Chief, Giancarlo Cravotto, for their enthusiastic support of the Special Issue, as well as the editorial staff of *Processes* for their efforts, and the SI manger, Ella Qiao.

Author Contributions: Conceptualization, I.M.A.-R. and A.T.; methodology, I.M.A.-R. and A.T.; software, I.M.A.-R. and A.T.; validation, I.M.A.-R. and A.T.; investigation, I.M.A.-R. and A.T.; data curation, I.M.A.-R. and A.T.; writing—original draft preparation, I.M.A.-R. and A.T.; writing—review and editing, I.M.A.-R. and A.T.; project administration, I.M.A.-R. and A.T. All authors have read and agreed to the published version of the manuscript.

Funding: This research received no external funding.

Conflicts of Interest: The authors declare no conflict of interest.

References

1. Campos, M.G.; Frigerio, C.; Bobiş, O.; Urcan, A.C.; Gomes, N.G.M. Infrared Irradiation Drying Impact on Bee Pollen: Case Study on the Phenolic Composition of *Eucalyptus globulus* Labill and *Salix atrocinerea* Brot. Pollens. *Processes* **2021**, *9*, 890. [CrossRef]
2. Potter, C.; Jones, D. Polyphenolic Profiling of Green Waste Determined by UPLC-HDMSE. *Processes* **2021**, *9*, 824. [CrossRef]
3. Vukoja, J.; Buljeta, I.; Pichler, A.; Šimunović, J.; Kopjar, M. Formulation and Stability of Cellulose-Based Delivery Systems of Raspberry Phenolics. *Processes* **2021**, *9*, 90. [CrossRef]
4. Ivić, I.; Kopjar, M.; Jakobek, L.; Jukić, V.; Korbar, S.; Marić, B.; Mesić, J.; Pichler, A. Influence of Processing Parameters on Phenolic Compounds and Color of Cabernet Sauvignon Red Wine Concentrates Obtained by Reverse Osmosis and Nanofiltration. *Processes* **2021**, *9*, 89. [CrossRef]
5. Wang, S.; Lin, A.; Han, Q.; Xu, Q. Evaluation of Direct Ultrasound-Assisted Extraction of Phenolic Compounds from Potato Peels. *Processes* **2020**, *8*, 1665. [CrossRef]
6. Puşcaş, A.; Mureşan, A.; Ranga, F.; Fetea, F.; Muste, S.; Socaciu, C.; Mureşan, V. Phenolics Dynamics and Infrared Fingerprints during the Storage of Pumpkin Seed Oil and Thereof Oleogel. *Processes* **2020**, *8*, 1412. [CrossRef]
7. Potter, C.; Jones, D. Polyphenolic Profiling of Forestry Waste by UPLC-HDMSE. *Processes* **2020**, *8*, 1411. [CrossRef]
8. Banica, F.; Bungau, S.; Tit, D.; Behl, T.; Otrisal, P.; Nechifor, A.; Gitea, D.; Pavel, F.M.; Nemeth, S. Determination of the Total Polyphenols Content and Antioxidant Activity of Echinacea Purpurea Extracts Using Newly Manufactured Glassy Carbon Electrodes Modified with Carbon Nanotubes. *Processes* **2020**, *8*, 833. [CrossRef]

9. Castro-López, C.; Gonçalves, C.; Ventura-Sobrevilla, J.; Pastrana, L.; Aguilar-González, C.; Martínez-Ávila, G. Moringa oleifera—Storage Stability, In Vitro-Simulated Digestion and Cytotoxicity Assessment of Microencapsulated Extract. *Processes* **2020**, *8*, 770. [CrossRef]
10. Hernández-Hernández, C.; Aguilar, C.; Flores-Gallegos, A.; Sepúlveda, L.; Rodríguez-Herrera, R.; Morlett-Chávez, J.; Govea-Salas, M.; Ascacio-Valdés, J. Preliminary Testing of Ultrasound/Microwave-Assisted Extraction (U/M-AE) for the Isolation of Geraniin from Nephelium lappaceum L. (Mexican Variety) Peel. *Processes* **2020**, *8*, 572. [CrossRef]
11. Jebabli, H.; Nsir, H.; Taamalli, A.; Abu-Reidah, I.; Álvarez-Martínez, F.J.; Losada-Echeberria, M.; Barrajón Catalán, E.; Mhamdi, R. Industrial-Scale Study of the Chemical Composition of Olive Oil Process-Derived Matrices. *Processes* **2020**, *8*, 701. [CrossRef]
12. Nguyen, T.T.; Doan, L.P.; Trinh Thi, T.H.; Tran, H.H.; Pham, Q.L.; Pham Thi, H.H.; Bach, L.G.; Matthäus, B.; Tran, Q.T. Fatty Acids, Tocopherols, and Phytosterol Composition of Seed Oil and Phenolic Compounds and Antioxidant Activity of Fresh Seeds from Three Dalbergia Species Grown in Vietnam. *Processes* **2020**, *8*, 542. [CrossRef]
13. Nasser, M.; Cheikh-Ali, H.; Hijazi, A.; Merah, O.; Al-Rekaby, A.; Awada, R. Phytochemical Profile, Antioxidant and Antitumor Activities of Green Grape Juice. *Processes* **2020**, *8*, 507. [CrossRef]
14. Wang, D.; Huang, J.; Yeung, A.W.K.; Tzvetkov, N.T.; Horbańczuk, J.O.; Willschke, H.; Gai, Z.; Atanasov, A.G. The Significance of Natural Product Derivatives and Traditional Medicine for COVID-19. *Processes* **2020**, *8*, 937. [CrossRef]
15. Chávez-González, M.; Sepúlveda, L.; Verma, D.; Luna-García, H.; Rodríguez-Durán, L.; Ilina, A.; Aguilar, C. Conventional and Emerging Extraction Processes of Flavonoids. *Processes* **2020**, *8*, 434. [CrossRef]

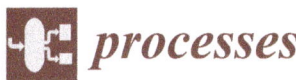 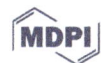

Article

Infrared Irradiation Drying Impact on Bee Pollen: Case Study on the Phenolic Composition of *Eucalyptus globulus* Labill and *Salix atrocinerea* Brot. Pollens

Maria G. Campos [1,2,*], Christian Frigerio [1], Otilia Bobiş [3], Adriana C. Urcan [4] and Nelson G. M. Gomes [5]

1. Laboratory of Pharmacognosy, Faculty of Pharmacy, Health Sciences Campus, University of Coimbra, Azinhaga de Santa Comba, 3000-548 Coimbra, Portugal; christian.frigerio.ff.up@gmail.com
2. CQ-Centre of Chemistry—Coimbra, Department of Chemistry, Faculty of Sciences and Technology, University of Coimbra, Rua Larga, 3004-535 Coimbra, Portugal
3. Life Science Institute, University of Agricultural Sciences and Veterinary Medicine Cluj-Napoca, 3-5 Mănăștur Street, 400372 Cluj-Napoca, Romania; obobis@usamvcluj.ro
4. Department of Microbiology and Immunology, Faculty of Animal Science and Biotechnologies, University of Agricultural Sciences and Veterinary Medicine, 3-5 Mănăștur Street, 400372 Cluj-Napoca, Romania; adriana.urcan@usamvcluj.ro
5. REQUIMTE/LAQV, Laboratório de Farmacognosia, Departamento de Química, Faculdade de Farmácia, Universidade do Porto, R. Jorge Viterbo Ferreira, nº 228, 4050-313 Porto, Portugal; ngomes@ff.up.pt
* Correspondence: mgcampos@ff.uc.pt

Abstract: Bee pollen is commonly reputed as a rich source of nutrients, both for bees and humans. Its composition is well balanced and can be taken as a stand-alone food or as supplement, including for the elderly owing its low caloric value. However, storage conditions frequently lead to product degradation, namely due to the high moisture content that enable the proliferation of molds and bacteria. Herein, an infrared (IR)-based technology is proposed as a mean to determine moisture content, setting also a new scalable approach for the development of a drying technology to be used for bee pollen processing, which can be carried out in a short time, without impacting the phenolic and flavonoid content and associated bioactive effects. Proof-of-concept was attained with an IR moisture analyzer, bee pollen samples from *Eucalyptus globulus* Labill and *Salix atrocinerea* Brot. being selected as models. Impact of the IR radiation towards the phenolic and flavonoid profiles was screened by HPLC/DAD profiling and radical scavenging ability by the DPPH assay. The IR-based approach shows good reproducibility while simultaneously reducing drying time and energy consumption, thus implying a low environmental impact and being suitable for industrial scale-up once no degradation has been found to occur during the radiation process.

Keywords: bee pollen; cinnamic acid derivatives; food processing; kaempferol glycosides; luteolin; quercetin glycosides; tricetin

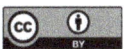

1. Introduction

Bee pollen is long known and classified as a food product [1], with a series of health benefits mainly attributed to a high content in phenolic constituents. While widely consumed, its preservation and quality control remain critical and call for further studies in this matter. Bee pollen is produced by the agglutination of selected flower pollens made by the worker bees, with nectar (and/or honey) and salivary substances, being collected at the entrance of the hive as small bolls, often named as pellets [2].

While scarce, currently available legislation defines bee pollen as a food, but some gaps dealing with its quality control remain to be filled, additional guidelines being currently proposed in the framework of an International Standard ISO normalization. The International Organization for Standardization includes the Working Group "TC 34/SC 19 Bee products, subgroup W3-Bee pollen", that intends to implement guidelines and procedures for the standardization of the processing and circulation of bee products. One of the main challenges is to ensure a convenient preservation of the nutrients along with the bioactive compounds, which prompted us to conceptualize the current study.

Bee pollen is mostly commercialized in a dehydrated form, major chemical modifications of the components being assured through an appropriate drying process, which is crucial, for example, to avoid mold contamination [2]. However, most of the currently available drying methods are characterized by high energy consumption and a concomitant environmental impact.

Indeed, several studies delivered experimental evidence on the nutritional value of bee pollen, being portrayed as a fine food supplement [3,4] due to its high content in macronutrients, with well-balanced proportions of proteins, lipids, and carbohydrates, along with micronutrients and bioactive compounds, namely simple phenolic constituents and a series of polyphenols, flavonoids being particularly reputed in this matter. Nowadays, there is a high demand for food sources with low caloric impact but with a high value in nutrients, and bee pollen is certainly one of the most popular food products amongst the elderly [5]. According to Peris [6], 15 g of bee pollen supplies the required daily dose of amino acids. The caloric value of bee pollen was estimated by others at 381.70 kcal (1595.51 Kj) for 100 g [7] which gives a significant additional value to hypocaloric diets. In addition to its nutritional value, a myriad of potential therapeutic properties of bee pollen have been also suggested based on an increasing number of studies being carried out in the last two decades (among many others [8–11]). However, it is worth to mention that only a few address the allergenicity of bee pollen and the storage of fresh and dry samples [12,13].

Besides the requirements dealing with the nutritional content and the possible presence of additives, such as pesticides or antibiotics, unequivocal identification of the floral origin of bee-pollen and the preservation process are of utmost importance.

The floral composition is affected by phytogeographical, genetic modifications and seasonal factors [14–16]. A consistent work being carried out by us delivering data on hand-collected pollen, herbarium specimens and bee pollen samples, gathered in different locations and years, to perform the identification of bee pollen floral origins [17–23]. The method previously described by Campos et al., [17,18] enables the identification of pollen *taxon* by the HPLC-DAD-based phenolic/polyphenolic profiling of hydroalcoholic extracts. Generation of a chemical fingerprint that is species-specific (specific for each species of pollen origin), was found to be more sensitive and precise than the microscopic analysis, as it allows the identification of each *taxon*, to genera and species. Nevertheless, pollen shells, obtained after centrifugation of the hydroalcoholic extracts should be further analyzed on their morphological features. Relevantly, cumulative evidence suggests that the profile of each *taxon* is independent of geographical or climatic factors, which makes this method universal. Considering the above, the current study aims (i) to unequivocally identify the floral source of the crude materials used in this "Case Study", and (ii) to investigate the impact of infrared (IR) radiation on the phenolic fingerprint in selected pollen samples. Radical scavenging ability was also assayed to further detail on the potential influence of IR on the extracts and the impact on the bioactive properties known to rely on phenolic compounds. The main end-point of the current work is to mimic a drying process with IR irradiation, with a low environmental impact due to the rapid, cheap, and accurate drying approach, thus setting a new perspective for further industrial drying applications.

2. Materials and Methods

2.1. Chemicals

Reference compounds were purchased from various suppliers: 2,2-diphenyl-1-picrylhydrazyl radical (DPPH), L-ascorbic acid and rutin were purchased from Sigma-Aldrich (St. Louis, MO, USA), ethanol 99% from Panreac (Castellar del Vallès, Spain), o-phosphoric acid and acetonitrile from Merck (Darmstradt, Germany). Water was treated in a Milli-Q (Millipore, Bedford, MA, USA) water purification system.

2.2. Bee Pollen Samples

Samples of bee pollen were collected in Lavos (Figueira da Foz, Portugal), immediately frozen and stored at −21 °C until analysis. Pollen pellets were separated by hand, according to their morphological features. Identification of each *taxon* was carried out by HPLC/DAD analysis of their hydroalcoholic extracts (details in the extraction section) according to [17,18]. Briefly, HPLC/DAD profiling delivers different phenolic fingerprints, their comparison with an internal database of floral pollen sources allowing the identification of the species of each *taxon* under analysis. The sediments, obtained after centrifugation of the hydroalcoholic extracts, were further analyzed on their morphological characters in a Leitz Laborlux microscope to further confirm the *taxon* of the separated *taxa* from the entire mixture [17]. After confirmation of the two main floral sources in a mixed sample, a representative amount of bee pollen pellets was separated, and identified as follows: *Eucalyptus globulus* Labill (sample 1) and *Salix atrocinerea* Brot. (sample 2).

2.3. Drying Process

The IR drying process has been performed with a moisture analyzer (Kern MLB 50-3) and optimized to reach a residual humidity of ca. 4% as recommended by others [2]. To determine the reproducibility of the IR method, five random samples of bee pollen with different water content were used. A standard drying process was also performed in an oven-drying system, operating at 40 °C, until constant weight was recorded. This procedure is done with a mean time of approximately 4 h and 45 min in a heater, until the relative humidity reached the required values.

2.4. Moisture Determination

Water content determination was also performed by two different methods. For the IR-based method the moisture analyzer (Kern MLB 50-3) was used. Five aliquots of 1 g of sample were dried at 50 °C until constant weight for three steps of 45 s.

The methods described on the Codex Alimentarius, European Pharmacopoeia and Portuguese Pharmacopoeia, are very similar, and were used as references [24].

2.5. Extracts Preparation

Fresh and dry samples of the two different *taxa* (*E. globulus* and *S. atrocinerea*) were extracted with a mixture of ethanol:water (1:1, v/v) at the concentration of 20 mg/mL and 10 mg/mL, respectively, using ultrasonication (30 min). Insoluble material was separated by centrifugation (6000 rpm/5 min) and used for microscopic analysis confirmation. The supernatant was immediately analyzed by HPLC/DAD for phenolic fingerprint and spectrophotometric analysis of free radical scavenging activity using the DPPH method, as below described.

2.6. Chromatographic Analysis

Chromatographic analyses were carried out by HPLC/DAD [18]. Briefly, 20 µL of fresh pollen extract and 10 µL of dried bee pollen extract were analyzed in a Gilson 170, separation being attained with a Waters Spherisorb ODS2 (5 mm) column (4.6 × 250 mm) by an acidified water-acetonitrile gradient with a flow rate of 0.8 mL/min, and a column temperature of 24 °C. Standard chromatograms were plotted at λ_{max} 260 and 340 nm. Spectral data for all peaks were accumulated in the range 220–400 nm using DAD (Gilson 170) and further analyzed with the software Unipoint. The suitability of the method was previously evaluated by Campos [17].

All the extracts were submitted to a qualitative and quantitative analysis of the main phenolic constituents. Structural determination of the phenolic compounds was performed according to the theoretical rules presented in Campos and Markham [25] and by comparison with our internal spectral database [25]. Concentrations were determined using the following standard curve equation obtained with rutin (1) (A = HPLC peak area):

$$y = 4.2159 \times 10^{-9} A + 0.0062 \; R^2 = 0.9996 \quad (1)$$

2.7. Free Radical Scavenging Activity

To evaluate the impact of IR radiation in the bioactivity of the extracts and the potential interference with the phenolic content, as phenolic constituents act as reference compounds in the preservation of the integrity of the samples, both pollen extracts were also used to determine the free radical scavenging activity upon the 2,2 diphenyl-picrylhydrazyl (DPPH) radical. The method was performed according to Campos et al., [19]. Measurements were carried out on a UV/VIS spectrophotometer Hitachi U-2000. Briefly, 2.5 mL of DPPH solution (5.96 mg in 250 mL of 1:1 ethanol/water solution) were mixed with an appropriate amount of extract (10, 20, 40, 60, 80, 100 µL), followed immediately by homogenization. After 10 min, quantification of the remaining DPPH radicals was recorded from the absorption at 517 nm. The reference standard was ascorbic acid with an EC_{50} value of 2.41 µg/mL.

2.8. Statistical Analysis

All determinations were performed in quintuplicate, for the moisture determination, or in triplicate, for the DPPH assay and chromatographic analysis. Graphics were created with STATISTICA 7 software. Classical statistical analysis was performed. DPPH test's results for the different drying methods were compared by t-test for variance ($p \leq 0.05$) with Microsoft Excel software. Validation of the moisture determination by Kern MLB 50-3 was done by Z-score test versus a standard method.

3. Results

3.1. Water Content Determination

The IR method reproducibility was studied using five bee pollen samples with a different water content (Table 1). The calculated relative standard deviation (RSD) ranged from 58.9%, determined for the fresh pollen (RH% = 27.77%), to 7.494% recorded with the dried samples (RH% = 2.25%). The method was validated by comparison with the standard methods described in the Portuguese Pharmacopoeia [24] using Z-score test. Admitting an error of the average of ±0.2% (the measurement uncertainty indicated by the Kern MLB 50-3 specifications) the moisture analyzer did not show any relevant differences comparing with the standard drying method.

Table 1. IR method reproducibility with different bee pollen samples containing different amounts of water.

	Sample 1	Sample 2	Sample 3	Sample 4	Sample 5
	11.79	27.82	26.1	2.26	22.34
	11.48	27.79	26.1	1.3	23.94
	11.08	27.88	25.88	2.19	22.05
	11.49	27.48	25.09	2.48	22.69
	11.61	27.86	25.86	2.08	22.79
Std deviation	0.26	0.16	0.42	0.17	0.34
Average	11.49	27.77	25.81	2.25	22.47
RSD%	2.27	0.59	1.61	7.49	1.51

Briefly, as evaluated with samples (1 g) of bee pollen, optimal drying performance was observed at 40 °C for 10 min. These parameters were optimized after a previous determination of the better conditions to be used in this IR-based drying process. No differences on the water content were observed between the two species under study, determined as 24.73 ± 0.21% for *E. globulus* and 24.77 ± 0.35% for *S. atrocinerea*.

3.2. Infrared Drying Process

The IR drying process was optimized considering the drying rate of different samples (1 g each), i.e., the time (in minutes) required to achieve a final moisture of 4%. As showed in Figure 1, a linear relationship was found between the IR exposure time and the relative humidity loss (ΔRH%) at 40 °C. This relationship is described by the equation:

$$Dt = 2.3172 \times \Delta RH\% + 0.2445; R^2 = 0.9776, \text{ where } Dt \text{ is the drying time (min)} \quad (2)$$

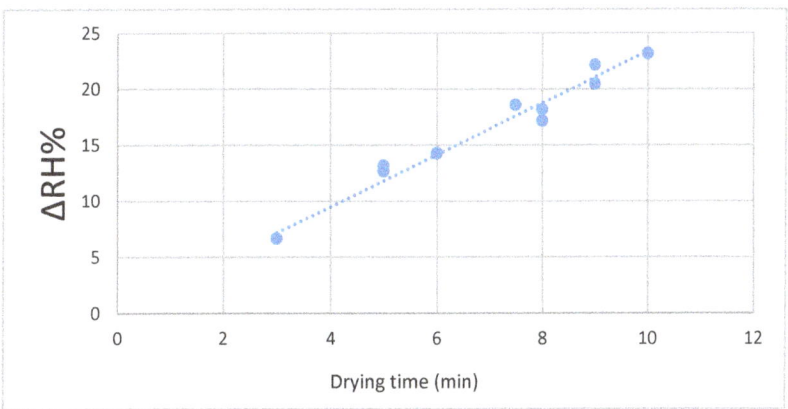

Figure 1. Relationship between the IR drying time and the relative humidity loss (ΔRH%) at 40 °C.

3.3. Pollen Phenolic/Flavonoid Profile

HPLC/DAD chromatographic analysis of the hydroethanolic pollen extracts was performed aiming to determine the pollen floral origin [18,26] and also to detect a possible interference with the qualitative and/or quantitative phenolic profiles (used as biomarkers) due to exposure to the IR radiation during the drying process. Phenolic profiles of the two samples, and the corresponding UV spectral data, are presented in Figure 2. The hydroethanolic extract obtained from *E. globulus* bee pollen (Figure 2a) was characterized by the occurrence quercetin-3-*O*-(β-D-glucopyranosyl-2-β-D-glucopyranoside) (namely quercetin-3-*O*-sophoroside) (RT 35.63), myricetin (RT 44.31), tricetin (RT 45.28), luteolin (RT 50.58) and 3-*O*-methylquercetin (RT 51.62), in addition to two cinnamic acid derivatives (RTs 57.11 and 57.67). These compounds were previously isolated from samples of *E. globulus* pollen, their structures being elucidated by NMR experiments (^{1}H and ^{13}C-NMR; ^{1}H,^{1}H-COSY; ^{1}H,^{13}C-COSY) [17,18]. Kaempferol-3-*O*-(β-D-rhamnopyranosyl-2-β-D-glucopyranoside) (namely kaempferol-3-*O*-neohesperoside) (RT 38.62) was detected as the main phenolic constituent on the hydroethanolic extract obtained from *S. atrocinerea* bee pollen samples, lower amounts of 3-*O*-glycosylated derivatives of quercetin (RT 37.04) and kaempferol (RT 39.26) being determined. Two caffeic acid derivatives (RT 45.31 and RT 46.52) were also identified. The profile (Figure 2b) was found to be identical to a previously described for *S. atrocinerea* in Campos et al. [18].

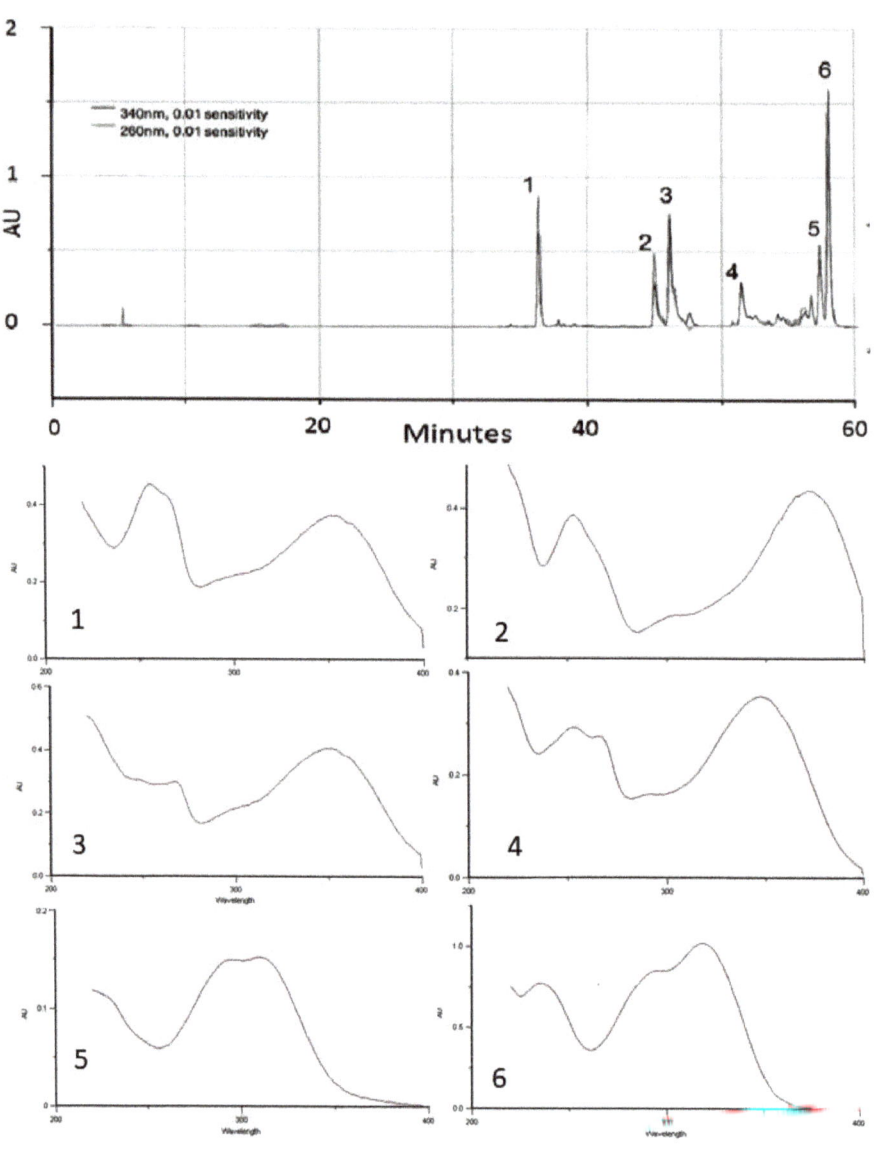

(a)

Figure 2. *Cont.*

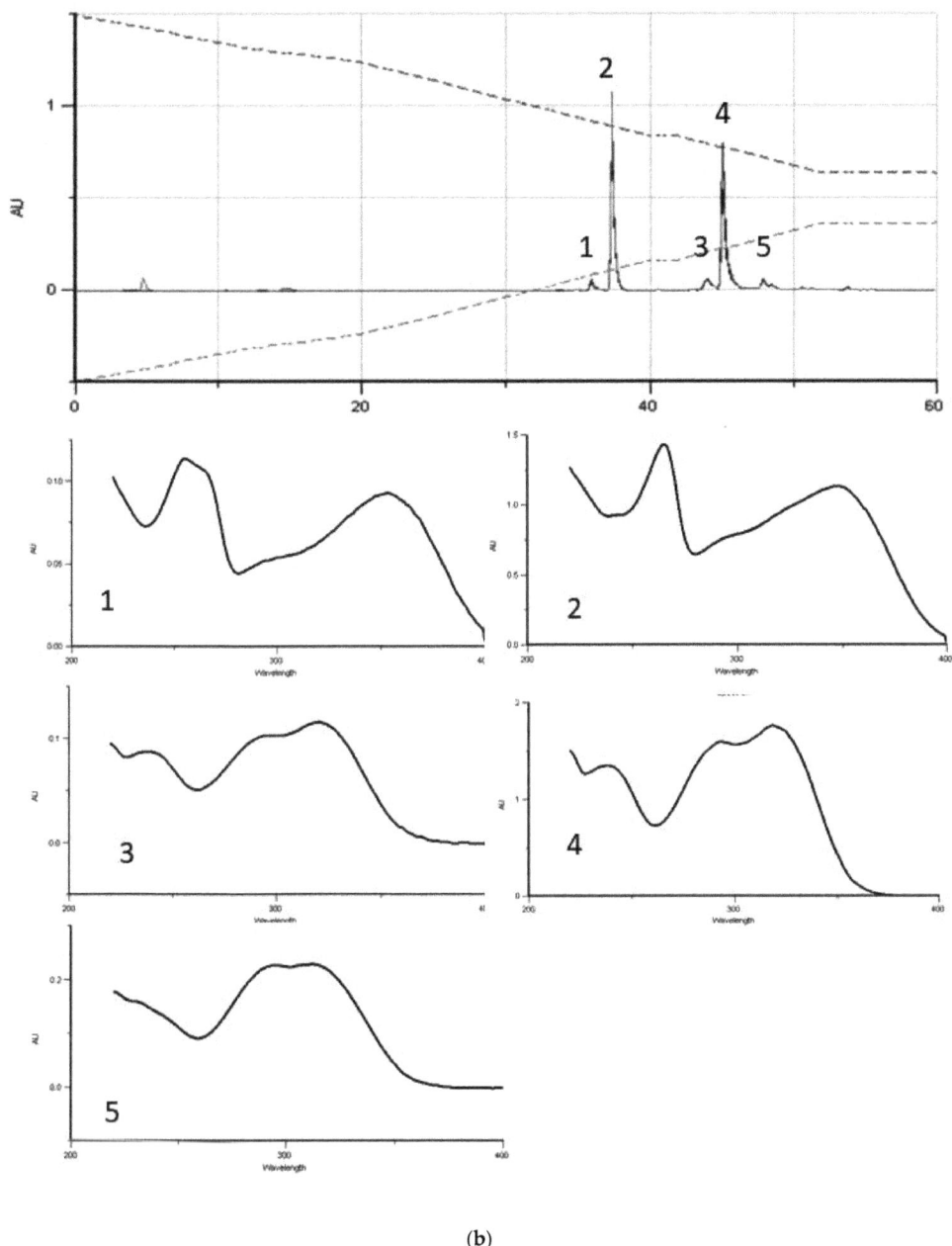

(b)

Figure 2. Phenolic/Flavonoidic profile of the two samples. (**a**) *E. globulus*; (**b**) *S. atrocinerea* obtained with HPLC/DAD analysis and plotted at 260 and 340 nm; Right side of the figure show the respective UV-spectra for each flavonoid and phenolic acid derivatives. (**a**) Compounds: 1. Quercetin-3-O-sophoroside; 2. myricitin; 3. tricetin; 4. luteolin; 5 and 6. derivatives of cinnamic acid-1 and 2 (spermidine); (**b**) Compounds: 1. Quercetin-3-O-sophoroside; 2. kaempferol-3-O-neohesperidoside; 3. 4 and 5. derivatives of caffeic acid.

The identification of each *taxon* was in agreement and further corroborated with the results obtained by microscopic analysis.

3.4. IR Radiation Effect on Phenolic Composition and on the Radical Scavenger Bioactivity

It is well known that bee pollen has a significant free radical scavenging activity [19,27–29], which is normally species-specific, dependent on similar phenolic/flavonoid profiles [19], and independent from exogenous parameters (geographical origin, climate, etc.). As such, these two parameters can be used as biomarkers of quality for bee pollen. As expected, the free radical scavenger activity of bee pollen is time-dependent and decreases with prolonged storage time [17,19].

Currently, there is no data dealing with the influence of post harvesting processing, namely with the drying processes by irradiation with IR, on the radical scavenging properties and/or in the HPLC/DAD profile of the phenolic/flavonoid compounds from bee pollen. The DPPH radical scavenging activity, expressed in EC_{50}, was assayed to evaluate the impact of the IR radiation.

All samples exhibited antiradical activity (Figure 3) with a linear concentration-dependency. Samples of *E. globulus* bee pollen showed EC_{50} values slightly above from those of previously reported data, suggesting a slight decrease in the antiradical ability [17,19]. Comparison of the EC_{50} values determined for the fresh pollen samples and the dried ones (by T-test for variance; $p \leq 0.05$) denotes a small decrease in the scavenging activity of the IR dried samples. No statistically relevant variation was detected in comparison with the traditional (standard) drying method. Fresh samples of *S. atrocinera* bee pollen showed high scavenging activity (around 100 µg/mL DPPH solution). As show in Figure 3, the activity remained unchanged with both drying processes.

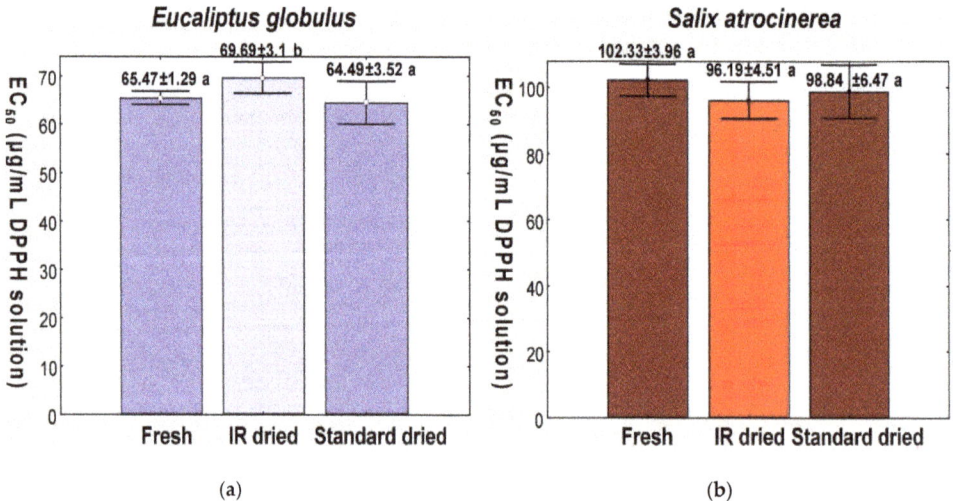

Figure 3. DPPH assay results for different drying methods expressed as EC50 (µg/mL DPPH solution). Results represents means ± SD (n = 3) (**a**,**b**) groups concordance by *t*-test analysis for variance ($p \leq 0.05$): (**a**) Data from *Eucalyptus globulus* bee pollen samples; (**b**) Data from *Salix atrocinera* bee pollen samples.

Subsequently, the profile obtained by HPLC-DAD was used to study the influence of the drying process on the qualitative and quantitative profiles of the major phenolic constituents. Pollen samples were submitted to two distinct drying procedures, the standard drying method in oven-drying at 40 °C until the RH% reached 4%, and the optimized IR drying process. Then, hydroethanolic extracts obtained with the dried pollen samples were analyzed by HPLC-DAD and assessed on their radical scavenging activity (DPPH-method), to further investigate the impact of the IR radiation in the drying processing.

Chromatographic profiles of extracts obtained from the dried samples of E. globulus (IR and standard drying methods) matched perfectly with the phenolic profile of the extract obtained from fresh bee pollen samples (Figure 4), attesting the absence of any qualitative modification on the phenolic/flavonoidic profile. To assess the possible influence on the quantitative profile, quercetin-3-O-sophoroside (used as biomarker) was quantitated. As observed in Figure 4, no differences on the amounts of the glycosylated quercetin derivative were recorded between the samples.

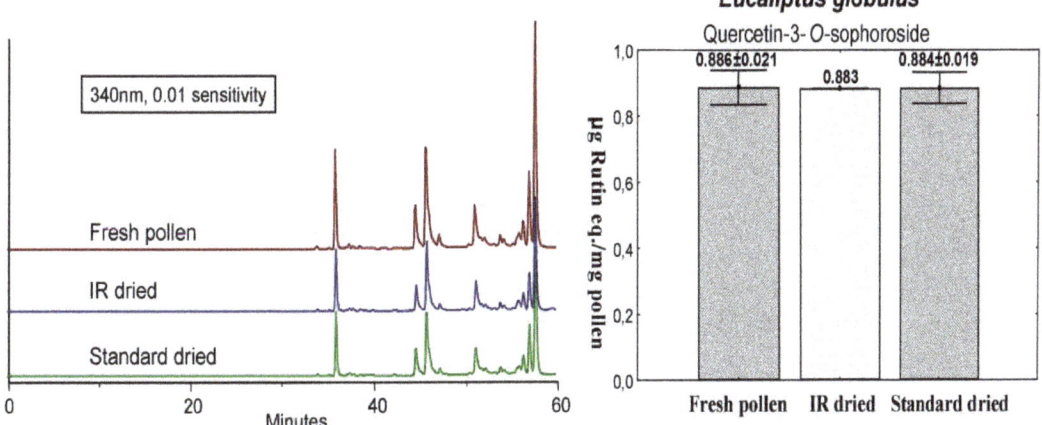

Figure 4. Chromatogram of E. globulus fresh and dried pollen extract and quercetin-3-O-sophoroside quantification, expressed as rutin equivalent mg/g of dry pollen. Results represents means ± SD (n = 3).

Likewise, the chromatographic profile of S. atrocinera bee pollen dried samples did not reveal any difference comparing to fresh pollen chromatographic profile (Figure 5). As seen in Figure 5, no difference in the concentration of the major flavonoid kaempferol-3-O-neohesperidoside (biomarker), was noted within the three samples.

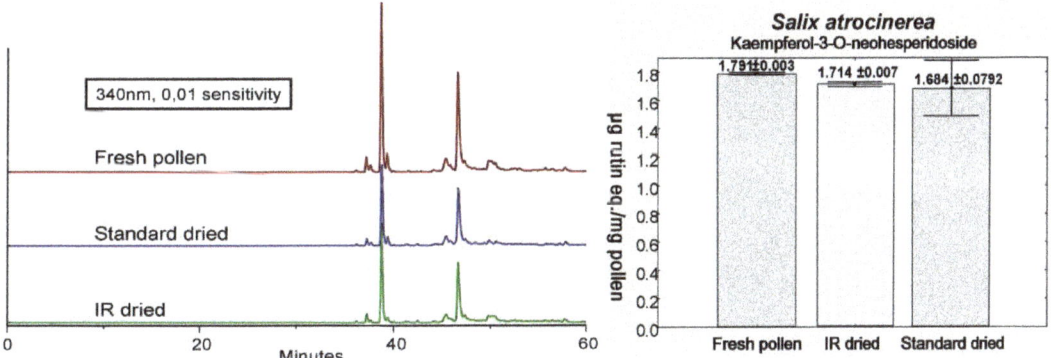

Figure 5. Chromatogram of S. atrocinerea fresh and dried pollen extract and kaempferol-3-O-neohesperidoside quantification, expressed as rutin equivalent mg/g dry pollen. Results are expressed as means ± SD (n = 3).

To further corroborate the absence of degradation, extracts (fresh and dried samples) were assayed on their free radical scavenging activity.

The extract obtained from E. globulus (Figure 4) fresh bee pollen samples was found to exhibit significant antiradical activity, an EC_{50} value of 65.47 ± 1.29 µg/mg, being recorded. No significant differences have been recorded in comparison with the extract obtained from samples dried under the standard approach (EC_{50} = 64.49 ± 3.52 µg/mL). The EC_{50} value estimated for the IR-based dried samples (EC_{50} of 69.69 ± 3.10 µg/mL) suggested a statistically significant, but slight, decrease on the antiradical activity. As no qualitative or quantitative differences have been observed in regard to the phenolic profiles of E. globulus pollen samples, the recorded decrease on the radical scavenging activity might be related with the occurrence of other, non-phenolic, constituents such has carotenoids. In contrast, the radical scavenging ability of the extracts obtained from fresh and dried samples of S. atrocinera bee pollen remained similar, as shown in Figure 5. Antiradical activity of the extracts obtained from samples of fresh pollen and dried samples (IR-based and standard method) was estimated at EC_{50} values of 102.33 ± 3.96, 96.19 ± 4.51) and 98.84 ± 6.47 µg/mL, respectively.

Considering the above, it is evident that neither of the drying methods elicited changes on the phenolic profiles (biomarkers) as well as on the derived free radical scavenging properties.

4. Discussion

Bee pollen is widely popular as a food supplement due to its equilibrate composition of proteins, lipids and sugars [4,23], high content in vitamins, as well all essential amino acids and unsaturated fatty acids (ω-3, ω-6, ω-9) [30–33].

Despite its widespread use, both due to the nutritional value and biological properties, water content determination and management are items of capital significance for the quality control and a safe consumption. Due to its richness in several nutrients, bee pollen is an ideal substrate for the development of microorganisms, especially mycotoxins-producing fungi, such as Aspergillus ochraceus Wilh, a frequent producer of ochratoxin A [34,35]. Various preservation methods have been proposed to avoid microbial contamination and growth, but drying processes remain the most convenient and appropriate if a RH% of ca. 4% is obtained. Recalling in mind the absence of a specific legislation in various countries, the routinely used methods for relative humidity determination (among others, AOAC or Pharmacopoeia methods) are generally time-consuming and susceptible to operator errors. In addition, the amount of energy being consumed has an environmental impact that must be considered.

To overcome such limitations, we propose a new IR-based drying method. Based on the obtained results (Table 1), it is clear that this method revealed to be reproducible in all the range of RH% assessed (±2–28%). Through Z-score test, the IR drying procedure was also compared with the official method [24] (which is similar to other Pharmacopoeias and Codex Alimentarius) and did not show any relevant performance difference. As such, while the methods are equivalent on their performance, the IR method greatly reduced the drying time (ca. 15 min for the moisture determination in samples) in comparison with standard methods requiring nearly 5 h to ensure the convenient reduction in RH%.

Drying conditions herein optimized in an IR moisture analyzer (Kern MLB 50-3), are scalable and guarantee the preservation of the matrix under these conditions. IR radiation did not affect phenolic biomarkers, but other structural classes such as proteins, lipids and vitamins, should be screened.

The HPLC/DAD profiles of the extracts, the quantification of the selected biomarkers and the reference bioactivity, as it is the radical free scavenging activity, were the preliminary models used in this study, and successfully applied to the different botanical origin samples. As showed in Figure 1, the IR dryer performance revealed an evident linear relationship between the amount of removed water (ΔRH%) and the drying time, and as seen in Figures 4 and 5, the phenolic/flavonoid profiles of fresh and dried pollen samples, show a stable correlation with the biomarker used for these *taxon*. These results reveal the high potential of this method for further development of a dry methodology in industrial settings.

Despite previous approaches dealing with water content determination [36–41], the effects of IR radiation in the bioactivity and chemical stability of the bee pollen samples are herein reported for the first time. The current methodology might well be used in other edible products of plant origin, thus calling for further studies in this matter.

Recently, experimental data came to light associating the evidence that Far IR (FIR) is efficient in drying processes due to its energy-saving performance, mainly because energy is directly supplied to the object to be heated without dispersing energy to unnecessary objects, and in the case of certain phenolic compounds, an increase of the total amount and even in the free radical scavenging effect was observed [42].

Once, bee pollen is mainly rich in phenolic compounds, that frequently underlie its biological properties, in particular the free radical scavenging and antioxidant activities [8,9,17,19,43–45], it is relevant to understand the influence of IR radiation in the processed product if used for these further purposes.

Such data will be crucial for the development of further studies with foods and medicinal plants, that are frequently required to be dry for preservation.

5. Conclusions

The traditional procedure to dry bee pollen samples consists in simple convective drying, being time and energy-consuming and requires large dryers with a negative environmental impact. The prolonged exposure to heat can also promote chemical modifications, namely on the content of metabolites that are responsible for the biological activity of this matrix. In the present study, an IR-based drying method is optimized, discussed and provided the basis for an accurate drying process. The results from this IR-based method are of utmost importance, especially due to its low time- and energy-consumption when compared with the standard drying method. No impact being caused by IR has been observed with the samples under study, namely on their phenolic profiles and selected biomarkers. Complementary methodologies (morphological analysis and antiradical activity) further corroborated that this technology as the potential to be developed in a large scale for industrial applications.

Author Contributions: Conceptualization, M.G.C.; methodology, M.G.C., C.F. and N.G.M.G.; software, M.G.C., C.F. and N.G.M.G.; validation, C.F. and N.G.M.G.; formal analysis, C.F. and N.G.M.G.; investigation, M.G.C., C.F. and N.G.M.G.; resources, M.G.C.; data curation, M.G.C.; writing—original draft preparation, M.G.C., C.F., N.G.M.G., O.B. and A.C.U.; writing—review and editing, O.B. and A.C.U.; supervision, M.G.C.; project administration, M.G.C.; funding acquisition, M.G.C. All authors have read and agreed to the published version of the manuscript.

Funding: The authors wish to thank to "Projeto Estratégico—(UI0204): UIDB/00313/2020 (Portugal).

Institutional Review Board Statement: Not applicable.

Informed Consent Statement: Not applicable.

Conflicts of Interest: The authors declare that they have no conflict of interest.

References

1. EFSA Supporting Pub. Technical Report. *EN-1234*. 2017; Volume 14. Available online: https://efsa.onlinelibrary.wiley.com/doi/abs/10.2903/sp.efsa.2017.EN-1234 (accessed on 1 April 2021). [CrossRef]
2. Campos, M.G.; Bogdanov, S.; Almeida-Muradian, L.B.; Szczesna, T.; Mancebo, Y.; Frigerio, C.; Ferreira, F. Pollen composition and standardisation of analytical methods. *J. Apic. Res.* **2008**, *47*, 154–161. [CrossRef]
3. Kroyer, G.; Hegedus, N. Evaluation of bioactive properties of pollen extracts as functional dietary food supplement. *Innov. Food Sci. Emerg. Technol.* **2001**, *2*, 171–174. [CrossRef]
4. Mărgăoan, R.; Mărghitas, L.A.; Dezmirean, D.S.; Dulf, F.V.; Bunea, A.; Socaci, S.A.; Bobiş, O. Predominant and secondary pollen botanical origins influence the carotenoid and fatty acid profile in fresh honeybee-collected pollen. *J. Agric. Food Chem.* **2014**, *62*, 6306–6316. [CrossRef] [PubMed]
5. Figueiredo, F.; Encarnação, T.; Campos, M.G. Algae as functional foods for the elderly. *Food Nut. Sci.* **2016**, *7*, 1122–1148. [CrossRef]

6. Peris, M.J. Producción y comércio de los produtos apícolas en España. 1º Congreso Nacional de Apicultura (Madrid). El Campo del Banco de Bilbao. *Apicultura* **1984**, *93*, 40–68.
7. Orzaez-Villanueva, M.T.; Diaz-Marquina, A.; Bravo-Serrano, R.; Blazquez-Abellan, G. The importance of bee-collected pollen in the diet: A study of its composition. *Int. J. Food Sci. Nut.* **2002**, *53*, 217–224. [CrossRef] [PubMed]
8. Leja, M.A.; Mareczek, G.; Wyżgolik, J.; Klepacz-Baniak, K.C. Antioxidative properties of bee pollen in selected plant species. *Food Chem.* **2007**, *100*, 237–240. [CrossRef]
9. Pascoal, A.; Rodrigues, S.; Teixeira, A.; Feásc, X.; Estevinho, L.M. Biological activities of commercial bee pollens: Antimicrobial, antimutagenic, antioxidant and anti-inflammatory. *Food Chem. Toxic.* **2014**, *63*, 233–239. [CrossRef]
10. Silva, D.N.A.; João, J.S.S.; Campos, M.G. Biological and Functional Properties of Bee Products for Medicinal Purposes. In *Traditional and Folk Herbal Medicine: Recent Researches*, 1st ed.; Gupta, V.K., Ed.; Daya Publishing House: New Delhi, India, 2014; Chapter 18; pp. 541–562, ISBN-10: 8170358744.
11. Mărgăoan, R.; Stranț, M.; Varadi, A.; Topal, E.; Yücel, B.; Cornea-Cipcigan, M.; Campos, M.G.; Vodnar, D.C. Bee pollen and bee bread: Bioactive constituents and health benefits. *Antioxidants* **2019**, *8*, 568. [CrossRef]
12. Anjos, O.; Paula, V.; Delgado, T.; Estevinho, L. Influence of the storage conditions on the quality of bee pollen. *Zemdirb. Agric.* **2019**, *106*, 87–94. [CrossRef]
13. Jagdis, A.; Sussman, G. Anaphylaxis from bee pollen supplement. *Canadian Med. Assoc. J.* **2012**, *184*, 1167–1169. [CrossRef]
14. EFSA Panel on Genetically Modified Organisms (GMO). Statement on the safety of MON810 maize pollen occurring in or as food. panel on genetically modified organisms (GMO). *EFSA J.* **2011**, *11*, 2434.
15. EFSA. Scientific opinion on an application (EFSA-GMO-NL-2012-107) for the placing on the market of maize MON 810 pollen under Regulation (EC) No 1829/2003 from Monsanto. *EFSA J.* **2012**, *10*, 3022. [CrossRef]
16. Szczesna, T.; Rybak-Chimielewska, H.; Chmielewsky, W. Sugar composition of pollen loads harvested at different periods of the beekeeping season. *J. Apic. Sci.* **2002**, *46*, 107–115.
17. Campos, M.G. Caracterização do Pólen Apícola Pelo Seu Perfil em Compostos Fenólicos e Pesquisa de Algumas Actividades Biologicas. Ph.D. Thesis, Faculty of Pharmacy, University of Coimbra, Coimbra, Portugal, 1997.
18. Campos, M.G.; Mitchel, K.; Cunha, A.; Markham, K.R. A systematic approach to the characterisation of bee pollens via their flavonoid/phenolic profiles. *Phytochem. Anal.* **1997**, *8*, 181–185. [CrossRef]
19. Campos, M.G.; Webby, R.F.; Markham, K.R.; Mitchell, K.A.; Cunha, A.P. Age-induced diminution of free radical scavenging capacity in bee pollens and the contribution of constituent flavonoids. *J. Agric. Food Chem.* **2003**, *51*, 742–745. [CrossRef]
20. Bakour, M.; Campos, M.G.; Imtara, H.; Lyoussi, B. Antioxidant content and identification of phenolic/flavonoid compounds in the pollen of fourteen plants using HPLC-DAD. *J. Apic. Res.* **2020**, *59*, 35–41. [CrossRef]
21. Bovi, T.S.; Caeiro, A.; Santos, S.A.; Zaluski, R.; Shinohara, A.J.; Lima, G.P.P.; Campos, M.G.; Junior, A.J.; Orsi, R.O. Flavonoid content in bee bread suffers seasonal variation and affects hypopharyngeal gland development in Apis mellifera honey bees. *J. Apic. Res.* **2019**, *20*, 1–8.
22. Negri, G.; Barreto, L.M.R.C.; Sper, F.L.; Carvalho, C.D.; Campos, M.G. Phytochemical analysis and botanical origin of *Apis mellifera* bee pollen from the municipality of Canavieiras, Bahia State, Brazil. *Braz. J. Food Techn.* **2018**, *21*, 1–16. [CrossRef]
23. Urcan, A.C.; Criste, A.D.; Dezmirean, D.S.; Mărgăoan, R.; Caeiro, A.; Campos, M.G. Similarity of data from bee bread with the same *taxa* collected in India and Romania. *Molecules* **2018**, *23*, 2491. [CrossRef]
24. Infarmed-National Authority of Medicines and Health Products. I.P. Perda Por Secagem. In *Portuguese Pharmacopoeia*, 7th ed; Infarmed, Ed.; Imprensa Nacional: Lisboa, Portugal, 2005; Chapter 2.2.32.d; pp. 49–50.
25. Campos, M.G.; Markham, K.R. *Structure Information from HPLC and on-Line Measured Absorption Spectra: Flavones, Flavonols and Phenolic Acids*, 1st ed.; Imprensa da Universidade de Coimbra: Coimbra, Portugal, 2007; pp. 14, 26–29, 91, 104, ISBN 978-989-8074-05-8.
26. Almaraz-Abarca, N.; Campos, M.G.; Delgado-Alvarado, E.A.; Ávila-Reyes, J.A.; Herrera-Corral, J.; González-Valdez, L.S.; Naranjo-Jiménez, N.; Frigerio, C.; Tomatas, A.F.; Almeida, A.J.; et al. Pollen flavonoid/phenolic acid composition of four species of cactaceae and its taxonomic significance. *Am. J. Agric. Biol. Sci.* **2008**, *3*, 534–543.
27. LeBlanc, B.W.; Davis, O.K.; Boue, S.; DeLucca, A.; Deeby, T. Antioxidant activity of Sonoran Desert bee pollen. *Food Chem.* **2009**, *115*, 1299–1305. [CrossRef]
28. Rebiai, A.; Lanez, T. Chemical composition and antioxidant activity of *Apis mellifera* bee pollen from northwest Algeria. *J. Fund. Appl. Sci.* **2012**, *4*, 155–163. [CrossRef]
29. Šaric, A.; Balog, T.; Sobočanec, S.; Kušić, B.; Šverko, V.; Rusak, G.; Likić, S.; Bubalo, D.; Pinto, B.; Reali, D.; et al. Antioxidant effects of flavonoid from Croatian *Cystus incanus* L. rich bee pollen. *Food Chem. Toxic.* **2009**, *47*, 547–554. [CrossRef] [PubMed]
30. Almeida-Muradian, L.B.; Pamplona, L.C.; Coimbra, S.; Barth, O.M. Chemical composition and botanical evaluation of dried bee pollen pellets. *J. Food Comp. Anal.* **2005**, *18*, 106–111. [CrossRef]
31. Conte, G.; Bednelli, G.; Serra, A.; Signorini, F.; Bientinesi, M.; Nicolella, C.; Mele, M.; Canale, M. Lipid characterization of chestnut and willow honeybee-collectged pollen: Impact of freeze-drying and microwave-assisted drying. *J. Food Comp. Anal.* **2016**. [CrossRef]
32. Gardana, C.; Del Bo', C.; Quicazán, M.C.; Correa, A.R.; Simonetti, P. Nutrients, phytochemicals and botanical origin of commercial bee pollen from different geographical areas. *J. Food Comp. Anal.* **2018**, *73*, 29–38. [CrossRef]

33. Bedlina-Aldemita, D.; Opper, C.; Schreiner, M.; D'Amico, S. Nutritional composition of pot-pollen produced by stingless bees (*Tetragona biroi* Friese) from the Philippines. *J. Food Comp. Anal.* **2019**, *82*, 103215. [CrossRef]
34. Medina, A.; Gonzalez, G.; Saez, J.M.; Mateo, R.; Jimenez, M. Bee pollen, a substrate that stimulates Ochratoxin A production by *Aspergillus ochraceus* Wilh. *Syst. Appl. Microb.* **2004**, *27*, 261–267. [CrossRef]
35. Rodríguez-Carrasco, Y.; Font, G.; Mañes, J.; Berrada, H. Determination of mycotoxins in bee pollen by gas chromatography–tandem mass spectrometry. *J. Agric. Food Chem.* **2013**, *61*, 1999–2005. [CrossRef]
36. Melo, I.; Almeida-Muradian, L. Comparison of methodologies for moisture determination on dried bee pollen samples. *Food Sci. Techn.* **2011**, *31*, 194–197. [CrossRef]
37. Arruda, V.A.S.; Pereira, A.A.S.; de Freitas, A.S.; Barth, O.M.; Almeida-Muradian, L.B. Dried bee pollen: B complex vitamins, physicochemical and botanical composition. *J. Food Comp. Anal.* **2013**, *29*, 100–105. [CrossRef]
38. Isik, A.; Ozdemir, M.; Doymaz, I. Infrared drying of bee pollen: Effects and impacts on food components. *Czech J. Food Sci.* **2019**, *37*, 69–74. [CrossRef]
39. Isik, A.; Ozdemir, M.; Doymaz, I. Effect of hot air drying on quality characteristics and physicochemical properties of bee pollen. *Food Sci. Tech.* **2019**, *39*, 224–231. [CrossRef]
40. Kanar, Y.; Mazi, B.G. Effect of different drying methods on antioxidant characteristics of bee-pollen. *J. Food Measur. Charact.* **2019**, *13*, 3376–3386. [CrossRef]
41. Keskin, M.; Özkök, A. Effects of drying techniques on chemical composition and volatile constituents of bee pollen. *Czech J. Food Sci.* **2020**, *38*, 203–208. [CrossRef]
42. Azad, M.O.K.; Piao, J.P.; Park, C.H.; Cho, H.D. Far infrared irradiation enhances nutraceutical compounds and antioxidant properties in *Angelica gigas* nakai powder. *Antioxidants* **2018**, *7*, 189. [CrossRef]
43. Mărghitaş, L.A.; Stanciu, O.G.; Dezmirean, D.S.; Bobiş, O.; Popescu, O.; Bogdanov, S.; Campos, M.G. In-vitro antioxidant capacity of honeybee-collected pollen of selected floral origin harvested from Romania. *Food Chem* **2009**, *115*, 878–883. [CrossRef]
44. Rzepecka-Stojko, A.; Pilawa, B.; Ramos, P.; Stojko, J. Antioxidative properties of bee pollen extracts examined by EPR spectroscopy. *J. Apic. Sci.* **2012**, *56*, 23–30. [CrossRef]
45. Silva, T.M.S.; Câmara, C.A.; Silva Lins, A.C.; Barbosa-Filho, J.M.; Freitas da Silva, E.M.S.; Santos, F.B.M. Chemical composition and free radical scavenging activity of pollen loads from stingless bee *Melipona subnitida* Ducke. *J. Food Comp. Anal.* **2006**, *19*, 507–511. [CrossRef]

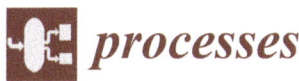

Article

Polyphenolic Profiling of Green Waste Determined by UPLC-HDMS^E

Colin M. Potter [1,*] and David L. Jones [1,2]

[1] Centre for Environmental Biotechnology, School of Natural Sciences, Bangor University, Bangor, Gwynedd LL57 2UW, UK; d.jones@bangor.ac.uk
[2] UWA School of Agriculture and Environment, The University of Western Australia, Perth, WA 6009, Australia
* Correspondence: colinmpotter@gmail.com

Abstract: Valorising green waste will greatly enhance and promote the sustainable management of this large volume resource. One potential way to achieve this is the extraction of high value human health promoting chemicals (e.g., polyphenols) from this material. Our primary aim was to identify the main polyphenols present in four contrasting green waste feedstocks, namely *Smyrnium olusatrum*, *Urtica dioica*, *Allium ursinum* and *Ulex europaeus*, using UPLC-HDMS^E. Polyphenol-rich *Camellia sinensis* (green tea) was used as a reference material. Samples were extracted and analysed by UPLC-HDMS^E, which was followed by data processing using Progenesis QI and EZ Info. A total of 77 high scoring polyphenolic compounds with reported benefits to human health were tentatively identified in the samples, with abundances varying across the plant types; *A. ursinum* was seen to be the least abundant in respect to the polyphenols identified, whereas *U. europaeus* was the most abundant. Important components with a diverse range of bioactivity, such as procyanidins, (−)-epigallocatechin, naringenin, eriodictyol and *iso*-liquiritigenin, were observed, plus a number of phytoestrogens such as daidzein, glycitin and genistein. This research provides a route to valorise green waste through the creation of nutritional supplements which may aid in the prevention of disease.

Keywords: TWIMS; polyphenols; phenol-explorer database; UPLC-MS-MS; Synapt G2-Si; phenolomics

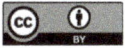

1. Introduction

In most countries, green waste typically represents a high volume, low value resource, with most of this material being composted and subsequently spread back to agricultural land to improve soil quality [1]. However, green waste also represents a promising starting material for the direct extraction of valuable compounds and for the chemical and fermentative conversion of this waste into basic chemicals [2]. One of the main issues in valorising this resource, however, is knowledge of what high value products can be obtained in sufficient quantities from different types of green wastes to make it commercially viable. One area that has drawn particular interest has been the extraction of polyphenols [3]. These plant species may also contain many other non-polyphenolic bioactive chemicals which are also worthy of attention. Co-extraction of these would, of course, further enhance the value of waste materials, though this research was focused on polyphenols. A full cost–benefit analysis and life cycle assessment are required to determine the valorisation benefits relative to other synthesis or extraction procedures.

Polyphenols are a naturally occurring group of secondary metabolites which are relatively abundant in plants and which are purported to have many health benefits [4–6]. For example, they are thought to play an important role in disease prevention, resulting not only from their antioxidant ability but also their epigenetic influence and their positive impact on the composition of gut microbiota. Due to their complex chemical structures, many of these plant-derived bioactive polyphenols can be difficult to synthesize in large quantities [7]. Green waste offers a potentially cheap feedstock to extract and purify these compounds; however, this necessitates good knowledge of the polyphenols present in different source materials [2].

Green waste is expected to contain many thousands of chemicals. Consequently, high resolution analytical approaches are needed to enable separation and identification of the myriad chemicals present. One potential solution is the use of ultra-performance liquid chromatography (UPLC) linked to an ion mobility time-of-flight high-definition/high-resolution mass spectrometer (UPLC-HDMS^E). Recent work characterising phenolic compounds in forestry waste has shown that UPLC-HDMS^E can provide an in-depth analysis of the wide suite of phenolics present [8]. This is also supported by the use of UPLC-HDMS^E for the detection and characterisation of bioactive compounds in complex medicinal mixtures and urine [9,10]. The characterisation of polyphenolics in agricultural or municipal green waste via UPLC-HDMS^E has not, to the best of our knowledge, been previously undertaken. The aim of this study was therefore to analyse the diversity of polyphenols in four contrasting but common green waste materials generated in municipal or agricultural settings. These plant-based feedstocks have previously been characterised by a range of analytical techniques, but they have not been subject to the potential benefits of the detailed characterisation provided by UPLC-HDMS^E. As a broad reference material, green tea (*Camellia sinensis*) was also included in the study. The phenolic chemistry of this plant material has been well characterised [6,11,12], and can therefore act as a validation of this discovery workflow, i.e., the expected polyphenols associated with green tea should be observed.

2. Materials and Methods

2.1. Sample Collection

Representative samples of Alexanders (*Smyrnium olusatrum*), Stinging Nettle (*Urtica dioica*), Wild garlic (*Allium ursinum*) and Gorse (*Ulex europaeus*) were collected from the Lligwy Bay area of Anglesey, Wales, UK (53°21′14″ N, 4°15′47″ W) in April 2019. The sample of *U. europaeus* was separated into separate flower and stem samples in order to observe whether there were any significant differences in the characterisation of these two physically connected structures. These plants were chosen due to their contrasting phylogenies and their frequent presence in municipal and agricultural green waste streams.

2.2. Sample Preparation

After collection, each sample was thoroughly washed in LC-MS grade water (Optima) and then freeze-dried (48 h) before being ground to a fine powder. A total of 0.5 g of powder was then placed in a glass beaker containing 10 mL of ethanol and sonicated in an ultrasonic water bath for 30 min before being left to stand for 24 h at 4 °C before being sonicated again for a further 30 min. After the solids had settled out, the supernatant was transferred to a polypropylene tube and centrifuged (10,000 rev min^{-1}, 30 min). Through heating to 60 °C, the resultant ethanol solution of extracted components was concentrated to 1 mL; that is to say that 1 mL of extract was equivalent to 1 g of initial sample. The sample produced was stored at −20 °C. The plant samples were prepared in quadruplicate.

2.3. Analytical Instrumentation

HDMS^E mode is a data-independent acquisition in which data for all gas phase parent ions, and also fragments (product ions) created, are recorded. This was recorded and saved as continuum data. In addition, a drift cell was used to collect ion mobility data. The Synapt G2-Si (Waters UK, Wilmslow, Cheshire, UK) can be described as a quadrupole time-of-flight mass spectrometer (Q-ToF) which has ion mobility capability added to the ion path. Analytes, which have been separated by the UPLC, were infused into a Z-Spray^{TM} source (Waters UK, Wilmslow, Cheshire, UK). Simultaneously, leucine enkephalin (Tyr-Gly Gly Phe-Leu) was infused via a separate probe, which provided the lock mass data to correct the mass axis drift which occurs during an acquisition. Baffle switching allowed for the selection of which infusion, analyte or lock mass entered the MS.

2.4. UPLC Conditions

A Waters I-class UPLC was used for analyte separation with a Waters Cortecs Shield RP18 (2.7 µm × 2.1 mm × 100 mm, Waters UK, Wilmslow, Cheshire, UK) solid core column installed. This column provides high selectivity for phenolic compounds due to the use of imbedded polar carbamate technology. A guard column of the same stationary phase was used for protection of the analytical column. Water with 0.1% acetic acid in reservoir A and MeOH with 0.1% acetic acid in reservoir B were used as the mobile phase. The flow rate, column temperature and injection volume were 0.5 mL min^{-1}, 40 °C and 1.0 µL, respectively. The starting composition for this eluent was 90% A and 10% B, with a linear change to 1% A with 99% B over the course of 4 min. At the end point, the initial conditions were returned to over a time of 0.2 min.

2.5. Synapt G2-Si Conditions

Negative ion data, in a mass range of 50 to 1200 Da, was acquired using resolution mode. The scan time was 0.2 s, with an average of 3 scans and a mass window of ±0.5 Da. mode. The cone voltage was 40 V. The method was set to acquire the lockmass (leucine enkephalin, 554.2615 Da) at regular intervals (30 s). This was not used for immediate mass correction throughout the run but stored for later use in the data processing phase.

2.6. Data Processing

Progenesis QI software (NonLinear Dynamics Ltd., Newcastle upon Tyne, UK) was used to process these data. An experimental design was chosen (between subjects) by creating individual groups for the various plant extracts, plus one for the reference (green tea) and one group for blank extracts. As this detail has previously been published [8], only a brief overview is provided here. Post deconvolution, a 5 ppm precursor tolerance was used to compare ions to the ChemSpider Polyphenols database [13] using isotope similarity scores above 90%, an elemental composition of C, O, H only and in an silico fragmentation tolerance of 90%. Similarly, filters were used to reveal only analytes with ANOVA p values ≤0.01 and where blanks were the lowest mean, and, also, scores with a value above 40 were selected for further evaluation. Multivariate analysis (MVA) was conducted through the use of EZInfo (Umetrics, Umeå, Sweden). Matlab (MatWorks Inc., Natlick, MA, USA) was used to create the heat map.

3. Results and Discussion

3.1. Bioactive Phenolic Compounds in the Green Waste Extracts

An Excel file in the supplementary materials (plant extracts XL SM v6) provides a detailed summary of the 77 high-scoring components elucidated through this analysis of green waste. Details such as retention time (min.), normalised abundance, drift time (ms) and accurate mass values are provided for parent ions and their main product ions. Very low ANOVA-p and q values are seen, which indicates a false discovery rate (FDR) close to zero. Mass errors of ≤5 ppm are observed in these data, plus scores of over 80 for isotope similarity.

In cases where it was not possible to distinguish analytes from species of the same accurate mass, the various possibilities are listed. Examples of total ion chromatograms (Figures S1–S6) and example molecular structures of the 29 identified components, with scores of 50.0 and above, are shown in Figure S7. Mass spectra (Figure S8) are available in the supplementary materials.

Green tea, which was used as a reference material, exhibited the expected polyphenols generally associated with this plant in the published literature. These include (−)-epigallocatechin, (−)-epigallocatechin gallate, theaflavin and procyanidin (B1, B2, B3 or B4). Another key component of green tea's polyphenol profile, (−)-epicatechin, was also observed at 1.23 min and m/z 289.0732, with an average abundance of score of 38.1, 6782 average abundance, a mass error of 4.8 ppm and very low ANOVA-p and q values (1.31×10^{-8} and 3.47×10^{-9}). A confirmatory product ion at m/z 245.0808, due to the loss of 44 Da (CH$_3$CHO), was observed [14]. This added further validity to this discovery method. An abundance profile of (−)-epicatechin across the plant extracts can be seen in the supplementary materials showing the greatest abundance in the green tea extract (Figure S9).

A heat map was created using averaged abundances for each sample type over the 77 identified polyphenol components (Figure 1). This visual overview of polyphenol identifications shows that abundances are higher in *U. europaeus* flower and stem extracts than they are in the extracts of *S. olusatrum*, *U. dioica* and *A. ursinum*. Furthermore, it can be seen that *A. ursinum* leaf has the lowest abundance of the components identified here. It is also noted that individual plant extracts have their own pattern or fingerprint of abundances, with components showing much variation been plant types.

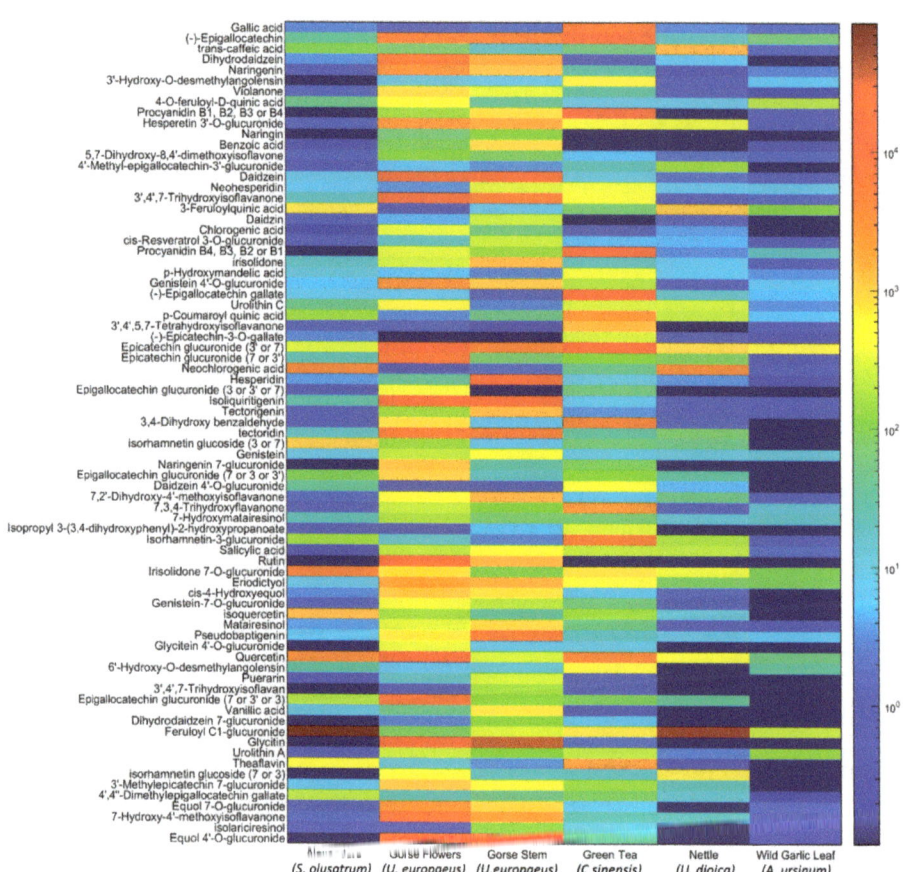

Figure 1. Heat map, using averaged abundances, created for each sample type across the 77 observed polyphenols.

A loadings bi-plot was created as another overview of the data. Pareto scaling was used in this unsupervised principal component analysis (PCA). Sample replicates are tightly clustered and sample types show clear separation. The relationship between sample types and the data swarm of m/z values (x-variables) can also be seen (Figure 2).

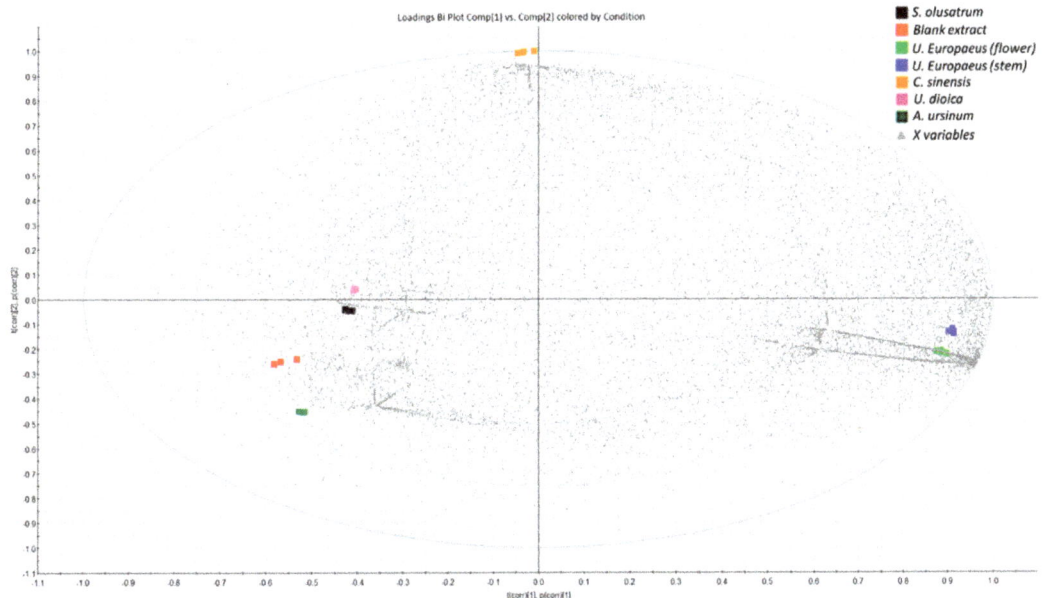

Figure 2. Loadings bi-plot showing tight clustering of sample types within the data swarm.

3.2. Tentative Identification of Polyphenols

Due to the lack of fragmentation data contained in databases, in silico predication has been used here. As the fragmentation mechanisms of polyphenols are well documented, this can be quite an effective approach. Retro-Diels-Alder (RDA) reactions [15] are the general category here, which also applies to the sugar moiety, which is often seen in polyphenols. Additionally, the mass spectra of conjugated phenolic compounds showed the aglycone ion as result of the loss of sugar moieties such as hexosyl ([M−162]$^-$) or pentosyl ([M−132]$^-$). An example of this is seen with the two isomers of isorhamnetin glucoside (3 or 7) that are identified at 1.81 and 2.63 min. Their [M-H]$^-$ ions undergo the loss of the hexoside moiety to create product ions of m/z 315.0503 and m/z 315.0508. It is also noted that these isobaric species are not only separated by chromatographic retention time but also by drift time, further confirming that these molecules are different in terms of their collision cross section (CCS). The isomer at 1.81 min is seen in high abundance in *U. dioica* and the other isomer at 2.63 min is high in *S. olusatrum*. Both are also fairly abundant in the *U. europaeus* flower extract. Isorhamnetin-3-glucoside is a major component of *Salicornia herbacea*, which is traditionally used in Asian medicine and is thought to exhibit multiple nutraceutical and pharmaceutical properties [16]. Isorhamnetin-7-glucoside is suggested to have antitumour activity in a review of topopoisons from weeds [17].

The highest scoring component, gallic acid, was identified by its [M-H]$^-$ ion at 1.43 min and the loss of 44 Da to create the product ion m/z 125.0238 [M-H-CH$_3$CHO]$^-$. Although this had an expected high abundance in the green tea extract, it was only present at low abundance in the plant extracts. The identification of (−)-epigallocatechin was achieved by observation of the [M-H$_2$O-H]$^-$ adduct at m/z 287.0562, eluting at 1.41 min and the main MS/MS fragments of m/z 257.0437 [C$_{14}$H$_{10}$O$_5$-H]$^-$ and m/z 151.0387 [C$_8$H$_8$O$_3$-H]$^-$. This is one of the key health components of green tea [18] and was present in this extract in high abundance. Although (−)-epigallocatechin was detected in all extracts, it was found to be in particularly high abundance in the *U. europaeus* flower and stem extracts. At m/z 179.0343 and 1.76 min, *trans*-caffeic acid was identified. The product ion m/z 135.0441 [C$_8$H$_7$O$_2$+e]$^-$ was used for additional confirmation. This component is well documented in the literature as a potent antioxidant which can aid in the fight against cellular injury due to reactive oxygen species [19], and was present in this study, with the highest abundance being in *U. dioica* and, to a lesser degree, in *S. olusatrum*.

To link together some key phytoestrogens, dihydrodaidzein (CSID154076) was elucidated via its [M-H]$^-$ adduct (m/z 255.0663) at 1.87 min. Major fragments of m/z 121.0282 [C$_7$H$_6$O$_2$-H]$^-$ and m/z 119.0495 [C$_8$H$_8$O-H]$^-$ were observed in the high energy MS/MS signal, although other product ions were apparent. Daidzein was observed at 2.58 min and m/z 253.0515, with confirmatory fragments m/z 224.0465 [C$_{14}$H$_9$O$_3$-H]$^-$ and m/z 208.0520 [C$_{14}$H$_8$O$_2$+e]$^-$ and genistein eluted at 2.73 min, with a parent ion at m/z 251.0336 [M-H$_2$O-H]$^-$ and primary fragment at m/z 223.0396 [C$_{14}$H$_{10}$O$_4$-H$_2$O-H]$^-$. The [2M-H]$^-$ ion revealed glycitin with an m/z ratio of 891.2362 and an MS/MS fragment at m/z 729.1821 [C$_{18}$H$_{11}$O$_5$+M+e]$^-$. These components, which were shown to be highly abundant in *U. europaeus* flower, *U. europaeus* stem and *U. dioica*, have been associated with protection against major adverse cardiac events in women [20]. The findings support the use of a plant-based diet and the need for future randomized prospective studies examining the influence of glycitin and genistein, as well as daidzein and dihydrodaidzein diets on cardiovascular outcomes. A literature review on the benefits of phytoestrogen supplementation on human cognition was conflicting, with less than half of the included studies showing beneficial effects, though supplementation with soy isoflavones for less than 6 months, irrespective of dose and mode, can improve cognitive performance, with greater impact on women than men. Equol is seen as an important product of daidzein metabolism in this process, though only 30%–50% of the general population are equol producers. This is thought to affect individual responses to isoflavone intervention [21]. Two isomeric glucosides of daidzein, which are known as daidzin (m/z 397.0933, 3.15 min) and puerarin (m/z 397.0938, 2.97 min), are also a soy isoflavones known to convert to equol. On top of this, identified at a lower score, is cis-4-hydroxyequol (m/z 257.0807, 2.32 min) which has activity similar to that of equol itself. Detail is available on glucuronidation via microbial metabolic processes, providing a possible route for how polyphenol glucuronides are formed outside of mammalian metabolism [22,23]. Though the 2 isomers of equol O-glucuronide (7 and 4') were identified at 1.43 and 2.18 min with m/z 417.1198 and m/z 835.2454 parent ions, respectively, literature is scarce on how these two components, found in high amounts in *U. europaeus* stem and flower extracts, would contribute to overall blood plasma equol levels post transformation via gut microbial enzymes.

Naringenin, a flavonoid common in citrus fruits, was found to be another high scoring component, with high abundance in the *U. europaeus* flower and stem extracts. Identified by its [M-H]$^-$ adduct (m/z 271.0617) at 1.31 min and MS/MS product ion at m/z 243.0654 [C$_{14}$H$_{12}$O$_4$-H]$^-$, many beneficial biological effects have been linked to naringenin, including antioxidant, cardioprotective, antitumor, antiadipogenic, antiviral, antibacterial and anti-inflammatory effects [24]. In light of the current global pandemic, positive claims have been made as to the therapeutic potential of naringenin in the treatment of COVID-19 [25,26]. Two positional isomers of naringenin were also observed: 3',4',7-trihydroxyisoflavanone ([M-H$_2$O-H]$^-$, m/z 253.0518, 1.79 min, dt 2.3370 ms) and 3',6,4'-trihydroxyflavanone, also known as butin ([M-H]$^-$, m/z 271.0604, 1.76 min, dt 2.5498 ms), the former being prominent in *U. europaeus* flower and stem and the latter being of greatest abundance in green tea, but also present in smaller amounts in the other extracts. These had similar retention times but were clearly separated by drift time, and are therefore different molecules. Molecules of this type are often associated with red wine as a contribution from the barrel wood [27] and have been shown to have potential health benefits [28]. In the context of this, naringin, the rhamnoglucoside of naringenin, was likewise identified in *U. europaeus* flowers and stem samples ([M-H$_2$O-H]$^-$, m/z 561.1596, 2.00 min), but at much lower abundance than naringenin. The major confirmatory MS/MS fragment was observed at m/z 515.1190 [C$_{25}$H$_{26}$O$_{13}$-H$_2$O-H]$^-$, showing partial fragmentation of the rhamnoglucoside group. The sugar moiety is a major determinant of the absorption of dietary flavonoid glycosides in mammals [29] and future research into comparative potency would be of interest here. The identification of naringenin 7-glucuronide ([2M-H]$^-$, m/z 895.1921, 2.32 min) in high abundance in *U. europaeus* flower extract brings to mind a similar question focused on the potency of the glucuronides of polyphenols.

Tetrahydroxyflavanones have been shown to reduce the heme group in cytochrome c, which is a necessary component of the electron transport system and is also involved in apoptotic pathways. The oxidation state of the iron in the heme group is crucial to its specific functions [30]. These compounds can be seen as the addition of a phenol group to naringenin, with two being observed in these data: 3′,4′,5,7-tetrahydroxyisoflavanone ([2M-H]$^-$, m/z 575.1184, 1.20 min) and eriodictyol ([M-H]$^-$, m/z 287.0554, 2.19 min). 3′,4′,5,7-tetrahydroxyisoflavanone was seen significantly only in the reference green tea extract and will therefore receive no further discussion. On the other hand, eriodictyol was present in all of the extracts analysed, with a high abundance in *U. europaeus* flower and stem, but reasonable amounts were also present in *U. dioica* and *A. ursinum* leaf. The potential health benefits of eriodictyol are plentiful [8], with further research showing increasing evidence of its function and benefits. For example, eriodictyol may have therapeutic potential for the treatment of rheumatoid arthritis [31], and a study also shows that eriodictyol may provide a new therapeutic strategy for the management of diabetic retinopathy through the inhibition of high glucose-induced oxidative stress and inflammation in retinal ganglial cells [32].

3′-Hydroxy-O-desmethylangolensin was identified by its [M-H]$^-$ adduct, m/z 273.0770, at 1.95 min and confirmed by its MS/MS fragment m/z 119.0497 [C_8H_8O-H]$^-$. This was only seen in significant amounts in the green tea reference and therefore will not be discussed in further detail. This was also the case for 6′-hydroxy-O-desmethylangolensin, which was identified by its [M-H]$^-$ adduct, m/z 273.0758, at 1.77 min, p-hydroxymandelic acid ([M-H]$^-$, m/z 167.0344, 1.18 min), (−)-epigallocatechin gallate ([M-H$_2$O-H]$^-$, m/z 439.0679, 1.76 min), (−)-epicatechin-3-O-gallate ([M-H$_2$O-H]$^-$, m/z 423.0708, 1.95 min), daidzein 4′-O-glucuronide ([M-H$_2$O-H]$^-$, m/z 411.0700, 1.42 min) and isopropyl 3-(3,4-dihydroxyphenyl)-2-hydroxypropanoate ([M-H$_2$O-H]$^-$, m/z 221.0812, 1.77 min). The strong presence of the heavily documented component of green tea, (−)-epigallocatechin gallate, further validates this discovery workflow [6,27,28]. Furthermore, the product ions m/z 289.0727 [$C_{15}H_{13}O_6$–H]$^-$, m/z 169.0146 [$C_7H_5O_5$+e]$^-$ and m/z 125.0242 [$C_6H_5O_3$+e]$^-$ were consistent with the loss of gallate (169 Da), producing an epigallocatechin minus the C-ring hydroxyl group (289 Da), with further fragmentation causing the loss of the B-ring (125 Da), which was also confirmed by library spectra [33].

Violanone was observed via its [M-H$_2$O-H]$^-$ adduct, with a score of 55.8 at m/z 297.0759 and 1.87 min. The main product ion m/z 121.0282 was due to [$C_7H_6O_2$+e]$^-$. Violanone was predominant in *U. europaeus* flower and stem extracts, but is also an important component of the fragrant Chinese rosewood (*Dalbergia odorifera*), which is used in traditional medicine, with claims broadly relating to its antioxidant qualities [34]. Furthermore, it is shown to selectively inhibit phytopathogenic fungi [35] and to be key component in the roots of *Pongamia pinnata*, which exhibits antioxidant, anticancer, antimicrobial and anti-inflammatory properties through its use in folk medicine [36]. It is noted, too, that the references to violanone in traditional medicinal plants, found in South Asia and China [34–36], also encompass the benefits of many other components identified in these plant extracts from Britain, including daidzein, eriodictyol, naringenin, genistein, isoliquiritigenin ([M-H]$^-$, m/z 255.0671, 2.72 min) and tectorigenin ([M-H$_2$O-H]$^-$, m/z 281.0454, 2.35 min). This begs the question as to whether the published benefits of polyphenols are plant specific, specific to certain phytochemical combinations or specific to a particular molecule in isolation? Isoliquiritigenin is found in very high abundance in *U. europaeus* flower and, to a lesser extent, in *U. europaeus* stem and *S. olusatrum*, with tectorigenin being high in *U. europaeus* stem and lower amounts in *U. europaeus* flower. Isoliquiritigenin is an important bioactive ingredient of traditional Chinese medicine, often extracted from the roots of liquorice plant species, including *Glycyrrhiza uralensis*, Mongolian glycyrrhiza and *Glycyrrhiza glabra*, with research exhibiting significant pharmacological properties, including both the prevention and treatment of tumours [37]. The transformation of tectoridin ([M-H]$^-$, m/z 461.1107, 1.55 min), also found in high abundance in *U. europaeus* flower and stem, to the bioactive compound tectorigenin is efficiently achieved by gut microflora, resulting in anaphylaxis inhibitory action [38]. Additionally, recent research suggests that tectorigenin inhibits airway inflammation and pulmonary fibrosis in allergic asthma [39].

4-*O*-Feruloyl-D-quinic acid was identified by its [M-H]$^-$ adduct and parent ion m/z 367.1050 at 0.43 min. The product ion m/z 291.0883 was explained by the fragment [C$_{15}$H$_{16}$O$_6$–H]$^-$. 3-Feruloylquinic acid was identified by its [M-H]$^-$ adduct and parent ion m/z 367.1024 at 1.60 min. The product ion m/z 295.0802 was explained by the fragment [C$_{14}$H$_{15}$O$_7$+e]$^-$. Chlorogenic acid (3-*O*-Caffeoylquinic acid) was identified by its [2M-H]$^-$ adduct and parent ion m/z 707.1802 at 2.47 min. The product ions m/z 663.1927 and m/z 459.1292 were explained by the fragment [C$_{15}$H$_{17}$O$_7$+e+M]$^-$ and [C$_7$H$_5$O+e+M]$^-$, respectively. *p*-Coumaroyl quinic acid was identified by its [M-H]$^-$ adduct and parent ion m/z 337.0923 at 1.54 min, and the product ion m/z 307.0820 was explained by the fragment [C$_{15}$H$_{16}$O$_7$-H]$^-$. These four molecules are known as chlorogenic acids, which are a polyphenolic family of quinic acid esters of hydroxyl-cinnamic acids such as *p*-coumaric acid, caffeic acid and ferulic acid. A placebo-controlled double-blind pilot study, conducted in Japan, found that chlorogenic acids decreased arterial stiffness, which is a characteristic of the progression of arteriosclerosis [40]. 4-*O*-Feruloyl-D-quinic acid was found in high amounts in *U. europaeus* flower and *A. ursinum* leaf extracts, whereas 3-feruloylquinic acid was found to be abundant in *S. olusatrum* and *U. dioica*. Chlorogenic acid was found to be most abundant in *U. europaeus* flower and *U. europaeus* stem, with its stereoisomer, neochlorogenic acid, also being observed ([M-H]$^-$, m/z 353.0876, 1.51 min), which was seen in high abundance in *S. olusatrum* and *U. dioica* as was *p*-coumaroyl quinic acid.

Theaflavin ([M-H]$^-$, m/z 563.1182, 2.56 min) is created when epicatechin and epigallocatechin come in contact with polyphenol oxidase. This analyte is used as an indicator of production quality in the tea industry, and can be present in low quality green tea but is more common in oolong and black teas. It is shown to be one of many components that are responsible for the antioxidant properties of tea [41]. Here, it is seen in the green tea reference but also in significant abundance in the alexander extract.

The two isomers of procyanidin were identified by their [M-H]$^-$ adduct, one at 1.18 min (m/z 577.1376) and the other at 1.30 min (m/z 577.1370), with drift times of 4.5570 ms and 4.6113 ms, respectively. These were either B1, B2, B3 or B4 isomers, but which two could not be determined by the technique as described, although, with external standards of the 4 isomers, retention time and drift time comparison could reveal which is which. Both isomers detected were described by the same three product ions, namely [C$_{22}$H$_{18}$O$_9$-H]$^-$, [C$_{22}$H$_{16}$O$_8$-H]$^-$ and [C$_{15}$H$_{13}$O$_6$+e]$^-$. As expected, these components were dominant in green tea [6,27,28], and both isomers were shown to be present in *U. europaeus* flower and stem extracts. These important phytochemicals, which give rise to the red positively charged cyanidin pigment associated with grapes and berries, exhibit beneficial health effects, including anti-inflammatory, anti-proliferative and antitumor activities, with many reports suggesting procyanidin as a promising lead compound for cancer prevention and treatment [42].

Many glucuronides of potent polyphenols have been identified and, as previously mentioned, most research relates to the creation of these via mammalian metabolism rather than their benefits as a result of ingestion. Of the remaining components, the highlights will be discussed, though further details can be found in the supplementary materials. *U. europaeus* flower extracts were found to have the highest abundance of hesperetin 3′-*O*-glucuronide and genistein 4′-*O*-glucuronide, to name but two examples of many. *U. europaeus* stem had a high abundance of the glucuronide of *cis*-resveratrol [43], which was the component that initially sparked great interest in polyphenols. Additionally, dihydrodaidzein 7-glucuronide was seen with the highest abundance in *U. europaeus* stem. 4′-Methyl epigallocatechin-3′-glucuronide was observed primarily in *U. dioica* extract, although the amount was fairly low. Irisolidone 7-*O*-glucuronide and feruloyl

C1-glucuronide were both seen in very high amounts in *S. olusatrum*, with lower amounts of both being detected in the *A. ursinum* leaf extract.

Benzoic acid (m/z 365.1031, 3.66 min) and salicylic acid (m/z 413.0867, 2.42 min) were both identified via their [3M-H]$^-$ adducts. Benzoic acid was further confirmed by its product ion m/z 347.0926 [C$_7$H$_5$O-H+2M]$^-$, as was the case for salicylic acid MS/MS fragment m/z 369.0980 [C$_6$H$_5$O-e+2M]$^-$. These analytes are commonplace in plants and have been used medicinally for many years, primarily for pain relief and as anti-inflammatory agents [44,45]. These analytes were seen in their highest abundance in *U. europaeus* stem and, to a lesser extent, *U. europaeus* flower. Additionally, *U. dioica* extract contained significant amounts of salicylic acid. Benzoic acid is the functional group in salicylic acid and its derivatives which are responsible for inducing stress tolerance in plants [46].

The high scoring component 5,7-Dihydroxy-8,4′-dimethoxyisoflavone (m/z 329.0660, 2.89 min) is seen as a bioactive component in mung beans (*Vigna radiata*) [47], although very little else is published on this specific methoxyisoflavone. The 2 product ions m/z 311.0552 ([C$_{17}$H$_{12}$O$_6$-H]$^-$) and m/z 293.0456 ([C$_{17}$H$_{11}$O$_5$-H]$^-$) helped to confirm the identity of this component. Although its score is high, its abundance is seen to be low across all of the extracts, with small amounts in *U. europaeus* flower and stem. On the other hand, the methoxyisoflavone, irisolidone (m/z 314.0786, 2.69 min), is well documented for health benefits, including anti-helicobacter pylori activity, inhibition of prostaglandin E2 production, hepatoprotective effects, anticancer, estrogenic activity, inhibition of JC-1 virus gene expression and anti-inflammatory activity. Irisolidone is created by the intestinal bacterial transformation of kakkalide (ChemSpider ID 4590337), which is a component of traditional medicine [48]. Irisolidone is evident in good abundance in *U. europaeus* stem and, to a lesser extent, *U. europaeus* flower. The product ion m/z 281.0451 ([C$_{16}$H$_9$O$_5$+e]$^-$) helped to confirm the identity of irisolidone. Two methoxyisoflavanones (without the double bond on the C-ring) were seen lower on the list of identifications ordered by score. 7,2′-Dihydroxy-4′-methoxyisoflavanone (m/z 267.0663, 2.41 min) and 7-Hydroxy-4′-methoxyisoflavanone (m/z 269.0829, 2.07 min) were seen mainly in *U. europaeus* flower, *U. europaeus* stem and *U. dioica* extracts. 7,2′-Dihydroxy-4′-methoxyisoflavanone has been shown to exist in many plants and is an important component of Tibetan medicine [49]. Isoflavanones are rare compared to isoflavones, with 7-Hydroxy-4′-methoxyisoflavanone being the focus of little research in recent years [50], but it could conceivably have similar activity to its more studied analogues.

The isomers, neohesperidin (m/z 591.1716, 2.77 min) and hesperidin (m/z 591.1724, 2.42 min) were identified with a high score by their [M-H$_2$O-H]$^-$ adducts. These are both derivatives of hesperetin, differing only in the configuration of their rhamnoglucoside moiety and, therefore, cannot, in truth, be specifically identified without external standards, which is made possible due to differences in chromatographic retention times, as well as drift time separation in ion mobility. Hesperidin and derivatives, which are commonly associated with citrus fruits, play an important role in plant defense systems to combat pathogens. It is thought that they may be useful for humans, as they possess antibacterial, antiviral and antifungal activities [51].

Furthermore, hesperidin and derivatives have been shown to have strong activity against the formation of advanced glycation end products which result in the accumulation of random damage in extracellular proteins. This process is known to have deleterious effects on biological functions which are associated with aging and diabetes, such as cataracts, nephropathy, vasculopathy, proliferative retinopathy and atherosclerosis [52]. Large amounts of hesperidin were observed in the *U. europaeus* stem extracts.

Urolithins have been shown to be effective in cancer chemoprevention [53] though, due to differences in gut microbiota, urolithin production capacity from ellagic acid varies amongst individuals [54]. Urolithin C ([M-H]$^-$, m/z 243.0288, 2.15 min) and urolithin A ([M-H]$^-$, m/z 227.0343, 1.75 min) were identified in the extracts studied, with both being significant in *U. europaeus* flowers and urolithin A being noticeably present in *A. ursinum* leaf.

Vanillin is an important flavour and fragrance component in the food industry, and is also used in the pharmaceutical and cosmetic industries. The two components, 3,4-dihydroxybenzadehyde ([2M-H]$^-$, m/z 275.0555, 1.18 min) and vanillic acid ([3M-H]$^-$, m/z 503.1197, 2.35 min), identified in this characterisation of plant extracts, play a key role in the biosynthetic pathway that produces vanillin [55]. 3,4-dihydroxybenzadehyde was found here in good abundance in *U. europaeus* flower, whereas vanillic acid was at its highest abundance in *U. europaeus* stem.

Lignans have been shown to have anticarcinogenic properties. 7-Hydroxymatairesinol has been shown to be effective in a prostate cancer model in vivo [56]. A study in the Netherlands showed that some plant lignans, including 7-hydroxymatairesinol ([M-H]$^-$, m/z 373.1285, 2.32 min), matairesinol ([M-H]$^-$, m/z 357.1336, 2.14 min) and *iso*-lariciresinol ([M-H]$^-$, m/z 359.1499, 1.90 min) can be converted by intestinal microflora into enterolignans, e.g., enterolactone and enterodiol, and may reduce the risk of certain types of cancer, as well as cardiovascular diseases, through anti-oxidant and anti-estrogenic actions [57]. Once again, their highest abundance was to be found in *U. europaeus* flower and stem.

The flavonoid, pseudobaptigenin, can be seen at [M-H]$^-$, m/z 281.0460, 3.10 min and was present in high abundance in *U. europaeus* stem and in lower quantities in *U. europaeus* flower. It is believed that this phytochemical could be used as a prototype for synthesizing new molecules against diabetic cataracts [58]. Although only observed at low abundance in *U. europaeus* stem, 3',4',7-trihydroxyisoflavan ([3M-H]$^-$, m/z 773.2626, 2.50 min) was present, but little is published about this trihydroxyisoflavan, which can be produced microbially but is included here for completeness. Found to be high in *S. olusatrum*, 4',4''-dimethylepigallocatechin gallate was observed via its [M-H]$^-$ adduct at m/z 485.1076 and 1.46 min. Research shows that methylation of epigallocatechin gallate alters its potency, with a study showing reduced inhibitory effects in macrophages [59], with a further study on cell surface binding abilities showing that dimethylation prevented surface binding completely, suggesting that the hydroxyl groups on the 4'-position in the B ring and the 4''-position in the gallate are crucial for the cell surface binding activity of epigallocatechin gallate [60].

Finally, we observed three related phytochemicals which all contain the chromone structure and that are very prominent in the polyphenol literature. Firstly, quercetin ([M-H]$^-$, m/z 301.0363, 2.30 min), secondly, isoquercetin ([M-H$_2$O-H]$^-$, m/z 445.0772, 2.40 min) and, finally, rutin ([M-H]$^-$, m/z 609.1482, 1.43 min). Isoquercetin is quercetin 3-*O*-glucoside and rutin is quercetin 3-*O*-rhamnoglucoside, with the sugar moiety being an important determinant in dietary flavonoid glycosides absorption in humans [29]. Quercetin is present in all the plant samples analysed here, with very high amounts in *U. europaeus* flower and high amounts in *S. olusatrum*. Quercetin is a powerful antioxidant that has a well-documented role in reducing different human cancers, and is one of the most abundant antioxidants in the human diet [61]. In fact, isoquercetin, which was found to be most abundant in *S. olusatrum*, and rutin, which was found in very high amounts in *U. europaeus* flowers, have also been shown to have powerful anti-mutagenic activity [6].

It is noted from a review relating to the drug discovery potential of these components that the chromones of the previous paragraph have large differences in their chemistry and bioactivity compared to the chroman-4-ones, all due to the C_2–C_3 double bond [62]. Naturally occurring chroman-4-ones, such as naringenin, naringin and eriodictyol, were evident in abundance across these plant extracts, providing, together with the other identified polyphenols, a diverse range of bioactivity, with much potential to benefit human and animal health [63].

4. Conclusions

The effective use of UPLC-HDMS^E for the detailed analysis of four common, but low value, green waste materials is demonstrated here. This discovery mode characterisation, which led to the identification of 77 polyphenols with well-documented health potential, opens the door for these plants to provide naturally occurring treatments for disease.

Supplementary Materials: The following are available online at https://www.mdpi.com/article/10.3390/pr9050824/s1. Figure S1: Total ion chromatogram of Alexanders (green) and the alignment reference (magenta), Figure S2: Total ion chromatogram of Gorse Flowers (green) and the alignment reference (magenta), Figure S3: Total ion chromatogram of Gorse Stem (green) and the alignment reference (magenta), Figure S4: Total ion chromatogram of Nettle (green) and the alignment reference (magenta), Figure S5: Total ion chromatogram of Wild Garlic Leaf (green) and the alignment reference (magenta), Figure S6: Total ion chromatogram of Green Tea (green) and the alignment reference (magenta), Figure S7: Molecular structures of identified polyphenolic components, Figure S8: Example mass spectra of identifications ordered from high to low score value, Figure S9: Abundance profile of (−)-epicatechin (CSID65230), m/z 289.0732, score 38.1, Figure S10: Alexanders, Smyrnium olusatrum, Figure S11: Stinging Nettle, Urtica dioica, Figure S12: Wild garlic, Allium ursinum, Figure S13: Gorse, Ulex europaeus, Green Waste extracts XL SM v7 is a spreadsheet of identifications and abundances.

Author Contributions: This research was conceptualized by C.M.P., who was also responsible for methodology and formal analysis. The samples were collected, prepared and analysed by C.M.P. The first draft of this manuscript was written by C.M.P. and reviewed and edited by D.L.J. and C.M.P. All authors have read and agreed to the published version of the manuscript.

Funding: This research received no external funding.

Institutional Review Board Statement: Not applicable.

Informed Consent Statement: Not applicable.

Data Availability Statement: Data available on request.

Acknowledgments: The authors are highly appreciative to the Welsh European Funding Office (WEFO) in respect to their funding of the Centre for Environmental Technology at Bangor University. The excellent assistance of E.S. Potter is acknowledged for the creation of the heat map.

Conflicts of Interest: The authors declare that they have no known competing financial interests or personal relationships that could have appeared to influence the work reported in this paper.

References

1. Sheldon, R.A. Green and sustainable manufacture of chemicals from biomass: State of the art. *Green Chem.* **2014**, *16*, 950–963. [CrossRef]
2. Langsdorf, A.; Volkmar, M.; Holtmann, D.; Ulber, R. Material utilization of green waste: A review on potential valorization methods. *Bioresourc Bioprocess.* **2021**, *8*, 19. [CrossRef]
3. Barba, F.J.; Zhu, Z.Z.; Koubaa, M.; Sant'Ana, A.S.; Orlien, V. Green alternative methods for the extraction of antioxidant bioactive compounds from winery wastes and by-products: A review. *Trends Food Sci. Technol.* **2016**, *49*, 96–109. [CrossRef]
4. De La Iglesia, R.; Milagro, F.I.; Campión, J.; Boqué, N.; Martínez, J.A. Healthy properties of proanthocyanidins. *BioFactors* **2010**, *36*, 159–168. [CrossRef]
5. Krikorian, R.; Kalt, W.; Mcdonald, J.E.; Shidler, M.D.; Summer, S.S.; Stein, A.L. Cognitive performance in relation to urinary anthocyanins and their flavonoid-based products following blueberry supplementation in older adults at risk for dementia. *J. Funct. Foods* **2019**, 103667. [CrossRef]
6. Preedy, V.; Zibadi, S.; Watson, R. *Polyphenols in Human Health and Disease*; Academic Press: New York, NY, USA, 2014; Volume 1, ISBN 9780123984562.
7. Uyama, H.; Kobayashi, S. Enzymatic synthesis of polyphenols. *Curr. Org. Chem.* **2003**, *7*, 1387–1397. [CrossRef]
8. Potter, C.M.; Jones, D.L. Polyphenolic Profiling of Forestry Waste by UPLC-HDMSe. *Processes* **2020**, *8*, 1411. [CrossRef]
9. Wu, F.F.; Sun, H.; Wei, W.F.; Han, Y.; Wang, P.; Dong, T.W.; Yan, G.L.; Wang, X.J. Rapid and global detection and characterization of the constituents in ShengMai San by ultra-performance liquid chromatography-high-definition mass spectrometry. *J. Sep. Sci.* **2011**, *34*, 3194–3199. [CrossRef]
10. Wang, P.; Sun, H.; Lv, H.; Sun, W.; Yuan, Y.; Han, Y.; Wang, D.W.; Zhang, A.H.; Wang, X.J. Thyroxine and reserpine-induced changes in metabolic profiles of rat urine and the therapeutic effect of Liu Wei Di Huang Wan detected by UPLC-HDMS. *J. Pharm. Biomed. Anal.* **2010**, *53*, 631–645. [CrossRef]
11. Da Silva Pinto, M. Tea: A new perspective on health benefits. *Food Res. Int.* **2013**, *53*, 558–567. [CrossRef]
12. Sapozhnikova, Y. Development of liquid chromatography-tandem mass spectrometry method for analysis of polyphenolic compounds in liquid samples of grape juice, green tea and coffee. *Food Chem.* **2014**, *150*, 87–93. [CrossRef]
13. Vos, F.; Crespy, V.; Chaffaut, L.; Mennen, L.; Knox, C.; Neveu, V. Phenol-Explorer: An online comprehensive database on polyphenol contents in foods. *Database* **2010**, *2010*, 1–9. [CrossRef]

14. Pandey, R.; Chandra, P.; Arya, K.R.; Kumar, B. Development and validation of an ultra high performance liquid chromatography electrospray ionization tandem mass spectrometry method for the simultaneous determination of selected flavonoids in Ginkgo biloba. *J. Sep. Sci.* **2014**, *37*, 3610–3618. [CrossRef]
15. Lopes, N.P.; Demarque, D.P.; Crotti, A.E.M.; Vessecchi, R.; Lopes, J. Fragmentation reactions using electrospray ionization mass spectrometry: An important tool for the structural elucidation and characterization of synthetic and natural products. *RSC-Nat. Prod. Rep.* **2016**, *33*, 432. [CrossRef]
16. Ahn, H.J.; You, J.; Park, S.; Li, Z.; Choe, D. RSC Advances and their contribution to improved anti-inflammatory activity. *RSC Adv.* **2020**, *10*, 5339–5350. [CrossRef]
17. Chaitanya, M.V.N.L.; Suresh, P.; Dhanabal, P.; Jubie, S. Human Topopoisons From Weeds: A Review. *Curr. Tradit. Med.* **2018**, *4*, 4–15. [CrossRef]
18. Andersen Oyvind, M.; Dersen Markham, K.R. *Flavonoids: Chemistry, Biochemistry and Applications*; CRC Press: Boca Raton, FL, USA, 2006; Volume 45, ISBN 9780849320217.
19. Gülçin, I. Antioxidant activity of caffeic acid (3,4-dihydroxycinnamic acid). *Toxicology* **2006**, *217*, 213–220. [CrossRef] [PubMed]
20. Barsky, L.; Cook-Wiens, G.; Doyle, M.; Shufelt, C.; Rogers, W.; Reis, S.; Pepine, C.J.; Noel Bairey Merz, C. Phytoestrogen blood levels and adverse outcomes in women with suspected ischemic heart disease. *Eur. J. Clin. Nutr.* **2020**. [CrossRef] [PubMed]
21. Zaw, J.J.T.; Howe, P.R.C.; Wong, R.H.X. Does phytoestrogen supplementation improve cognition in humans? A systematic review. *Ann. N. Y. Acad. Sci.* **2017**, *1403*, 150–163. [CrossRef]
22. Costa, E.M.D.M.B.; Pimenta, F.C.; Luz, W.C.; De Oliveira, V. Selection of filamentous fungi of the Beauveria genus able to metabolize quercetin like mammalian cells. *Braz. J. Microbiol.* **2008**, *39*, 405–408. [CrossRef]
23. Marvalin, C.; Azerad, R. Microbial glucuronidation of polyphenols. *J. Mol. Catal. B Enzym.* **2011**, *73*, 43–52. [CrossRef]
24. Salehi, B.; Fokou, P.V.T.; Sharifi-Rad, M.; Zucca, P.; Pezzani, R.; Martins, N.; Sharifi-Rad, J. The therapeutic potential of naringenin: A review of clinical trials. *Pharmaceuticals* **2019**, *12*, 11. [CrossRef] [PubMed]
25. Tutunchi, H.; Naeini, F.; Ostadrahimi, A.; Hosseinzadeh-Attar, M.J. Naringenin, a flavanone with antiviral and anti-inflammatory effects: A promising treatment strategy against COVID-19. *Phyther. Res.* **2020**, *1*, 1–11. [CrossRef]
26. Alberca, R.W.; Teixeira, F.M.E.; Beserra, D.R.; de Oliveira, E.A.; de Andrade, M.M.S.; Pietrobon, A.J.; Sato, M.N. Perspective: The Potential Effects of Naringenin in COVID-19. *Front. Immunol.* **2020**, *11*, 1–9. [CrossRef] [PubMed]
27. Sanz, M.; Fernández de Simón, B.; Esteruelas, E.; Muñoz, Á.M.; Cadahía, E.; Hernández, M.T.; Estrella, I.; Martinez, J. Polyphenols in red wine aged in acacia (Robinia pseudoacacia) and oak (Quercus petraea) wood barrels. *Anal. Chim. Acta* **2012**, *732*, 83–90. [CrossRef]
28. Duan, J.; Guan, Y.; Mu, F.; Guo, C.; Zhang, E.; Yin, Y.; Wei, G.; Zhu, Y.; Cui, J.; Cao, J.; et al. Protective effect of butin against ischemia/reperfusion-induced myocardial injury in diabetic mice: Involvement of the AMPK/GSK-3β/Nrf2 signaling pathway. *Sci. Rep.* **2017**, *7*, 1–14. [CrossRef] [PubMed]
29. Hollman, P.C.H.; Bijsman, M.N.C.P.; Van Gameren, Y.; Cnossen, E.P.J.; De Vries, J.H.M.; Katan, M.B. The sugar moiety is a major determinant of the absorption of dietary flavonoid glycosides in man. *Free Radic. Res.* **1999**, *31*, 569–573. [CrossRef]
30. Rabago Smith, M.; Kindl, E.D.; Williams, I.R.; Moorman, V.R. 5,7,3′,4′-Hydroxy substituted flavonoids reduce the heme of cytochrome c with a range of rate constants. *Biochimie* **2019**, *162*, 167–175. [CrossRef]
31. Liu, Y.C.; Yan, X.N. Eriodictyol inhibits survival and inflammatory responses and promotes apoptosis in rheumatoid arthritis fibroblast-like synoviocytes through AKT/FOXO1 signaling. *J. Cell. Biochem.* **2019**, *120*, 14628–14635. [CrossRef]
32. Lv, P.; Yu, J.; Xu, X.; Lu, T.; Xu, F. Eriodictyol inhibits high glucose-induced oxidative stress and inflammation in retinal ganglial cells. *J. Cell. Biochem.* **2019**, *120*, 5644–5651. [CrossRef]
33. HighChem LLC mzCloud. Available online: https://www.mzcloud.org/ (accessed on 1 December 2020).
34. The, S.N. A Review on the Medicinal Plant Dalbergia odorifera Species: Phytochemistry and Biological Activity. *Evid.-Based Complement. Altern. Med.* **2017**, *1*. [CrossRef]
35. Deesamer, S.; Kokpol, U.; Chavasiri, W.; Douillard, S.; Peyrot, V.; Vidal, N.; Combes, S.; Finet, J.P. Synthesis and biological evaluation of isoflavone analogues from Dalbergia oliveri. *Tetrahedron* **2007**, *63*, 12986–12993. [CrossRef]
36. Wen, R.; Lv, H.; Jiang, Y.; Tu, P. Anti-inflammatory isoflavones and isoflavanones from the roots of Pongamia pinnata (L.) Pierre. *Bioorganic Med. Chem. Lett.* **2018**, *28*, 1050–1055. [CrossRef]
37. Peng, F.; Du, Q.; Peng, C.; Wang, N.; Tang, H.; Xie, X.; Shen, J.; Chen, J. A Review: The Pharmacology of Isoliquiritigenin. *Phyther. Res.* **2015**, *29*, 969–977. [CrossRef]
38. Park, E.-K.; Shin, Y.-W.; Lee, H.-U.; Lee, C.S.; Kim, D. Passive Cutaneous Anaphylaxis-Inhibitory Action of Tectorigenin, a Metabolite of Tectridin by Intestinal Microflora. *Biol. Pharm. Bull.* **2004**, *27*, 1099–1102. [CrossRef] [PubMed]
39. Wang, Y.; Jing, W.; Qu, W.; Liu, Z.; Zhang, D.; Qi, X.; Liu, L. Tectorigenin inhibits inflammation and pulmonary fibrosis in allergic asthma model of ovalbumin-sensitized guinea pigs. *J. Pharm. Pharmacol.* **2020**, *72*, 956–968. [CrossRef] [PubMed]
40. Suzuki, A.; Nomura, T.; Jokura, H.; Kitamura, N.; Saiki, A.; Fujii, A. Chlorogenic acid-enriched green coffee bean extract affects arterial stiffness assessed by the cardio-ankle vascular index in healthy men: A pilot study. *Int. J. Food Sci. Nutr.* **2019**, *70*, 901–908. [CrossRef]
41. Drynan, J.W.; Clifford, M.N.; Obuchowicz, J.; Kuhnert, N. The chemistry of low molecular weight black tea polyphenols. *Nat. Prod. Rep.* **2010**, *27*, 417–462. [CrossRef] [PubMed]
42. Lee, Y. Cancer chemopreventive potential of procyanidin. *Toxicol. Res.* **2017**, *33*, 273–282. [CrossRef]

43. Wiciski, M.; Leis, K.; Szyperski, P.; Wcelewicz, M.M.; Mazur, E.; Pawlak-Osiska, K. ARTICLE IN PRESS Impact of resveratrol on exercise performance: A review Effet du resveratrol sur la performance physique: Revue générale. *Sci. Sport.* **2018**, *1*. [CrossRef]
44. Qualley, A.V.; Widhalm, J.R.; Adebesin, F.; Kish, C.M.; Dudareva, N. Completion of the core β-oxidative pathway of benzoic acid biosynthesis in plants. *Proc. Natl. Acad. Sci. USA* **2012**, *109*, 16383–16388. [CrossRef]
45. Raskin, I. Role of salicylic acid in plants. *Annu. Rev. Plant Physiol. Plant Mol. Biol.* **1992**, *43*, 439–463. [CrossRef]
46. Senaratna, T.; Merritt, D.; Dixon, K.; Bunn, E.; Touchell, D.; Sivasithamparam, K. Benzoic acid may act as the functional group in salicylic acid and derivatives in the induction of multiple stress tolerance in plants. *Plant Growth Regul.* **2003**, *39*, 77–81. [CrossRef]
47. Ganesan, K.; Xu, B. A critical review on phytochemical profile and health promoting effects of mung bean (Vigna radiata). *Food Sci. Hum. Wellness* **2018**, *7*, 11–33. [CrossRef]
48. Kang, K.A.; Zhang, R.; Piao, M.J.; Ko, D.O.; Wang, Z.H.; Kim, B.J.; Park, J.W.; Kim, H.S.; Kim, D.H.; Hyun, J.W. Protective effect of irisolidone, a metabolite of kakkalide, against hydrogen peroxide induced cell damage via antioxidant effect. *Bioorganic Med. Chem.* **2008**, *16*, 1133–1141. [CrossRef] [PubMed]
49. Wang, Q.; Wu, X.; Yang, X.; Zhang, Y.; Wang, L.; Li, X.; Qiu, Y. Comprehensive quality evaluation of Lignum Caraganae and rapid discrimination of Caragana jubata and Caragana changduensis based on characteristic compound fingerprints by HPLC-UV and HPLC-MS/MS coupled with chemometrics analysis. *Phytochem. Anal.* **2020**, *31*, 846–860. [CrossRef]
50. Al-Maharik, N. Isolation of naturally occurring novel isoflavonoids: An update. *Nat. Prod. Rep.* **2019**, *36*, 1156–1195. [CrossRef]
51. Iranshahi, M.; Rezaee, R.; Parhiz, H.; Roohbakhsh, A.; Soltani, F. Protective effects of flavonoids against microbes and toxins: The cases of hesperidin and hesperetin. *Life Sci.* **2015**, *137*, 125–132. [CrossRef]
52. Li, D.; Mitsuhashi, S.; Ubukata, M. Protective effects of hesperidin derivatives and their stereoisomers against advanced glycation end-products formation. *Pharm. Biol.* **2012**, *50*, 1531–1535. [CrossRef] [PubMed]
53. Stanisławska, I.J.; Piwowarski, J.P.; Granica, S.; Kiss, A.K. The effects of urolithins on the response of prostate cancer cells to non-steroidal antiandrogen bicalutamide. *Phytomedicine* **2018**, *1*. [CrossRef]
54. García-Villalba, R.; Beltrán, D.; Espín, J.C.; Selma, M.V.; Tomás-Barberán, F.A. Time course production of urolithins from ellagic acid by human gut microbiota. *J. Agric. Food Chem.* **2013**, *61*, 8797–8806. [CrossRef]
55. Kundu, A. Vanillin biosynthetic pathways in plants. *Planta* **2017**, *245*, 1069–1078. [CrossRef]
56. Bylund, A.; Saarinen, N.; Zhang, J.X.; Bergh, A.; Widmark, A.; Johansson, A.; Lundin, E.; Adlercreutz, H.; Hallmans, G.; Stattin, P.; et al. Anticancer effects of a plant lignan 7-hydroxymatairesinol on a prostate cancer model in vivo. *Urol. Oncol. Semin. Orig. Investig.* **2005**, *23*, 380–381. [CrossRef]
57. Milder, I.E.J.; Feskens, E.J.M.; Arts, I.C.W.; De Mesquita, H.B.B.; Hollman, P.C.H.; Kromhout, D. Intake of the Plant Lignans Secoisolariciresinol, Matairesinol, Lariciresinol, and Pinoresinol in Dutch Men and Women 1. *Nutr. Epidemiol.* **2005**, *135*, 1202–1207. [CrossRef] [PubMed]
58. Jeevanandam, J.; Madhumitha, R.; Saraswathi, N.T. Identification of potential phytochemical lead against diabetic cataract: An in silico approach. *J. Mol. Struct.* **2020**, *1226*, 129428. [CrossRef]
59. Chiu, F.L.; Lin, J.K. HPLC analysis of naturally occurring methylated catechins, 3"- and 4"-methyl-epigallocatechin gallate, in various fresh tea leaves and commercial teas and their potent inhibitory effects on inducible nitric oxide synthase in macrophages. *J. Agric. Food Chem.* **2005**, *53*, 7035–7042. [CrossRef]
60. Yano, S.; Fujimura, Y.; Umeda, D.; Miyase, T.; Yamada, K.; Tachibana, H. Relationship between the biological activities of methylated derivatives of (-)-epigallocatechin-3-O-gallate (EGCG) and their cell surface binding activities. *J. Agric. Food Chem.* **2007**, *55*, 7144–7148. [CrossRef]
61. Rauf, A.; Imran, M.; Khan, I.A.; ur-Rehman, M.; Gilani, S.A.; Mehmood, Z.; Mubarak, M.S. Anticancer potential of quercetin: A comprehensive review. *Phyther. Res.* **2018**, *32*, 2109–2130. [CrossRef] [PubMed]
62. Emami, S.; Ghanbarimasir, Z. Recent advances of chroman-4-one derivatives: Synthetic approaches and bioactivities. *Eur. J. Med. Chem.* **2015**, *93*, 539–563. [CrossRef]
63. Shyamal, K.; Jash, G.B. Recent progress in the research of naturally occurring flavonoids: A look through. *Signpost Open Access J. Org. Biomol. Chem.* **2013**, *1*, 65–168.

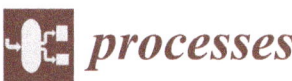

Article

Formulation and Stability of Cellulose-Based Delivery Systems of Raspberry Phenolics

Josipa Vukoja [1], Ivana Buljeta [1], Anita Pichler [1], Josip Šimunović [2] and Mirela Kopjar [1,*]

1. Faculty of Food Technology, Josip Juraj Strosmayer University, F. Kuhača 18, 31000 Osijek, Croatia; jjosipa.vukoja@gmail.com (J.V.); ivana.buljeta@ptfos.hr (I.B.); anita.pichler@ptfos.hr (A.P.)
2. Department of Food, Bioprocessing and Nutrition Sciences, North Carolina State University, Raleigh, NC 27695, USA; simun@ncsu.edu
* Correspondence: mirela.kopjar@ptfos.hr

Abstract: Encapsulation of bioactives is a tool to prepare their suitable delivery systems and ensure their stability. For this purpose, cellulose was selected as carrier of raspberry juice phenolics and freeze-dried cellulose/raspberry encapsulates (C/R_Es) were formulated. Influence of cellulose amount (2.5%, 5%, 7.5% and 10%) and time (15 or 60 min) on the complexation of cellulose and raspberry juice was investigated. Obtained C/R_Es were evaluated for total phenolics, anthocyanins, antioxidant activity, inhibition of α-amylase and color. Additionally, encapsulation was confirmed by FTIR. Stability of C/R_Es was examined after 12 months of storage at room temperature. Increasing the amount of cellulose during formulation of C/R_E from 2.5% to 10%, resulted in the decrease of content of total phenolics and anthocyanins. Additionally, encapsulates formulated by 15 min of complexation had a higher amount of investigated compounds. This tendency was retained after storage. The highest antioxidant activities were determined for C/R_E with 2.5% of cellulose and the lowest for those with 10% of cellulose, regardless of the methods used for its evaluation. After storage of 12 months, antioxidant activity slightly increased. Encapsulates with 2.5% of cellulose had the highest and those with 10% of cellulose the lowest capability for inhibition of α-amylase. The amount of cellulose also had an impact on color of C/R_Es. Results of this study suggest that cellulose could be a good encapsulation polymer for delivering raspberry bioactives, especially when cellulose was used in lower percentages for formulation of encapsulates.

Keywords: cellulose/raspberry encapsulates; phenolics; anthocyanins; antioxidant activity; inhibition of α-amylase

Citation: Vukoja, J.; Buljeta, I.; Pichler, A.; Šimunović, J.; Kopjar, M. Formulation and Stability of Cellulose-Based Delivery Systems of Raspberry Phenolics. Processes 2021, 9, 90. https://doi.org/10.3390/pr9010090

Received: 30 November 2020
Accepted: 30 December 2020
Published: 4 January 2021

Publisher's Note: MDPI stays neutral with regard to jurisdictional claims in published maps and institutional affiliations.

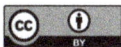

Copyright: © 2021 by the authors. Licensee MDPI, Basel, Switzerland. This article is an open access article distributed under the terms and conditions of the Creative Commons Attribution (CC BY) license (https://creativecommons.org/licenses/by/4.0/).

1. Introduction

Recommendations of nutritionists are consumption of plant-based foods since this type of diet has been linked with a lowered occurrence of various types of degenerative diseases. Over the years, phenolic compounds and fibers have been highlighted as two major functional compounds responsible for prevention of different diseases [1]. Polyphenols were put forward as components that are related with antioxidant, anti-inflammatory, antimicrobial and antiproliferation activity as well as with reduction of diverse chronic diseases such as cardiovascular and neurodegenerative diseases, certain cancers, type II diabetes and osteoporosis [2–4]. The diverse effects of secondary plant metabolites are connected with different chemical structures of those compounds and their major categories include flavonoids, phenolic acids, lignans, coumarins, stilbenes and quinones [2]. Consumption of dietary fibers has been also related with various health benefits such as decrease of risk of development of coronary heart disease, hypertension, diabetes, obesity as well as some gastrointestinal disorders [5]. In plant cells, polyphenols are primarily located in the vacuoles but throughout harvesting, processing and consumption, they can interact with components of plant cell walls (PCWs). Cellulose, hemicellulose and pectin are dominant components of PCWs, with cellulose portion of approximately 35% on a dry weight basis [6,7].

The aim of this study was the preparation of encapsulates based on raspberry phenolics and cellulose to obtain functional food ingredients combining two components with potential health benefits. As a phenolic source we selected raspberries since they are grown worldwide, and are known for their pleasant and favorable flavors as well as for bioactive compounds with potential health benefits [4,8,9]. As far as we know, most of the studies related to phenolics/PCWs were designed to explore release of phenolics bounded on PCWs in gastrointestinal tract under different conditions and examination of influence of type of bonding between phenolics and PCWs. Binding of phenolics to PCWs can significantly affect release of these compounds from the food matrix for potential absorption in the gastrointestinal tract. Studying the effects of the interaction of phenolics and PCWs is challenging due to the complexity of both type of components and those interactions are playing an important role in the bioaccessibility and bioavailability of phenolics [10,11]. Through studies, non-covalent interactions like hydrogen bonds and hydrophobic interactions were emphasized as main mechanisms of complex interaction between phenolics and plant PCWs [12–17]. It was observed that these interactions depended on the chemical characteristics (such as molecular structure and molecular weight) as well as on the physical properties and initial concentration of both, phenolic compounds and PCWs [18,19]. Additionally, for these interactions environmental factors like pH, ionic strength, and temperature should not be neglected [20,21]. The aim of our study was to use this knowledge for the preparation of functional food ingredients i.e., to explore the possibility of application of cellulose as a tool for the preparation of functional food additives. Obtained functional food ingredients could be used for enrichment of bakery products, dairy products, fruit products with fibers and phenolics, as well as increase of antioxidant activity and color modification. Nsor–Atindana et al. [22] in their review demonstrated that cellulose has been extensively explored as a functional ingredient in food industry from meat products, emulsions, beverages, dairy products, bakery to confectionary and different types of fillings. They emphasized that this polymer has many promising applications in functional and nutraceutical food industries and can contribute to positive effects on gastrointestinal physiology, and hypolipidemic effects, influencing the expression of enzymes involved in lipid metabolism [22]. In our previous study, we emphasized the possibility of cellulose application as carrier of raspberry volatiles [23] for modification of flavor in added products as another possible application of obtained cellulose/raspberry encapsulates. Therefore, encapsulates were formulated by complexation of cellulose and raspberry juice. Different cellulose/raspberry encapsulates were formulated with constant amount of juice, while the cellulose amounts varied (2.5%, 5%, 7.5% and 10%), and the complexation of cellulose and raspberry juice was carried out for 15 and 60 min. In addition, stability of encapsulates over the time is also a very important quality factor. In order to investigate this, encapsulates were stored for 12 months at room temperature. The amounts of total phenolics content, anthocyanins, antioxidant activity, inhibition of α-amylase and color of the complexes after formulation and during storage were investigated.

2. Materials and Methods

2.1. Materials

Cellulose (microcrystalline) was obtained from Kemika (Zagreb, Croatia). Potassium chloride, sodium acetate, methanol and sodium carbonate, were purchased from Kemika (Zagreb, Croatia). [1]Trolox, [1]2,2-diphenyl-1-picrylhydrazil (DPPH) and [2]α-amylase from porcine pancreas (type VI-B, ≥5 units/mg solid) were purchased from Sigma-Aldrich ([1]St. Louis, MO, USA; [2]Germany). Starch soluble, iron (III) chloride hexahydrate, sodium acetate, ethanol, ammonium acetate and Folin–Ciocalteu reagent were bought from Grammol (Zagreb, Croatia). Then, 3,5-dinitrosalicylic acid was from Alfa Aesar (Kandel, Germany). Sodium hydroxide and potassium sodium tartarate tetrahydrate were from T.T.T. (Sveta nedjelja, Croatia). Potassium dihydrogen phosphate was from BDH Prolabo (UK).

[3]Neocuproine, [4]2,4,6-tripyridyl-s-tirazine (TPTZ) and [5]copper (II) chloride were bought from Acros Organics ([3]Geel, Belgium; [4]China; [5]SAD). Acetic acid (min 99.5%) was from Alkaloid (Skopje, North Macedonia) and hydrochloric acid (37%) from Carlo Erba Reagents (Val de Reuil, France).

2.2. Formulation of Cellulose/Raspberry Encapsulates

Formulation of cellulose/raspberry encapsulates was described in detail in our previous study [23]. Briefly, cellulose (2.5%, 5%, 7.5% and 10%) and raspberry juice were mixed on a magnetic stirrer for 15 or 60 min at room temperature. Obtained mixtures were centrifuged for 15 min at 4000 rpm, followed by separation of the liquid part and precipitate was freeze-dried to obtain dry powder. Freeze-drying was conducted in a laboratory freeze-dryer (Christ Freeze Dryer, Alpha 1-4, Germany) under following conditions: Freezing temperature was adjusted at −55 °C; the temperature of sublimation from −35 to 0 °C; and the vacuum level 0.220 mbar. The temperature of the isothermal desorption varied from 0 to 21 °C under the vacuum of 0.060 mbar. Obtained freeze-dried encapsulates were used immediately for determination of selected parameters. For evaluation of stability, encapsulates were packed in sealed bags and stored at room temperature for 12 months.

2.3. Preparation of Extracts

First, 0.8 g of the freeze-dried cellulose/raspberry encapsulate was extracted with 5 mL of acidified methanol (HCl:methanol ratio was 1:99) in an ultrasonic bath for 15 min, after which the mixture was allowed to stand for 15 min to separate the solid and liquid phases. The liquid extract was decanted and centrifuged for 10 min at 10,000 rpm. The resulting liquid extract was separated into a plastic tube. Solid phase was extracted two more times with an additional volume of solvent (5 mL), as described above. A new 5 mL of acidified methanol was added to the residue for the fourth time and extracted for 15 min. The whole mixture was centrifuged for 15 min at 4000 rpm. The obtained extract was used for evaluation of total phenols, anthocyanins, inhibition of α-amylase and antioxidant activity.

2.4. Determination of Total Phenolic Content

The total phenolic content was determined according to the modified colorimetric Folin–Ciocalteu method [24]. Briefly, 0.2 mL of extracted sample and 1.8 mL of deionized water were added to the test tube, followed by 10 mL of Folin–Ciocalteu reagent (1:10) and finally 8 mL of 7.5% sodium carbonate (Na_2CO_3). After development of color (for 120 min), absorbance was read at 765 nm using a spectrophotometer. A gallic acid calibration curve was used for expression of total phenolics and results were expressed as grams of gallic acid equivalents per kilogram of sample (g GAE/kg). Measurements were performed in triplicates.

2.5. Determination of Monomeric Anthocyanin Content

Determination of monomeric anthocyanins was performed by pH-differential method [25]. Briefly, 0.2 mL of extract was mixed with 2.8 mL of 0.025 M KCl (pH 1) and 0.4 M sodium acetate (pH 4.5), respectively. After 15 min, absorbance of mixture was read at two wavelengths ($A_{\lambda vis}$ = 515 nm and 700 nm) against a blank cell containing distilled water. The absorbance (A) of the sample was calculated according to the following formula [25]:

$$A = (A_{\lambda vis} - A_{700})_{pH1.0} - (A_{\lambda vis} - A_{700})_{pH4.5}$$

The monomeric anthocyanin content (AC) was calculated according to the following formula:

$$AC = (A \times MW \times DF \times 1000) \div (\varepsilon \times l)$$

where, AC was expressed in mg of cyanidin-3-glucoside/kg, MW was the molecular weight of cyanidin-3-glucoside (449.2), DF was the dilution factor, ε was the molar absorptivity (26,900) and l was the cuvette length (1 cm). All measurements were done in triplicate.

2.6. Inhibition of α-amylase

The experiment was performed according to slightly modified method described by da Silva et al. [26] and Kellogg et al. [27]. Briefly, 0.2 mL of sample was mixed with 0.4 mL of α-amylase solution (1 mg/mL) and mixture was incubated for 10 min at 37 °C. Afterwards, 0.2 mL of 1% starch solution was added and the mixture was incubated for another 10 min at 37 °C. Further, 1 mL of 3,5-dinitrosallicylic acid (DNS) reagent was added and boiled for 5 min to stop the reaction. Mixture was quickly cooled in ice bath to room temperature, and 10 mL of distilled water was added to the mixture. Absorbance was read at wavelength of 540 nm. A control sample represented the uninhibited reaction, and a blank (without the enzyme present) was also measured for each sample. The percentage of inhibition was calculated according to the following formula:

$$\%Control = \frac{(A_{inh} - A_{blank})}{A_{con}} \times 100\%$$

where A_{inh} was absorbance of the inhibited reaction, A_{blank} absorbance of the extract with substrate (no enzyme present) and A_{con} absorbance of the uninhibited enzyme. All measurements were done in triplicate.

2.7. Antioxidant Activity

The antioxidant activity of the samples was determined by the radical scavenging activity method using 2,2-diphenyl-1-picrylhydrazyl radical as previously described by Brand–Williams et al. [28]. Briefly, 0.2 mL of extract was mixed with 3 mL of DPPH solution (0.5 mM). Absorbance was measured at 517 nm after mixture was incubated 15 min. Cupric reducing antioxidant capacity assay was carried out according to the method of Apak et al. [29]. Briefly, mixture of copper chloride (1 mL), neocuproine (1 mL) and ammonium acetate buffer (1 mL) was prepared, and then 0.2 mL of sample extract and 0.9 mL distilled water were added. Absorbance was measured at 450 nm after mixture was incubated for 30 min. The antioxidant capacity of samples was determined by the method of Benzie and Strain [30]. Briefly, 0.2 mL of sample was mixed with 3 mL of FRAP reagent. Absorbance was measured at 593 nm after mixture was incubated for 30 min. In all cases, measurements were done against a blank that was prepared using distilled water. As a standard for expression of antioxidant activity (DPPH, FRAP and CUPRAC), calibration curve of trolox was prepared and results were expressed as μmol of trolox equivalents per 100 g of sample (μmol TE/100 g). All measurements were done in triplicate.

2.8. Color Measurement and Color Change

Color measurements were carried out with a chromometer Minolta CR-400 (Minolta; Osaka, Japan) with recording of L^*, a^*, b^*, C^* and h parameters. Measurements were performed in triplicates. Numerical values of L^*, a^* and b^* were used to calculate the total color change (ΔE).

2.9. Analysis by Fourier Transform Infrared (FTIR) Spectroscopy

For recording of infra-red spectra, FTIR-ATR (Cary 630, Agilent, Santa Clara, CA, USA) was used by the attenuated total reflection method. Screening of samples through the range from 4000 cm^{-1} to 600 cm^{-1} was carried out to obtain IR spectra.

2.10. Statistical Analysis

Analysis of variance (ANOVA) and Fisher's least significant difference (LSD) with the significance defined at $p < 0.05$ were applied for statistical evaluation of obtained results using software program STATISTICA 13.1 (StatSoft Inc, Tulsa, OK, USA). All results were presented as the mean values ± standard deviation.

3. Results and Discussion

In order to evaluate the possibility of preparation of freeze-dried cellulose-based encapsulates as delivery systems of raspberry phenolics, encapsulates were prepared by complexation of various amounts of cellulose with constant amount of raspberry juice. On the basis of previous studies [7,10,11] of potential absorption of phenolics onto plant cell wall material in the gastrointestinal tract it was observed that interactions occurred rapidly thus we selected shorter and prolonged time of preparation of encapsulates. Therefore, complexation was performed for 15 min and 60 min in order to investigate influence of complexation time on investigated parameters. Stability of freeze-dried encapsulates after 12 months of storage was also evaluated.

3.1. Total Phenolics Content and Anthocyanins Content

Total phenolics content of cellulose/raspberry encapsulates after formulation and 12 months storage are presented in Table 1 while results of anthocyanins content are presented in Table 2. Complexation time and the amount of used cellulose for formulation of cellulose/raspberry encapsulates (C/R_Es) had an impact on the amount of both investigated parameters, total phenolics and anthocyanins content. C/R_E formulated for 15 min of complexation with the addition of 2.5% of cellulose had the highest total phenolics (2.43 g/kg). Increasing the amount of cellulose from 2.5% to 10%, the content of total phenolics decreased. Encapsulates formulated throughout shorter time of complexation (15 min) had a higher amount of total phenolics in comparison to encapsulates formulated for 60 min. This trend was also observed for anthocyanins content. C/R_E formulated by 15 min of complexation with the addition of 2.5% of cellulose had the highest anthocyanins content (429.40 mg/kg). Encapsulates obtained with prolonged complexation had lower anthocyanins content and with the increase of cellulose amount, content of anthocyanins decreased. Study of the interaction between phenolics and cellulose showed that maximum binding capacity depended on molecular structure of these compounds and it ranged from 0.4 to 1.4 g per g of cellulose [7]. Interaction between different phenolics (catechin, ferulic acid, chlorogenic acid, gallic acid and cyanidin-3-glucoside) and cellulose occurred spontaneously, within 1 min, and rapidly increased over 30 min [7]. Up to 2 h, further slow binding occurred but after that time plateau was reached. In addition, it was determined that chlorogenic acid had different behavior then other investigated phenolics. While all other phenolics bonded similarly on a molar basis, binding of chlorogenic acid was lower [7]. Investigation of binding of anthocyanins and phenolic acids from purple carrot juice to cell wall polysaccharides occurred within 30 s and it was observed that binding was rapid within 10 min, while afterwards a relatively slow increase in binding was observed [10,11]. As authors stated [7], those results were beneficial for predication of phenolics behavior during food consumption since it is likely that phenolics would bind to fibers during mastication in the mouth or later in the stomach and small intestine. Our results also support this binding tendency i.e., with prolonged time of complexation lower amount of phenolics was determined on formulated encapsulates. Consequently, we can conclude that complexation of cellulose-based encapsulates would not be time consuming. Liu et al. [1] predicted that initial binding occurred due to adsorption of phenolics on the binding sites of cellulose surface due to presence of labile hydroxyl groups. Additional interaction occurred due to non-covalent binding i.e., hydrogen bonding and hydrophobic interactions [1]. Important factors for non-covalent binding were also phenolic rings i.e., their number and their conformational flexibility [31]. Since non-covalent binding was included in the adsorption process of phenolics onto cellulose, probably prolonged complexation time which included stirring resulted in breaking of hydrogen bonds and hydrophobic interactions therefore lower contents of phenolics on C/R_Es were detected.

Table 1. Total phenolics content (g/kg) on cellulose/raspberry encapsulates (C/R_Es) prepared by 15 or 60 min of complexation, after formulation and after storage.

	Complexation Time (min)	
Samples	15	60
	After preparation	
C/R_E_2.5%	2.43 ± 0.03 [a]	1.96 ± 0.01 [a]
C/R_E_5%	1.70 ± 0.25 [c]	1.54 ± 0.03 [b]
C/R_E_7.5%	1.38 ± 0.02 [d]	1.23 ± 0.01 [c]
C/R_E_10%	1.26 ± 0.27 [e]	1.16 ± 0.04 [c]
	After 12 months of storage	
C/R_E_2.5%	2.08 ± 0.11 [b]	1.67 ± 0.15 [b]
C/R_E_5%	1.76 ± 0.22 [c]	1.50 ± 0.11 [b]
C/R_E_7.5%	1.47 ± 0.14 [d]	1.19 ± 0.29 [c]
C/R_E_10%	0.96 ± 0.17 [e]	0.72 ± 0.06 [d]

Results in the same column marked with the same letters were not significantly different ($p \leq 0.05$); Statistical differences between results are presented in the tables in the following increasing order: a > b > c > d > e; 2.5%, 5%, 7.5% and 10%—the amounts of used cellulose for formulation of C/R_Es.

Table 2. Anthocyanin content (mg/kg) on C/R_Es prepared by 15 or 60 min of complexation, after formulation and after storage.

Samples	Complexation Time (min)	
	15	60
	After formulation	
C/R_E_2.5%	429.40 ± 2.98 [a]	411.88 ± 1.12 [a]
C/R_E_5%	392.04 ± 5.84 [b]	374.02 ± 2.37 [b]
C/R_E_7.5%	356.83 ± 4.10 [c]	337.35 ± 4.09 [c]
C/R_E_10%	320.19 ± 2.50 [d]	274.10 ± 0.00 [d]
	After 12 months of storage	
C/R_E_2.5%	280.75 ± 5.58 [e]	237.06 ± 5.64 [e]
C/R_E_5%	243.01 ± 2.41 [f]	221.08 ± 2.98 [f]
C/R_E_7.5%	209.79 ± 4.85 [g]	192.40 ± 0.00 [g]
C/R_E_10%	175.43 ± 3.21 [h]	166.36 ± 0.37 [h]

Results in the same column marked with the same letters were not significantly different ($p \leq 0.05$); Statistical differences between results are presented in the tables in the following increasing order: a > b > c > d > e > f > g > h; 2.5%, 5%, 7.5% and 10%—the amounts of used cellulose for formulation of C/R_Es.

During storage, the same tendency as after preparation regarding total phenolics and anthocyanins was observed. Encapsulates with the lowest amount of cellulose addition had the highest amount of phenolics and anthocyanins (respectively). Stability of the obtained encapsulates i.e., retention of components was also evaluated during storage over 12 months period. The highest retention of phenolics was on the encapsulates formulated with 5% and 7.5% of cellulose (complete retention) using 15 min of complexation, as well as in encapsulates with the same amount of cellulose formulated for 60 min of complexation (from 90 to 96%). Samples with 2.5% of cellulose formulated by 15 min and 60 min of complexation had 85% and 70 % of phenolic retention. The lowest retention was on encapsulates formulated with 10% of cellulose (76% in encapsulates formulated for 15 min and 62% on encapsulates formulated for 60 min of complexation). Retention of anthocyanins on encapsulates formulated by 15 min of complexation decreased with the increase of cellulose amounts (65%, 62%, 59% and 55% for encapsulates formulated with 2.5%, 5%, 7.5% and 10% of cellulose, respectively). On encapsulates obtained by prolonged complexation, retention of anthocyanins ranged from 57% to 60%.

3.2. Total Antioxidant Activity and Inhibition of α-amylase

Evaluation of the antioxidant activity was carried out by application of DPPH, FRAP and CUPRAC methods. DPPH method is the most common method for in vitro antioxidant activity evaluation, and it is based on free radical scavenging activity, while FRAP and CUPRAC methods are used for measurement of the ability of antioxidants to reduce ferric iron and cupric ion, respectively [32]. Obtained results of antioxidant activity of C/R_Es are presented in Table 3. Antioxidant activity of C/R_E determined by DPPH method ranged from 23.51 to 20.01 µmol TE/100 g for C/R_Es formulated by 15 min of complexation, and it was determined that with the increase of cellulose amounts, a decrease of antioxidant activity occurred. Statistically significant difference between C/R_Es formulated by 60 min of complexation was not detected. After 12 months of storage, antioxidant activity in all C/R_Es slightly increased but there was no significant difference between C/R_Es with different amounts of cellulose regardless of complexation time. Values of antioxidant activity obtained by FRAP method ranged from 2.81 to 1.79 µmol TE/100 g. C/R_E formulated with 2.5% of cellulose throughout 15 min and 60 min of complexation had the highest antioxidant activity. By increasing the amount of cellulose from 2.5% to 10%, values of antioxidant activity decreased. After storage, the same tendency was retained. Similar results as with the DPPH and FRAP methods, were also obtained by CUPRAC method. C/R_E prepared with 2.5% of cellulose had the highest antioxidant activity and with the increase of cellulose amounts, a decrease in antioxidant activity occurred. After storage, the value of antioxidant activity increased in all encapsulates. C/R_E with 2.5% of cellulose that had the highest phenolic content also had the highest antioxidant activity, while C/R_E with 10% of cellulose, with the lowest phenolic content, had the lowest antioxidant activity. After 12 months of storage, antioxidant activity in most cases was higher than in the C/R_Es after formulation, that was probably a consequence of structural changes of phenolics since formation of polymerized phenols as well as oxidized ones can occur which can exhibit higher antioxidant activity than non-polymerized and non-oxidized phenols [33–35].

Table 3. Antioxidant activity (µmol TE/100 g) of C/R_Es prepared by 15 or 60 min of complexation, after formulation and after storage.

Samples	DPPH		FRAP		CUPRAC	
	Complexation Time (min)					
	15	60	15	60	15	60
	After formulation					
C/R_E_2.5%	23.51 ± 0.56 [b]	22.86 ± 0.15 [b]	2.81 ± 0.02 [b]	2.56 ± 0.15 [a]	103.20 ± 0.19 [b]	82.94 ± 5.14 [b]
C/R_E_5%	22.83 ± 0.31 [b]	23.10 ± 0.15 [b]	2.40 ± 0.05 [d]	2.50 ± 0.14 [a]	79.61 ± 0.43 [c]	84.84 ± 2.53 [b]
C/R_E_7.5%	22.24 ± 0.19 [c]	22.79 ± 0.02 [b]	2.29 ± 0.03 [d]	2.09 ± 0.04 [b]	69.19 ± 1.60 [e]	70.19 ± 0.04 [c]
C/R_E_10%	20.01 ± 0.78 [d]	22.73 ± 0.17 [b]	2.02 ± 0.02 [e]	1.79 ± 0.06 [c]	54.47 ± 5.91 [f]	55.48 ± 2.80 [e]
	After storage					
C/R_E_2.5%	25.68 ± 0.27 [a]	25.89 ± 0.36 [a]	3.08 ± 0.08 [a]	2.52 ± 0.08 [a]	127.30 ± 0.20 [a]	97.59 ± 3.81 [a]
C/R_E_5%	24.96 ± 1.32 [a,b]	26.52 ± 0.31 [a]	2.36 ± 0.05 [d]	2.46 ± 0.03 [a]	100 70 ± 3.30 [b]	97.88 ± 2.53 [a]
C/R_E_7.5%	26.54 ± 0.64 [a]	25.15 ± 0.59 [a]	2.59 ± 0.04 [c]	2.01 ± 0.00 [b]	92.26 ± 0.20 [c]	85.02 ± 0.96 [b]
C/R_E_10%	25.64 ± 0.16 [a]	25.29 ± 0.83 [a]	1.76 ± 0.00 [f]	1.72 ± 0.02 [c]	81.54 ± 1.50 [c]	66.65 ± 1.22 [d]

Results in the same column marked with the same letters were not significantly different ($p \leq 0.05$); Statistical differences between results are presented in the tables in the following increasing order: a > b > c > d > e > f; 2.5%, 5%, 7.5% and 10%—the amounts of used cellulose for formulation of C/R_Es.

Inhibition (%) of α-amylase by application of C/R_Es is presented in Table 4. C/R_Es formulated with lower amounts of cellulose had higher capability of inhibition of α-amylase, regardless of time of complexation. After storage, percentage of inhibition of this enzyme decreased. In contrast to the results after formulation, a difference was observed after storage between encapsulates prepared for 15 and 60 min of complexation.

Table 4. Inhibition (%) of α-amylase by application C/R_Es prepared by 15 or 60 min of complexation, after formulation and after storage.

Samples	Complexation Time (min)	
	15	60
	After preparation	
C/R_E_2.5%	56.07 ± 0.18 [a]	57.40 ± 0.58 [a]
C/R_E_5%	54.84 ± 0.50 [b]	57.15 ± 0.52 [a]
C/R_E_7.5%	53.43 ± 0.21 [c]	54.90 ± 0.39 [b]
C/R_E_10%	53.69 ± 0.14 [c]	52.40 ± 0.25 [c]
	After 12 months of storage	
C/R_E_2.5%	45.84 ± 0.24 [b]	48.40 ± 0.66 [c]
C/R_E_5%	45.54 ± 0.41 [b]	48.26 ± 0.03 [c]
C/R_E_7.5%	45.63 ± 0.25 [b]	48.87 ± 0.22 [b]
C/R_E_10%	45.32 ± 0.41 [b]	48.43 ± 0.47 [a]

Results in the same column marked with the same letters were not significantly different ($p \leq 0.05$); Statistical differences between results are presented in the tables in the following increasing order: a > b > c; 2.5%, 5%, 7.5% and 10%—the amounts of used cellulose for formulation of C/R_Es.

3.3. Color Parameters of Encapsulates

CIE Lab color parameters L*, a*, b*, C* and °h measured for C/R_Es after formulation and after storage at room temperature for 12 months are shown in Tables 5 and 6. L* value defines lightness of sample (0 is black and 100 is white); a* redness (redness (+) and greenness (-)) and b* yellowness (yellowness (+) and blueness (-)). C* or chroma defines the color saturation value and °h is the hue angle (from 0° for red, over 90° for yellow and 180° for green, up to 270° for blue and back to 0°)).

Table 5. Color parameters of C/R_Es prepared by 15 or 60 min of complexation after formulation.

	L*	a*	b*	°h	C*
	15 min of complexation				
C/R_E_2.5%	68.93 ± 0.03 [f]	34.42 ± 0.09 [a]	2.28 ± 0.06 [a]	3.79 ± 0.11 [a]	34.50 ± 0.09 [a]
C/R_E_5%	70.71 ± 0.02 [d]	32.88 ± 0.06 [b]	1.52 ± 0.04 [b,c]	2.64 ± 0.07 [c]	32.92 ± 0.05 [b]
C/R_E_7.5%	71.14 ± 0.02 [c]	32.39 ± 0.03 [b,c]	1.25 ± 0.01 [d]	2.21 ± 0.03 [d]	32.41 ± 0.03 [c]
C/R_E_10%	73.57 ± 0.01 [b]	30.38 ± 0.03 [e]	1.46 ± 0.02 [c]	2.75 ± 0.04 [c]	30.42 ± 0.03 [e]
	60 min of complexation				
C/R_E_2.5%	69.25 ± 0.02 [e]	34.18 ± 0.05 [a]	2.29 ± 0.04 [a]	3.83 ± 0.06 [a]	34.26 ± 0.05 [a]
C/R_E_5%	71.58 ± 0.02 [c]	32.14 ± 0.06 [c]	1.44 ± 0.04 [c]	2.57 ± 0.07 [c]	32.17 ± 0.06 [c]
C/R_E_7.5%	71.60 ± 0.01 [c]	31.92 ± 0.02 [d]	1.78 ± 0.02 [b]	3.20 ± 0.02 [b]	31.97 ± 0.02 [d]
C/R_E_10%	74.09 ± 0.02 [a]	29.94 ± 0.04 [f]	1.11 ± 0.04 [d]	2.13 ± 0.07 [d]	29.96 ± 0.04 [f]

Results in the same column marked with the same letters were not significantly different ($p \leq 0.05$); Statistical differences between results are presented in the tables in the following increasing order: a > b > c > d > e > f; 2.5%, 5%, 7.5% and 10%—the amounts of used cellulose for formulation of C/R_Es.

On C/R_Es after formulation, lightness fluctuated from 68.93 to 74.09. The highest L* value was associated to C/R_E formulated with 10% of cellulose and the lowest with 2.5% of cellulose, regardless of complexation time. In C/R_Es analyzed after storage of 12 months, L* value increased. Increasing of L* value in the C/R_Es after storage could be because of their exposure to light during the storage period. The highest a* value was observed on C/R_E formulated with 2.5% of cellulose and the lowest when 10% of cellulose was used for complexation. These results could be correlated to the anthocyanins content since those C/R_Es also had the highest anthocyanin content. After storage, decrease of a* value occurred but the tendency remained. The same trend was observed for b*, °h and C* values. Total color change was calculated after storage of C/R_Es. The highest total color change was calculated for C/R_E formulated with 7.5% of cellulose and the lowest for C/R_E with 10% of cellulose, regardless of the complexation time.

Table 6. Color parameters of C/R_Es prepared by 15 or 60 min of complexation after storage.

	L*	a*	b*	ΔE	°h	C*
			15 min of complexation			
C/R_E_2.5%	73.37 ± 0.05 [e]	27.23 ± 0.01 [a]	2.47 ± 0.04 [a]	8.45	5.18 ± 0.08 [b]	27.34 ± 0.01 [a]
C/R_E_5%	74.17 ± 0.05 [d]	26.76 ± 0.05 [b]	2.13 ± 0.01 [c]	7.06	4.55 ± 0.03 [c]	26.85 ± 0.05 [b]
C/R_E_7.5%	76.30 ± 0.02 [b]	24.42 ± 0.02 [c]	1.89 ± 0.01 [d]	9.52	4.43 ± 0.02 [c]	24.49 ± 0.02 [c]
C/R_E_10%	76.60 ± 0.02 [b]	24.67 ± 0.02 [c]	1.57 ± 0.01 [e]	6.47	3.63 ± 0.03 [c]	24.72 ± 0.02 [c]
			60 min of complexation			
C/R_E_2.5%	73.62 ± 0.02 [e]	27.41 ± 0.03 [a]	2.03 ± 0.03 [c]	8.06	4.24 ± 0.07 [c]	27.48 ± 0.03 [a]
C/R_E_5%	75.41 ± 0.01 [c]	24.67 ± 0.02 [c]	2.36 ± 0.00 [b]	8.44	5.47 ± 0.01 [a]	24.78 ± 0.02 [c]
C/R_E_7.5%	76.39 ± 0.02 [b]	24.17 ± 0.02 [d]	2.07 ± 0.01 [c]	9.12	4.89 ± 0.07 [b]	24.26 ± 0.02 [c]
C/R_E_10%	77.05 ± 0.01 [a]	23.73 ± 0.01 [e]	1.86 ± 0.03 [d]	6.21	4.47 ± 0.07 [c]	23.80 ± 0.01 [d]

Results in the same column marked with the same letters were not significantly different ($p \leq 0.05$); Statistical differences between results are presented in the tables in the following increasing order: a > b > c > d > e; 2.5%, 5%, 7.5% and 10%—the amounts of used cellulose for formulation of C/R_Es.

3.4. IR Spectra of Encaptulates

Comparison of IR spectra of cellulose with C/R_Es after formulation and after storage is presented by Figure 1. Since all C/R_Es had identical spectra and identical differences were observed, only one encapsulate was presented. IR spectra of cellulose and C/R_Es overlapped in region from 3400 cm^{-1} to 3200 cm^{-1} that can be assigned to stretching of O-H and in several bands. Overlapping bands were at 2900 cm^{-1} assigned to CH_3 symmetric stretch, 1640 cm^{-1} that defines H-O-H deformation of water, 1431 cm^{-1} and 1364 cm^{-1} both assigned to CH_2. Furthermore, overlapping was observed on bands at 1312 cm^{-1} which can be assigned to C-H deformation vibration, 1200 cm^{-1} assigned to C-O-C, C-O dominated by the ring vibrations of polysaccharides, 1150 cm^{-1} assigned to C-O stretching vibrations, 1103 cm^{-1} connected to CO, CC ring of polysaccharides, 1051 cm^{-1} assigned to C-O stretching and C-O bending of carbohydrates, 1028 cm^{-1} assigned to CH_2 groups and C-O stretching vibration coupled with C-O bending of the C-OH groups of carbohydrates and 894 cm^{-1} assigned to C-C [36]. In comparison to cellulose, C/R_Es had additional bands at 1714 cm^{-1}, 820 cm^{-1} and 780 cm^{-1} which are assigned to C=O stretching (associated with HC=O linked to aromatic or C=O in ketones or carboxyl group), ring CH deformation and out of plane bending vibrations. The decrease of OH stretching that can occur due to intramolecular hydrogen bonding can be interpreted by the ratio of $A_{4000-2995}/A_{1337}$. This ratio can be used as a criterion of hydrogen-bond intensity (HBI) [37]. HBI decreased in C/R_Es in comparison to cellulose, and the same trend was retained over the storage period. In the study of Abdelwahab and Amin [38] on adsorption of phenols from aqueous solutions by *Luffa cylindrica* fibers, it was observed that band intensities decreased on the IR spectra when phenols were adsorbed on investigated fibers. They emphasized that functional groups of the fibers surface have been occupied with phenols but also penetration into the interlayer fiber space occurred [38].

Combining results of this study and our previous study [23] it can be concluded that cellulose can be used for formulation of stable delivery systems of raspberry active ingredients i.e., phenolics, anthocyanins and volatiles. Obtained encapsulates could be used as functional additives to some products like dairy products, bakery products, fruit products, confectionary and different types of fillings. Encapsulates could be used in order to improve nutritional value of products throughout enrichment of those products with phenolic compounds and increase of their antioxidant potential. On the other hand, these functional additives can improve quality of products throughout color and flavor modification but also decrease of oxidation of labile components can be expected.

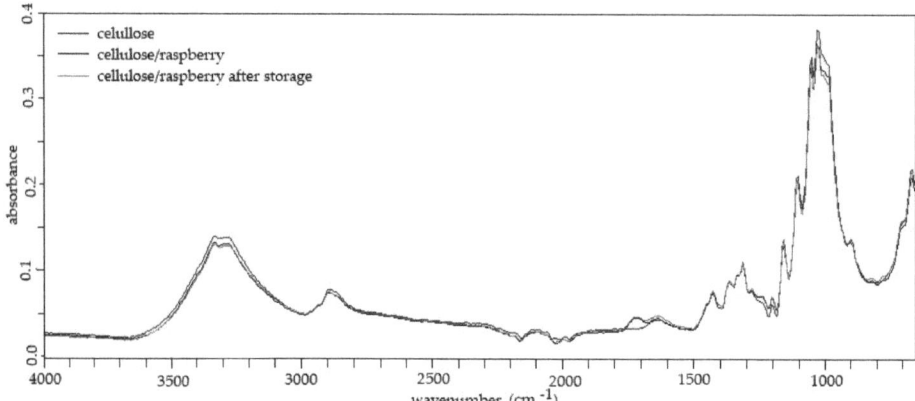

Figure 1. IR spectra of cellulose and cellulose/raspberry encapsulates after preparation and after storage.

4. Conclusions

Cellulose was chosen as the delivery system for raspberry bioactive compounds in order to formulate an ingredient that could be used for development and/or improvement of novel foods. Results of our study revealed that amount of cellulose and complexation time used for formulation of encapsulates had influence on the adsorption efficiency of raspberry bioactive compounds. Encapsulates formulated with lower amount of cellulose for 15 min of complexation had better binding of phenolic components. Therefore, we can conclude that formulation of cellulose-based encapsulates would not be time consuming. On the other hand, after the prolonged storage time, the highest phenolic retention was observed in the complexes prepared with 5% and 7.5% of cellulose. Encapsulates with 2.5% of cellulose also had the highest antioxidant activity, and those encapsulates had the highest capability of inhibition of α-amylase. This research is a good platform for development of new products as well as for improvement of existing ones. Future studies should be governed to formulation of the products with the addition of cellulose-based encapsulates and investigation of real effects of encapsulates on antioxidant potential, oxidative stability, color modification and flavor modification of products in which they were added. Stability of enriched products over the time would also give valuable insight on real effect of encapsulates on product quality. Moreover, sensory analysis of newly obtained products would be beneficial to obtain possible response of consumers on this type of enriched products.

Author Contributions: Conceptualization, M.K. and J.Š.; methodology, J.V., A.P. and M.K.; formal analysis, J.V., I.B.; investigation, J.V., I.B.; data curation, J.V., I.B.; writing—original draft preparation, J.V., I.B.; writing—review and editing, M.K., A.P., J.Š.; supervision, M.K., A.P.; project administration, M.K.; funding acquisition, M.K. All authors have read and agreed to the published version of the manuscript.

Funding: The work was part of PZS-2019-02-1595 project and it has been fully supported by the "Research Cooperability" Program of the Croatian Science Foundation funded by the European Union from the European Social Fund under the Operational Programme Efficient Human Resources 2014–2020.

Institutional Review Board Statement: Not applicable.

Informed Consent Statement: Not applicable.

Data Availability Statement: Not available.

Conflicts of Interest: The authors declare no conflict of interest.

References

1. Liu, D.; Martinez-Sanz, M.; Lopez-Sanchez, P.; Gilbert, E.P.; Gidley, M.J. Adsorption behavior of polyphenols on cellulose is affected by processing history. *Food Hydrocoll.* **2017**, *63*, 496–507. [CrossRef]
2. Cai, Y.Z.; Sun, M.; Xing, J.; Luo, Q.; Corke, H. Structure radical scavenging activity relationships of phenolic compounds from traditional Chinese medicinal plants. *Life Sci.* **2006**, *78*, 2872–2888. [CrossRef] [PubMed]
3. Velderrain-Rodríguez, G.R.; Palafox-Carlos, H.; Wall-Medrano, A.; Ayala-Zavala, J.F.; Chen, C.Y.; Robles-Sánchez, M.; Astiazaran-García, H.; Alvarez-Parrilla, E.; González-Aguilar, G.A. Phenolic compounds: Their journey after intake. *Food Func.* **2014**, *5*, 189–197. [CrossRef] [PubMed]
4. Carvalho, E.; Franceschi, P.; Feller, A.; Palmieri, L.; Wehrens, R.; Martens, S. A targeted metabolomics approach to understand differences in flavonoid biosynthesis in red and yellow raspberries. *Plant Physiol. Biochem.* **2013**, *72*, 79–86. [CrossRef] [PubMed]
5. Anderson, J.W.; Baird, P.; Davis, R.H., Jr.; Ferreri, S.; Knudtson, M.; Koraym, A.; Waters, V.; Williams, C.L. Health benefits of dietary fiber. *Nutr. Rev.* **2009**, *67*, 188–205. [CrossRef] [PubMed]
6. Brett, C.T.; Waldron, K.W. *Physiology and Biochemistry of Plant Cell Walls*, 2nd ed.; Chapman & Hall, Springer: Amsterdam, The Netherlands, 1996.
7. Phan, A.D.T.; Netzel, G.; Wang, D.; Flanagan, B.M.; D'Arcy, B.R.; Gidley, M.J. Binding of dietary polyphenols to cellulose: Structural and nutritional aspects. *Food Chem.* **2015**, *171*, 388–396. [CrossRef] [PubMed]
8. Battino, M.; Beekwilder, J.; Denoyes-Rothan, B.; Laimer, M.; McDougall, G.J.; Mezzetti, B. Bioactive compounds in berries relevant to human health. *Nutr. Rev.* **2009**, *67* (Suppl. 1), S145–S150. [CrossRef]
9. Durgo, K.; Belscak-Cvitanovic, A.; Stancic, A.; Franekic, J.; Komes, D. The bioactive potential of red raspberry (*Rubus idaeus* L.) leaves in exhibiting cytotoxic and cytoprotective activity on human laryngeal carcinoma and colon adenocarcinoma. *J. Med. Food* **2012**, *15*, 258–268. [CrossRef]
10. Padayachee, A.; Netzel, G.; Netzel, M.; Day, L.; Zabaras, D.; Mikkelsen, D. Binding of polyphenols to plant cell wall analogues—Part 1: Anthocyanins. *Food Chem.* **2012**, *134*, 155–161. [CrossRef]
11. Padayachee, A.; Netzel, G.; Netzel, M.; Day, L.; Zabaras, D.; Mikkelsen, D. Binding of polyphenols to plant cell wall analogues—Part 2: Phenolic acids. *Food Chem.* **2012**, *135*, 2287–2292. [CrossRef]
12. Phan, A.D.T.; Flanagan, B.M.; D'Arcy, B.R.; Gidley, M.J. Binding selectivity of dietary polyphenols to different plant cell wall components: Quantification and mechanism. *Food Chem.* **2017**, *233*, 216–227. [CrossRef] [PubMed]
13. Pinelo, M.; Arnous, A.; Meyer, A.S. Upgrading of grape skins: Significance of plant cell-wall structural components and extraction techniques for phenol release. *Trends Food Sci. Technol.* **2006**, *17*, 579–590. [CrossRef]
14. Le Bourvellec, C.; Renard, C. Interactions between polyphenols and macromolecules: Quantification methods and mechanisms. *Crit. Rev. Food Sci. Nutr.* **2012**, *52*, 213–248. [CrossRef] [PubMed]
15. Le Bourvellec, C.; Guyot, S.; Renard, C. Non-covalent interaction between procyanidins and apple cell wall material: Part I. Effect of some environmental parameters. *Biochim. Biophys. Acta Gen. Subj.* **2004**, *1672*, 192–202. [CrossRef] [PubMed]
16. Renard, C.M.; Baron, A.; Guyot, S.; Drilleau, J.-F. Interactions between apple cell walls and native apple polyphenols: Quantification and some consequences. *Int. J. Biol. Macromol.* **2001**, *29*, 115–125. [CrossRef]
17. Tang, H.R.; Covington, A.D.; Hancock, R.A. Structure-activity relationships in the hydrophobic interactions of polyphenols with cellulose and collagen. *Biopolymers* **2003**, *70*, 403–413. [CrossRef] [PubMed]
18. Le Bourvellec, C.; Renard, C. Non-covalent interaction between procyanidins and apple cell wall material. Part II: Quantification and impact of cell wall drying. *Biochim. Biophys. Acta Gen. Subj.* **2005**, *1725*, 1–9. [CrossRef]
19. Le Bourvellec, C.; Bouchet, B.; Renard, C. Non-covalent interaction between procyanidins and apple cell wall material. Part III: Study on model polysaccharides. *Biochim. Biophys. Acta Gen. Subj.* **2005**, *1725*, 10–18. [CrossRef]
20. Gao, R.P.; Liu, H.; Peng, Z.; Wu, Z.; Wang, Y.X.; Zhao, G.H. Adsorption of (−)-epigallocatechin-3-gallate (EGCG) onto oat beta-glucan. *Food Chem.* **2012**, *132*, 1936–1943. [CrossRef]
21. Wu, Z.; Ming, J.; Gao, R.; Wang, Y.; Liang, Q.; Yu, H. Characterization and antioxidant activity of the complex of tea polyphenols and oat β-glycan. *J. Agric. Food Chem.* **2011**, *59*, 10737–10746. [CrossRef]
22. Nsor-Atindana, J.; Chen, M.; Goff, H.D.; Zhong, F.; Sharif, H.R.; Li, Y. Functionality and nutritional aspects of microcrystalline cellulose in food. *Carbohydr. Polym.* **2017**, *172*, 159–174. [CrossRef] [PubMed]
23. Vukoja, J.; Pichler, A.; Ivić, I.; Šimunović, J.; Kopjar, M. Cellulose as a delivery system of raspberry juice volatiles and their stability. *Molecules* **2020**, *25*, 2624. [CrossRef] [PubMed]
24. Singleton, V.L.; Rossi, J.A. Colorimetry of total phenolics with phosphomolybdic-phosphotonutric acid reagents. *Am. J. Enol. Vitic.* **1965**, *16*, 144–158.
25. Giusti, M.M.; Wrolstad, R.E. Characterization and Measurement of Anthocyanins by UV-Visible Spectroscopy. In *Current Protocols in Food Analytical Chemistry Current Protocols*; John Wiley &Sons, Inc.: Hoboken, NJ, USA, 2001; pp. F1.2.1–F1.2.13.
26. da Silva, S.M.; Koehnlein, E.A.; Bracht, A.; Castoldi, R.; de Morais, G.R.; Baesso, M.L.; Peralta, R.A.; de Souza, C.G.M.; de Sá-Nakanishi, A.B.; Peralta, R.M. Inhibition of salivary and pancreatic α-amylases by a pinhão coat (*Araucaria angustifolia*) extract rich in condensed tannin. *Food Res. Int.* **2014**, *56*, 1–8. [CrossRef]
27. Kellogg, J.; Grace, M.H.; Lila, M.A. Phlorotannins from Alaskan seaweed inhibit carbolytic enzyme activity. *Mar. Drugs* **2014**, *12*, 5277–5294. [CrossRef]

28. Brand-Williams, W.; Cuvelier, M.E.; Berset, C. Use of a free radical method to evaluate antioxidant activity. *Lebensm. Wiss. Technol.* **1995**, *28*, 25–30. [CrossRef]
29. Apak, R.; Guculu, K.G.; Ozyurek, M.; Karademir, S.E. Novel total antioxidant capacity index for dietary polyphenols and vitamins C and E, using their cupric iron reducing capability in the presence of neocuproine: CUPRAC method. *J. Agric. Food Chem.* **2004**, *52*, 7970–7981. [CrossRef]
30. Benzie, I.F.; Strain, J.J. The ferric reducing ability of plasma (FRAP) as a measure of "antioxidant power": The FRAP assay. *Anal. Biochem.* **1996**, *239*, 70–79. [CrossRef]
31. Cartalade, D.; Vernhet, A. Polar interactions in flavan-3-ol adsorption on solid surfaces. *J. Agric. Food Chem.* **2006**, *54*, 3086–3094. [CrossRef]
32. Alam, M.N.; Bristi, N.J.; Rafiquzzaman, M. Review on in vivo and in vitro methods evaluation of antioxidant activity. *Saudi Pharm. J.* **2013**, *21*, 143–152. [CrossRef]
33. Da Porto, C.; Calligaris, S.; Celotti, E.; Nicoli, M.C. Antiradical properties of commercial cognacs assessed by the DPPH test. *J. Agric. Food Chem.* **2000**, *48*, 4241–4245. [CrossRef] [PubMed]
34. Manzocco, L.; Calligaris, S.; Mastrocola, D.; Nicoli, M.C.; Lerici, C.R. Review of nonenzymatic browning and antioxidant capacity in processed foods. *Trends Food Sci. Technol.* **2001**, *11*, 340–346. [CrossRef]
35. Nicoli, M.C.; Calligaris, S.; Manzocco, L. Effect of enzymatic and chemical oxidation on the antioxidant capacity of catechin model systems and apple derivatives. *J. Agric. Food Chem.* **2000**, *48*, 4576–4580. [CrossRef] [PubMed]
36. Movasaghi, Z.; Rehman, S.; Rehman, I. Fourier transform infrared (FTIR) spectroscopy of biological tissues. *Appl. Spectrosc. Rev.* **2008**, *43*, 134–179. [CrossRef]
37. Oh, S.Y.; Yoo, D.I.; Shinb, Y.; Seoc, G. FTIR analysis of cellulose treated with sodium hydroxide and carbon dioxide. *Carbohydr. Res.* **2005**, *340*, 417–428. [CrossRef]
38. Abdelwahab, O.; Amin, N.K. Adsorption of phenol from aqueous solutions by *Luffa cylindrica* fibers: Kinetics, isotherm and thermodynamic studies. *Egypt. J. Aquat. Res.* **2013**, *39*, 215–223. [CrossRef]

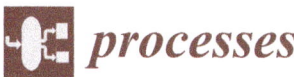

Article

Influence of Processing Parameters on Phenolic Compounds and Color of Cabernet Sauvignon Red Wine Concentrates Obtained by Reverse Osmosis and Nanofiltration

Ivana Ivić [1], Mirela Kopjar [1], Lidija Jakobek [1], Vladimir Jukić [2], Suzana Korbar [1], Barbara Marić [1], Josip Mesić [3] and Anita Pichler [1,*]

1. Faculty of Food Technology Osijek, Josip Juraj Strossmayer University, F. Kuhača 18, 31000 Osijek, Croatia; iivic@ptfos.hr (I.I.); mirela.kopjar@ptfos.hr (M.K.); lidija.jakobek@ptfos.hr (L.J.); skorbar@ptfos.hr (S.K.); bmaric@ptfos.hr (B.M.)
2. Faculty of Agrobiotechnical Sciences Osijek, Josip Juraj Strossmayer University, V. Preloga 1, 31000 Osijek, Croatia; vladimir.jukic@fazos.hr
3. Polytechnic in Požega, Vukovarska 17, 34000 Požega, Croatia; jmesic@vup.hr
* Correspondence: anita.pichler@ptfos.hr

Abstract: In this study, Cabernet Sauvignon red wine was subjected to reverse osmosis and nanofiltration processes at four different pressures (25, 35, 45, and 55 bar) and two temperature regimes (with and without cooling). The aim was to obtain concentrates with a higher content of phenolic compounds and antioxidant activity and to determine the influence of two membrane types (Alfa Laval RO98pHt M20 for reverse osmosis and NF M20 for nanofiltration) and different operating conditions on phenolics retention. Total polyphenol, flavonoid, monomeric anthocyanin contents, and antioxidant activity were determined spectrophotometrically. Flavan-3-ols and phenolic acids were analyzed on a high-performance liquid chromatography system and sample colour was measured by chromometer. The results showed that the increase in applied pressure and decrease in retentate temperature were favorable for higher phenolics retention. Retention of individual compounds depended on their chemical structure, membrane properties, membrane fouling, and operating conditions. Both types of membranes proved to be suitable for Cabernet Sauvignon red wine concentration. In all retentates, phenolic compounds content was higher than in the initial wine, but no visible color change ($\Delta E^* < 1$) was observed. The highest concentrations of phenolic compounds were detected in retentates obtained at 45 and 55 bar, especially with cooling.

Keywords: Cabernet Sauvignon concentrate; reverse osmosis; nanofiltration; phenolic compounds

1. Introduction

Wine is one of the most consumed alcoholic beverages, and its moderate consumption is recommended due to phenolic content and antioxidant activity, especially red wine varieties. The polyphenols are responsible for the colour, astringency, bitterness, and mouthfeel of the wine [1], but they are mostly known as strong antioxidants that protect the human body from the harmful effects of free radicals. Studies showed that their intake regulates oxidative stress in cells preventing cardiovascular, degenerative, and other chronic diseases [2,3]. Wine phenolics present a large group of several hundred compounds, including non-flavonoids (hydroxybenzoic acids, hydroxycinnamic acids, and stilbenes) and flavonoids (flavonols, dihydroflavonols, flavan-3-ols, tannins, and anthocyanins). They originate from grape skins and seeds from where they are extracted during crushing, maceration, and fermentation. Red wine contains a significantly higher concentration of phenolic compounds (1800–3000 mg/L) than white wine due to longer contact of skins and seeds with grape juice [4]. The concentrations of polyphenols in wine depend on several factors, such as grape variety, grape maturity and harvest date, climate, soil characteristics, pre-fermentation, fermentation, and aging conditions. The profile of

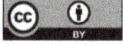

anthocyanins for each grape variety is usually stable, but they can vary due to different vintage or above-mentioned factors [5]. Vinification procedures have a great effect on the composition and concentration of wine polyphenols. Maceration is often conducted for better extraction of color and flavor compounds from grape skins and seeds to juice, mostly during red wine production. Clarification is an inevitable step in the winemaking process, but it usually results in a decrease in phenolic compound concentration, depending on the phenols' structure and clarifying agents [6]. Wine aging mainly affects the concentration of hydroxycinnamic esters, anthocyanidins, and tannins that are manifested through colour and astringency degree change [1].

Poor vintage, inadequate climate conditions, or winemaking procedures can result in a wine with phenolic compound content lower than desired. For that purpose, several techniques have been developed to extract, increase, or correct their quantity. Recently, membrane filtration stands out as a practical method due to low energy, low cost, mild temperatures, high efficiency, and no-additives requirement [7]. They imply pressure-driven membrane operations that are divided according to the membrane characteristics and pore size on microfiltration (MF), ultrafiltration (UF), nanofiltration (NF), and reverse osmosis (RO) [8].

Nanofiltration and reverse osmosis membranes are usually composite membranes with a high strength polymer as a supporting layer. That kind of arrangement provides the necessary permeability and selectivity, endurance, and ability to be back-flushed during cleaning [9]. During the filtration process, membranes split the main stream into two fractions: retentate that is retained on the membrane and permeate that is yielded through it. Wine permeate contains mostly water, ethanol, and small amounts of acetic acid, lactic acid, and several other low molecular weight compounds. This property enables the use of NF and RO membranes for wine dealcoholization under low-temperature conditions without any greater change in organoleptic properties of the initial wine [10–13]. On the other hand, membranes retain larger molecules, such as sugars, higher acids, and higher alcohols, phenolic and aroma compounds [14–16], that create osmotic pressure and concentration polarization on the membrane surface. Therefore, high transmembrane pressure should be applied to overcome the osmotic pressure and ensure optimal permeate flux. The most commonly used pressures are between 20 and 60 bar; today, even higher for the reverse osmosis process. The higher the pressure, the higher the permeate flux, although increased pressure can lead to faster membrane fouling and better bioactive compounds retention [17]. Those characteristics can be used for polyphenol extraction from wine industry wastewaters [18] or grape pomace extracts [19]. Bánvölgyi [20] used nanofiltration processes for red wine concentration to achieve higher concentrations of polyphenols in red wine. Such obtained wine concentrate can further be used as a drink or for wine color and aroma correction and low-alcohol wine production. Red wine concentrates with increased polyphenol content can also be used in the food and pharmaceutical industry as functional food [21].

This study aimed to obtain Cabernet Sauvignon red wine concentrates with increased polyphenol content and antioxidant activity. To establish optimal operating parameters, two types of membranes (RO98pHt for reverse osmosis and NF M20 for nanofiltration), four different pressures (25, 35, 45, and 55 bar), and two temperature regimes (with and without cooling) were applied for red wine concentration. The effect of different membranes and operating conditions on retention of total phenolic compounds, flavonoids, anthocyanins, and antioxidant activity in red wine concentrates was determined after each experimental run. Additionally, the color parameters of the obtained samples were determined.

2. Materials and Methods

2.1. Chemicals and Standards

Chemicals and standards used in this study were obtained as follows: gallic acid monohydrate, quercetin dihydrate, aluminum chloride, potassium persulfate, Trolox, 2,2′-azinobis(3-ethylbenzothiazoline sulfonic acid) (ABTS), 2,2-diphenyl-1-picrylhydrazil

(DPPH), 2,4,6-tripyridyl-s-triazine (TPTZ), gallic acid, caffeic acid, catechin, and epicatechin from Sigma-Aldrich (St. Lois, MO, USA); Folin-Ciocalteu reagent, sodium carbonate, sodium nitrite, sodium hydroxide, potassium bisulfite, potassium chloride, sodium acetate, and hydrochloric acid from Kemika (Zagreb, Croatia); sodium acetate trihydrate, ferric chloride hexahydrate, and ammonium acetate from Gram-Mol (Zagreb, Croatia); copper(II) chloride from Acros Organics (New Jersey, NJ, USA); HPLC grade methanol and neocuproine from Merck (Darmstadt, Germany) and phosphoric acid (HPLC grade) from Fluka (Buchs, Switzerland).

2.2. Wine

Wine samples of Cabernet Sauvignon grapewine variety were produced at the Faculty of Agrobiotechnical Sciences, experimental field Mandićevac, Đakovo vineyard, Croatia, vintage 2018.

2.3. Concentration of Cabernet Sauvignon Red Wine

The concentration of red wine was conducted on LabUnit M20 (De Danske Sukkerfabrikker, Denmark) with a plate-and-frame module equipped with six composite Alfa Laval flat sheet polyamide membranes. Two types of membranes were applied: RO98pHt M20 (pH range 2–11, maximum temperature 60 °C, maximum pressure 55 bar and NaCl rejection $\geq$98%) and NF M20 (pH range 3–10, maximum temperature 50 °C, maximum pressure 55 bar and $MgSO_4$ rejection $\geq$99%). The surface of one membrane was 0.0289 m^2. The concentration was carried out at four different pressures (25, 35, 45, and 55 bar) and two temperature regimes (with and without cooling) for each membrane type. For each experimental run, a 3 L of the initial feed was used. Every 4 min, the permeate volume, and retentate temperature were recorded. At the end of each process, 1.3 L of retentate and 1.7 L of permeate were obtained. Water flux was measured before and after each experimental run at the same pressures (25, 35, 45, and 55 bar).

2.4. Total Polyphenol Content (TPC) Determination

Total polyphenol content was determined according to the Folin-Ciocalteu method [22]. A sample (0.2 mL) was mixed with 1.8 mL of deionized water, 10 mL of 3.3% Folin-Ciocalteu solution, and 8 mL of sodium carbonate solution (7.5%). For blank, a sample was replaced with water. Prepared mixtures were left at least 2 h in the dark, and then absorbance was measured at 765 nm by spectrophotometer (Cary 60 UV-Vis, Agilent Technologies, Santa Clara, CA, USA). For the calculation of concentration, the gallic acid calibration curve was used (gallic acid was diluted in distilled water to yield 0.5–4.0 g/L), and results were expressed as its equivalents (g GAE/L). Three repetitions were made for each sample.

2.5. Total Flavonoid Content (TFC) Determination

The method for total flavonoids content determination was as follows [23]: 0.5 mL of sample was mixed with 4 mL of distilled water and 0.3 mL of 5% sodium nitrite solution. After 5 min, 1.5 mL of 2% aluminum chloride solution was pipetted. Five minutes later, 2 mL of 1 M sodium hydroxide and 1.7 mL of distilled water were added. Distilled water was used as blank, and the absorbance was measured at 510 nm. The calibration curve of catechin was made by diluting it in ethanol in a concentration in the range of 0.2 to 2.0 g/L. Results were expressed as catechin equivalents (g CE/L) and as average values of 3 repetitions for each sample.

2.6. Monomeric Anthocyanin Content (MAC) Determination

A pH-differential method [24] for MAC determination was used. Samples (0.2 mL) were mixed with 2.8 mL of potassium chloride buffer (pH 1.0) and 2.8 mL of sodium acetate buffer (pH 4.5). Three repetitions were prepared for each sample. The absorbance was measured after 15 min at 512 ($\lambda_{vis\text{-}max}$) nm and 700 nm, and the following formula was used for concentration calculation:

$$c_{(a)}(mg/L) = (A \times MW \times DF \times 1000)/(\varepsilon \times l), \tag{1}$$

where $c_{(a)}$ is the concentracion of anthocyanins (mg/L), A is the absorbance of a sample obtained from A = $(A_{512} - A_{700})_{(pH\ 1.0)} - (A_{512} - A_{700})_{(pH\ 4.5)}$, MW is the molecurar weight of predominant anthocyanin in the sample (cyanidin-3-glucoside, MW = 449.2), DF is the dilution factor, ε is the molar absorptivity (cyanidin-3-glucoside, ε = 26,900) and l-pathlength (1 cm).

2.7. Polymeric Color Determination

For polymeric color determination [24], in one test tube, 0.2 mL of sample and 3.0 mL of distilled water were added, and in another test tube, 0.2 mL of sample, 2.8 mL of water, and 0.2 mL of 20% potassium bisulfite solution were added. The absorbance was measured after 15 min at 420, 512, and 700 nm. For each sample, three parallels were made, and the following parameters were calculated:

Colour density calculation (samples treated with water):

$$\text{Color density} = [(A_{420\ nm} - A_{700\ nm}) + (A_{512\ nm} - A_{700\ nm})] \times DF \tag{2}$$

$$\text{Polymeric color} = [(A_{420\ nm} - A_{700\ nm}) + (A_{512\ nm} - A_{700\ nm})] \times DF \tag{3}$$

Polymeric color calculation (samples treated with potassium bisulfite):
Percent polymeric color calculation:

$$\text{Percent polymeric color (\%)} = (\text{polymeric color}/\text{color density}) \times 100 \tag{4}$$

2.8. Antioxidant Activity (AA) Determination

Four methods, DPPH, ABTS, ferric reducing/antioxidant power assay (FRAP), and cupric reducing antioxidant capacity (CUPRAC), were used for antioxidant activity determination. All results were expressed as Trolox equivalents (μmol TE/100 mL) as average values of three repetitions for each sample.

DPPH (2,2-diphenyl-1-picrylhydrazyl) free radicals [25] were dissolved in 96% ethanol, and 3 mL of that solution was mixed with 0.2 mL of sample. After 15 min, absorbance was measured at 517 nm. Water was used for blank trial.

ABTS or 2,2′-azinobis(3-ethyl-benzothiazoline-6-sulfonic acid) was dissolved in water to a 7 mM concentration, and 2.45 mM potassium persulfate was added to obtain a stock solution that was diluted in ethanol (96%) in a 2:70 ratio before analysis. Then, 0.2 mL of sample and 3.2 mL of ABTS were mixed and left in the dark for 95 min. The absorbance was measured at 734 nm [26]. For blank, the sample was replaced with distilled water.

FRAP (ferric reducing/antioxidant power assay) was conducted as follows [27]: 300 mM sodium acetate with pH 3.6, 10 mM TPTZ diluted in 40 mM hydrochloric acid, and 20 mM $FeCl_3 \times 6H_2O$ were mixed in 10:1:1 ratio, respectively and heated at 37 °C. Further, 3 mL of FRAP reagent was mixed with 0.2 L of sample (or water for blank). The absorbance was measured after 15 min at 593 nm.

CUPRAC (cupric reducing antioxidant capacity) method [28] is a simple method for antioxidant activity determination. Three reagents are needed: 10 mM $CuCl_2 \times 2H_2O$ solution, 7.5 mM neocuproine (Nc) solution, and 1 M ammonium acetate (NH_4Ac) solution, pH = 7 0. In a test tube, 0.2 mL of sample (water for blank) was mixed with 1 mL of each reagent and 3.9 mL of distilled water. The color change was measured at 450 nm after 30 min.

2.9. HPLC Determination of Phenolic Compounds

Individual phenolic components were identified by high-performance liquid chromatography (HPLC) system 1260 Infinity II (Agilent Technologies, Santa Clara, CA, USA), equipped with a quaternary pump and PDA (photodiode array) detector. A Poroshell 120 EC-C18 column (4.6 × 100 mm^2, 2.7 μm) and a Poroshell 120 EC-C18 guard column (4.6 × 5 mm^2, 2.7 μm) were used. Solutions 0.1% H_3PO_4 and 100% methanol were used as mobile phases A and B, respectively. The flow was set to 1 mL/min, and the injected sample volume was 10 μL. The gradient was used as follows: 0 min 5% B, 3 min 30% B, 15 min 35% B, 22 min 37% B, 30 min 41% B, 32 min 45% B, 40 min 49% B, 45 min 80% B, 48 min 80% B, 50 min 5% B, 53 min 5% B. For calibration curves, following stock solutions were diluted with methanol: 16–80 mg/L of gallic acid (r^2 = 1.0000), 8.5–125 mg/L of (+)-catechin (r^2 = 0.9956), 8.4–125 mg/L of (−)-epicatechin (r^2 = 0.9955) and 9.7–48.5 mg/L of caffeic acid (r^2 = 0.9911). Caftaric and coutaric acid were tentatively identified by comparing their retention times and peak spectrum with those of authentic standards and literature data. Hydroxycinnamic acids were identified at 320 nm, and gallic acid, catechin, and epicatechin were identified at 280 nm. Samples were analyzed in duplicates.

2.10. Color Parameters Measurement

Color measurement of the analyzed samples was conducted on a chromometer CR-400 (Konica Minolta, Inc., Osaka, Japan). For color evaluation, a Lab system was used, and the following parameters were determined: L* indicates lightness (0 is black, and 100 is white); a* is redness (+) or greenness (−); b* is yellowness (+) or blueness (−); C* represents color saturation or chroma, and °h is the hue angle [29]. All samples were measured three times, and results were expressed as the mean value. The color difference between the initial wine and obtained retentates was determined by ΔE* value calculated by the following formula:

$$\Delta E^* = [(\Delta L^*)^2 + (\Delta a^*)^2 + (\Delta b^*)^2]^{1/2}, \quad (5)$$

2.11. Membrane Performance Determination

To evaluate membrane performance under different operating conditions, the following parameters were calculated:

$$J = V_p/(A \times t), \quad (6)$$

where J is the permeate flux (L/m^{2}h), V_p is the permeate volume (L), A is the membrane surface (m^2), and t is time (hours). Further, the volume reduction factor (VRF) was calculated by:

$$VRF = V_f/V_{rt}, \quad (7)$$

where V_f is the initial feed volume (L) and V_R is the retentate volume (L). Water flux was measured before and after each experimental run, and the fouling index (%) was calculated:

$$FI = (1 - J_{W1}/J_{W0}) \times 100, \quad (8)$$

where J_{W0} and J_{W1} are the water fluxes (L/m^{2}h) before and after wine concentration, respectively.

2.12. Statistical Analysis

The results were expressed as the mean ± standard deviation. Analysis of variance (ANOVA) and Fisher's least significant difference (LSD) test ($p < 0.05$) were determined for statistical analyses in STATISTICA 13.1 (StatSoft Inc., Tulsa, OK, USA) software program.

3. Results and Discussion

3.1. Influence of Processing Parameters On Permeate Flux and Membrane Fouling

Four different transmembrane pressures (25, 35, 45, and 55 bar) and two temperature regimes (with and without cooling) were applied during reverse osmosis (RO) and nanofiltration (NF) of the Cabernet Sauvignon red wine variety. The initial temperature in all runs was 20 °C, but the final temperature of retentates depended on the applied pressure (the higher the pressure, the higher the retentate temperature). Higher retentate temperatures in all runs were achieved during the reverse osmosis process compared to the nanofiltration at the same pressures (Figure 1). The cooling regime resulted in lower temperatures than in the experiments without cooling, meaning that the lowest final retentate temperature was measured at 25 bar with cooling (35 °C for RO and 32 °C for NF processes), and the highest at 55 bar without cooling (56 °C for RO and 47 °C for NF processes). The increase in pressure and temperature also resulted in higher permeate flux. The pressure had the main influence, but the increase in permeate flux was also a result of a lower viscosity of the feed due to higher temperature [14,30]. The highest average permeate flux was recorded at 55 bar without cooling (17.75 L/m²h for RO and 39.45 L/m²h for NF processes), and the lowest one was measured at 25 bar with cooling (3.74 L/m²h during RO and 15.44 L/m²h during NF processes).

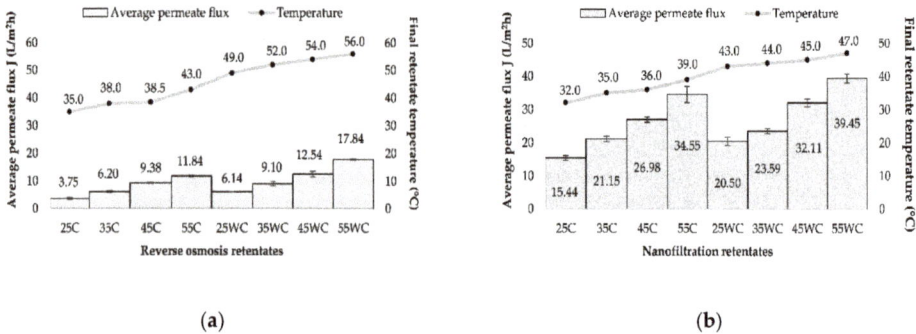

Figure 1. Influence of transmembrane pressure (25, 35, 45, and 55 bar) on the average permeate flux (L/m²h) and retentate temperature (°C) during concentration of Cabernet Sauvignon red wine by reverse osmosis (a) and nanofiltration (b), with (C) and without cooling (WC).

Several factors influence the membrane filtration processes, such as membrane type, the number of membranes used, module arrangement, operating time, applied pressure, and temperature [20,31]. The increase in feed concentration and membrane fouling during reverse osmosis and nanofiltration processes results in an increase in osmotic pressure on the membrane surface that leads to a permeate flux decrease [17,31,32]. In this study, the volume reduction factor (VRF) was calculated, and its influence on permeate flux was observed (Figure 2).

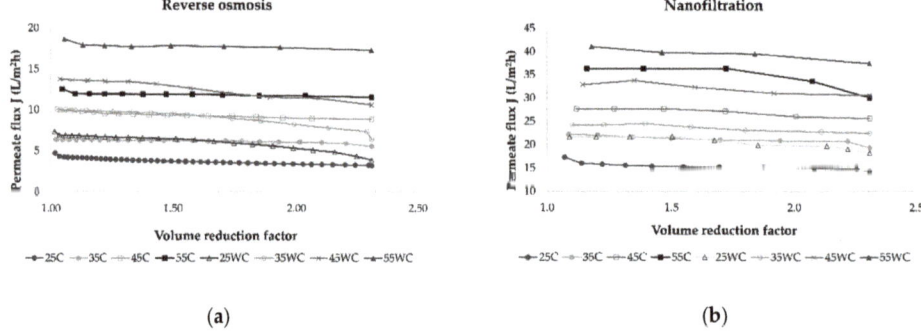

Figure 2. Influence of retentate concentration index (I_{rt}) on permeate flux (L/m²h) during concentration of Cabernet Sauvignon red wine by reverse osmosis (a) and nanofiltration (b) at 25, 35, 45, and 55 bar, with (C) and without cooling (WC).

In all experiments, the permeate flux decreased as the VRF value increased (2.31 was achieved at the end of each experiment), resulting in higher retention of bioactive compounds in the retentate. This behavior was a result of concentration polarization, fouling of the membrane, and osmotic pressure on the membrane surface [31,33,34]. The duration of each experimental run depended on applied pressure and temperature, and if these parameters were higher, the process took less time to obtain the desired volume of retentate and VRF. This is shown in Figure 3, where it can be observed that lower pressure and cooling regime resulted in a longer filtration process. Furthermore, the NF process was significantly shorter than RO at the same operating conditions.

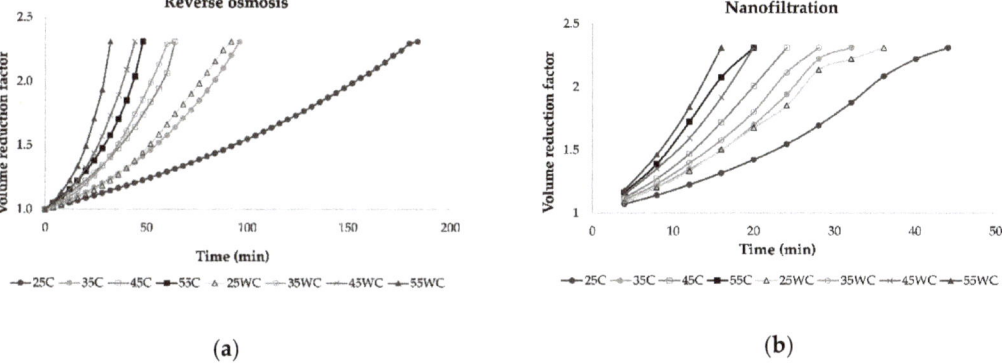

Figure 3. Influence of process duration (min) on volume reduction factor during concentration of Cabernet Sauvignon red wine by reverse osmosis (a) and nanofiltration (b) at 25, 35, 45, and 55 bar, with (C) and without cooling (WC).

Gurak et al. [34] used the LabUnit 20 system for reverse osmosis concentration of grape juice. They established that transmembrane pressure increased from 40 to 60 bar and temperature increased from 20 to 40 °C leading to higher permeate flux. In this study, permeate flux during reverse osmosis and nanofiltration was the highest at 55 bar when cooling was not applied. The use of NF membranes resulted in higher permeate flux than RO membranes due to larger pore size [31]. During both processes, the retentate volume was reduced, and the VRF increased through time, lowering the permeate flux and increasing the membrane fouling. A VRF value of 2.31 was achieved in all experiments, but it was achieved faster at higher pressures due to higher permeate flux. Yammine et al. [19] obtained similar results for VRF using three different pressures, 10, 20, and 30 bar.

The permeate flux decline under constant operating pressure occurred due to membrane fouling, as mentioned. However, if a constant flux is ensured, a pressure increase will occur [35]. It is a consequence of sealing or blocking of the membrane pores and cake formation [36]. In this study, the flux of pure water was measured before and after each wine concentration to establish flux decline due to membrane fouling. Average values were calculated and are presented in Figure 4. It can be observed that during NF processes before and after wine concentration, water flux was higher than the ones in RO processes. During both processes, the water flux significantly decreased after wine concentration, compared to the one before concentration.

According to the water flux before and after wine concentration, the fouling index (FI) for RO and NF membranes was calculated and is presented in Table 1. The fouling index was significantly higher for RO membranes (average FI was 55.66%) than for NF membranes (26.76%). This was expected because RO membranes retain smaller molecules and ions due to smaller pore size and molecular weight cut-off (MWCO) than the NF membranes.

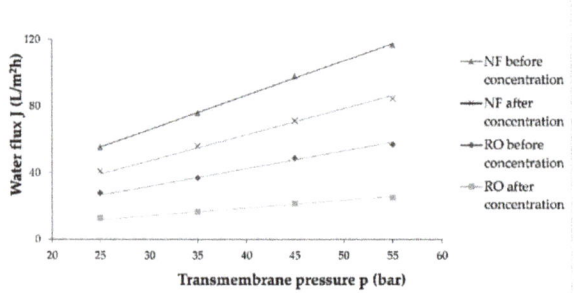

Figure 4. Influence of different transmembrane pressure (bar) on water flux (L/m^{2}h) before and after wine concentration by reverse osmosis (RO) and nanofiltration (NF) processes at 55 bar with cooling.

Table 1. Fouling index (%) of reverse osmosis (RO) and nanofiltration (NF) membranes at four different pressures.

Pressure (bar)	Fouling Index (%)	
	RO98pHt M20	NF M20
25	55.10	25.94
35	55.38	26.00
45	55.95	27.38
55	56.21	27.74

Membrane fouling and FI depend on the chemical composition of the feed, organic molecules, salt, and colloidal accumulation [35,37] and on the adsorption of organic compounds on the membrane surface. The adsorption of compounds on the membrane was a result of hydrophobic interactions [7]. Each compound contributes to the membrane fouling, depending on their chemical characteristics, such as molecular weight and polarity [38]. Increased adsorption of compounds and hydrophobic interactions on the membrane surface were correlated to higher flux decline [39]. Fouling of the membrane can increase the retention of bioactive compounds, but the permeate flux decline will eventually result in a slow concentration process, membrane deterioration, and high production costs [37].

3.2. Influence of Processing Parameters on Total Phenolic Compounds Retention

Total polyphenol content (TPC), total flavonoid content (TFC), monomeric anthocyanin content (MAC), and polymeric color (PC) of the initial wine and retentates obtained by reverse osmosis and nanofiltration are presented in Tables 2 and 3, respectively. The concentrations of total phenolic compounds increased during reverse osmosis treatment of Cabernet Sauvignon red wine, especially at higher pressures and lower temperatures. When cooling was not applied, slightly lower retention of TPC was observed due to the higher permeability of the membrane [33,34]. The results showed that the highest concentration of TPC was measured in the RO retentate at 45 bar (3.06 g/L) and 55 bar (3.11 g/L) with cooling, and the lowest at 25 and 35 bar without cooling (2.51 and 2.50 g/L, respectively). However, during the reverse osmosis process, their concentration increased compared to the initial wine (1.85 g/L). The concentration of TPC also increased during the nanofiltration process, and the highest concentrations were found in all retentates obtained with cooling (without significant difference among applied pressures) and the retentate obtained at 55 bar without cooling (around 3 g/L).

Table 2. Total polyphenol content (TPC), total flavonoid content (TFC), monomeric anthocyanin content (MAC), and polymeric color (PC) of an the initial Cabernet Sauvignon wine variety and retentates obtained by reverse osmosis at 25, 35, 45, and 55 bar with cooling (C) and without cooling (WC).

Sample	TPC (g GAE/L)	TFC (g CE/L)	MAC (mg CGE/L)	PC (%)
Wine	1.85 ± 0.01 [a]	0.71 ± 0.01 [a]	88.38 ± 0.87 [a]	54.77 ± 0.80 [a]
25C	2.99 ± 0.02 [d]	1.23 ± 0.07 [d]	156.05 ± 0.10 [d]	60.08 ± 0.84 [b]
35C	2.99 ± 0.03 [d]	1.22 ± 0.03 [d]	156.68 ± 0.05 [d]	60.35 ± 0.58 [b]
45C	3.06 ± 0.09 [de]	1.32 ± 0.03 [e]	167.91 ± 0.21 [e]	61.53 ± 0.12 [b]
55C	3.11 ± 0.05 [e]	1.39 ± 0.06 [e]	170.12 ± 0.39 [f]	61.25 ± 1.12 [b]
25WC	2.51 ± 0.02 [b]	1.10 ± 0.02 [b]	127.55 ± 0.01 [b]	60.12 ± 0.39 [b]
35WC	2.50 ± 0.02 [b]	1.10 ± 0.02 [b]	127.61 ± 0.02 [b]	60.51 ± 0.77 [b]
45WC	2.65 ± 0.04 [c]	1.15 ± 0.01 [c]	129.95 ± 0.30 [c]	61.78 ± 0.63 [b]
55WC	2.87 ± 0.08 [d]	1.30 ± 0.03 [e]	130.49 ± 0.21 [c]	61.17 ± 0.71 [b]

Different superscript letters indicate significant differences among samples within the column ($p < 0.05$; ANOVA, Fisher's LSD test).

Table 3. Total phenolic compounds of the initial Cabernet Sauvignon wine variety and retentates obtained by nanofiltration at 25, 35, 45, and 55 bar with cooling (C) and without cooling (WC).

Sample	TPC (g GAE/L)	TFC (g CE/L)	MAC (mg CGE/L)	PC (%)
Wine	1.85 ± 0.01 [a]	0.71 ± 0.01 [a]	88.38 ± 0.87 [a]	54.77 ± 0.80 [a]
25C	2.96 ± 0.04 [c]	1.16 ± 0.04 [b]	148.71 ± 0.26 [d]	60.56 ± 1.19 [b]
35C	2.94 ± 0.05 [c]	1.25 ± 0.02 [c]	149.04 ± 0.75 [d]	60.77 ± 0.75 [b]
45C	3.04 ± 0.07 [c]	1.33 ± 0.02 [d]	155.94 ± 0.27 [f]	60.83 ± 0.81 [b]
55C	3.11 ± 0.07 [c]	1.35 ± 0.01 [d]	162.48 ± 0.88 [g]	60.61 ± 1.73 [b]
25WC	2.77 ± 0.09 [b]	1.24 ± 0.01 [c]	130.09 ± 0.03 [b]	60.81 ± 0.71 [b]
35WC	2.81 ± 0.05 [b]	1.24 ± 0.02 [c]	137.99 ± 0.96 [c]	60.85 ± 0.44 [b]
45WC	2.82 ± 0.05 [b]	1.29 ± 0.05 [cd]	148.64 ± 0.03 [d]	60.87 ± 1.39 [b]
55WC	3.02 ± 0.02 [c]	1.31 ± 0.04 [d]	152.38 ± 0.06 [e]	60.77 ± 0.96 [b]

Different superscript letters indicate significant differences among samples within the column ($p < 0.05$; ANOVA, Fisher's LSD test).

The initial wine contained 0.71 g/L of TFC. The TFC content increased during the RO process, with the highest concentration at 45 bar (1.32 g/L) and 55 bar (1.39 g/L) with cooling, although there was no significant difference ($p > 0.05$) between those values and the one obtained at 55 bar without cooling (1.33 g/L). Nanofiltration processes at 45 and 55 bar resulted in similar TFC retention, and at those pressure, the highest concentrations (around 1.32 g/L) were measured with no significant difference between the two temperature regimes. The lowest concentrations of TFC in RO retentates were found at 25 and 35 bar without cooling (1.10 g/L for both) and in NF retentates at 25 bar with cooling (1.16 g/L).

Processes at 55 bar with cooling were the best in terms of monomeric anthocyanins retention, where the concentration was 170.12 mg/L in RO retentate and 162.48 mg/L in NF retentate, which is almost double the concentration found in the initial wine (88.38 mg/L). During processes without cooling, lower retention of MAC was observed compared to the processes with cooling. Compared to the RO membranes, NF membranes retained slightly higher concentrations of MAC when cooling was not applied at the same pressures.

Polymeric color represents the percentage of the color derived from polymerized material [33], and in the initial wine, 54.77% of polymeric color was measured. During the reverse osmosis process, an increase in polymeric color percentage was observed, but there was no significant difference among obtained retentates (average value was 60.85%). A similar trend for the polymeric color was observed during the nanofiltration process, where the average value among retentates was 60.75%, with no significant difference regarding pressure or temperature change.

Comparing two types of membranes, RO98pHt and NF M20, it was observed that both membranes retained phenolic compounds and both processes resulted in higher concentrations of TPC, TFC, and MAC than in the initial wine. RO processes with cooling resulted in retentates with similar content of TPC and TFC and higher concentrations of MAC in comparison to NF processes with cooling. However, when cooling was not applied, NF process retained slightly higher concentrations of total polyphenols, flavonoids, and monomeric anthocyanins. The highest difference was observed for MAC content at 55 bar without cooling (130.49 mg/L in RO retentate and 152.38 mg/L in NF retentate). Gurak et al. [34] established that higher pressure (60 bar) and lower temperature (20 °C) resulted in higher retention of MAC in grape juice. Reverse osmosis membranes retain smaller molecules and ions than nanofiltration ones, but this leads to faster membrane fouling and higher retentate temperature. Higher retentate temperature leads to higher membrane permeability and lower retention of phenolic compounds. Banvolgyi et al. [14] found that retention of resveratrol and anthocyanins during nanofiltration of red wine was higher at lower temperatures (20 °C). Similar results have been obtained during chokeberry juice concentration by reverse osmosis [33].

3.3. Influence of Processing Parameters on Individual Phenolic Compounds Retention

The concentrations of gallic acid, (+)-catechin, (−)-epicatechin, caffeic, caftaric, and coutaric acid in the initial Cabernet Sauvignon wine and retentates obtained by reverse osmosis and nanofiltration at 25, 35, 45, and 55 bar with and without cooling are presented in Tables 4 and 5.

Table 4. Concentration (mg/L) of individual phenolic compounds in the initial Cabernet Sauvignon wine variety and retentates obtained by reverse osmosis at 25, 35, 45, and 55 bar with cooling (C) and without cooling (WC).

Sample	Gallic Acid	(+)-Catechin	(−)-Epicatechin	Caffeic Acid	Caftaric Acid	Coutaric Acid
Wine	23.2 ± 0.0 [a]	54.7 ± 0.2 [a]	47.0 ± 0.3 [a]	13.0 ± 0.0 [a]	49.1 ± 0.2 [a]	16.8 ± 0.0 [a]
25C	31.2 ± 0.2 [c]	95.4 ± 0.2 [e]	60.9 ± 0.9 [c]	16.1 ± 0.0 [c]	65.4 ± 0.1 [c]	21.5 ± 0.0 [b]
35C	31.6 ± 0.0 [c]	95.8 ± 0.7 [e]	67.5 ± 0.7 [d]	15.8 ± 0.0 [b]	66.3 ± 0.1 [d]	21.7 ± 0.1 [b]
45C	34.1 ± 0.1 [d]	98.7 ± 0.3 [g]	69.1 ± 1.2 [d]	16.8 ± 0.0 [d]	72.7 ± 0.2 [g]	23.4 ± 0.1 [d]
55C	39.0 ± 0.1 [f]	99.2 ± 0.4 [g]	82.2 ± 0.5 [g]	18.2 ± 0.2 [f]	80.8 ± 0.5 [i]	25.6 ± 0.2 [f]
25WC	30.6 ± 0.2 [b]	90.2 ± 0.3 [b]	58.5 ± 0.7 [b]	15.7 ± 0.0 [b]	64.8 ± 0.0 [b]	21.5 ± 0.1 [b]
35WC	33.8 ± 0.5 [d]	92.3 ± 0.2 [c]	74.3 ± 0.7 [e]	15.8 ± 0.1 [b]	67.1 ± 0.5 [e]	22.7 ± 0.2 [c]
45WC	34.5 ± 0.6 [d]	94.4 ± 0.0 [d]	74.9 ± 0.3 [e]	16.7 ± 0.1 [d]	71.1 ± 0.9 [f]	22.7 ± 0.2 [c]
55WC	36.3 ± 0.1 [e]	97.5 ± 0.5 [f]	80.1 ± 0.6 [f]	17.2 ± 0.0 [e]	77.0 ± 0.2 [h]	24.1 ± 0.1 [e]

Significant differences ($p < 0.05$) between samples are indicated by different superscript letters within the column (ANOVA, Fisher's LSD test).

Table 5. Concentration (mg/L) of individual phenolic compounds in the initial Cabernet Sauvignon wine variety and retentates obtained by nanofiltration at 25, 35, 45, and 55 bar with cooling (C) and without cooling (WC).

Sample	Gallic Acid	(+)-Catechin	(−)-Epicatechin	Caffeic Acid	Caftaric Acid	Coutaric Acid
Wine	23.2 ± 0.1 [b]	54.7 ± 0.2 [a]	47.0 ± 0.3 [a]	13.0 ± 0.1 [a]	49.1 ± 0.2 [a]	16.8 ± 0.1 [a]
25C	29.6 ± 0.1 [e]	70.0 ± 0.1 [b]	53.3 ± 0.2 [c]	13.3 ± 0.1 [h]	71.9 ± 0.1 [f]	23.2 ± 0.1 [f]
35C	29.5 ± 0.2 [e]	71.2 ± 0.3 [c]	71.2 ± 0.4 [f]	13.5 ± 0.1 [c]	72.4 ± 0.1 [g]	23.3 ± 0.1 [f]
45C	29.1 ± 0.1 [e]	78.5 ± 0.8 [f]	72.0 ± 0.1 [fg]	13.4 ± 0.1 [bc]	72.2 ± 0.1 [fg]	23.3 ± 0.1 [f]
55C	29.8 ± 0.1 [e]	88.6 ± 0.7 [h]	73.0 ± 0.5 [g]	13.7 ± 0.1 [d]	73.9 ± 0.4 [h]	23.8 ± 0.1 [g]
25WC	22.0 ± 0.8 [a]	73.9 ± 0.1 [d]	49.9 ± 0.3 [b]	13.2 ± 0.1 [b]	66.6 ± 0.1 [b]	21.8 ± 0.1 [b]
35WC	23.9 ± 0.1 [c]	77.2 ± 0.2 [e]	56.0 ± 0.3 [d]	13.3 ± 0.1 [b]	68.3 ± 0.1 [c]	22.5 ± 0.1 [c]
45WC	25.4 ± 0.1 [d]	79.8 ± 0.5 [f]	52.4 ± 0.6 [c]	13.3 ± 0.1 [b]	69.4 ± 0.1 [d]	22.2 ± 0.1 [d]
55WC	25.8 ± 0.1 [d]	85.7 ± 0.7 [g]	60.6 ± 1.6 [e]	13.3 ± 0.1 [b]	71.1 ± 0.2 [e]	22.9 ± 0.1 [e]

Significant differences ($p < 0.05$) between samples are indicated by different superscript letters within the column (ANOVA, Fisher's LSD test).

One phenolic acid (gallic acid), two flavan-3-ols (catechin and epicatechin), and three hydroxycinnamic acids (caffeic, caftaric, and coutaric acid) were monitored in the initial red wine and retentates obtained by reverse osmosis and nanofiltration. Those components are characteristic of red wines, including the Cabernet Sauvignon wine variety [40–42]. The concentration of gallic acid in the initial wine was 23.2 mg/L, and after the reverse osmosis process, an increase in gallic acid concentration was observed, with the highest concentration at 55 bar with cooling (39.0 mg/L). The concentrations of catechin and epicatechin followed the same trend, increasing from 54.7 and 47.0 mg/L in the initial wine to 99.2 and 81.9 mg/L, respectively, in the RO retentate at 55 bar with cooling. The increase in transmembrane pressure had the same effect on the hydroxycinnamic acid retention, meaning that the highest concentrations of caffeic, caftaric, and coutaric acids were found in the retentate obtained at 55 bar with cooling. The increase in temperature in the RO process without cooling resulted in lower retention of all phenolic compounds compared to the regime with cooling. The change in applied pressure had the same influence in both temperature regimes.

The concentration of wine by nanofiltration resulted in an increase in all mentioned components, especially at 45 and 55 bar with cooling. The concentration of gallic acid increased from 23.2 mg/L in the initial wine to 29.5 mg/L in the NF retentates obtained with cooling, with no significant difference among pressures ($p > 0.05$). A small loss occurred when cooling was not applied. A similar trend was noticed for coutaric acid with the highest concentrations obtained with cooling (23.2–23.8 mg/L). The processes without cooling resulted in slightly higher retention of (+)-catechin than the regime with cooling at the same pressures, except for 55 bar with cooling where the concentration was highest (88.6 mg/L). Higher pressure and lower temperature were also beneficial for (−)-epicatechin, caffeic, and caftaric acid, with the highest concentrations obtained at 55 bar (73.0, 13.7, and 73.9 mg/L, respectively). The pressure change had no significant influence on caffeic acid concentration when cooling was not applied.

The retention of phenolic compounds depended on several factors. Membrane characteristics and operating conditions are the main ones. As stated before, pressure increase resulted in faster membrane fouling, increasing the retention of phenolic compounds. The retention of individual compounds depended on their molecular weight and polarity, membrane molecular weight cut-off (MWCO), membrane fouling index, and resistance [35]. In this study, the concentrations of individual phenolic compounds were slightly higher in the RO retentates than in the nanofiltration ones. Coutaric acid was an exception because its retention in NF retentates was similar to the one in RO retentates, even higher at lower pressures with cooling. It was expected that RO membranes show higher retention of phenolic compounds due to smaller pore size and MWCO value [43], but this was not the only parameter that affected phenolic retention. NF processes were significantly shorter, especially when cooling was not applied, compared to the RO processes. Long process duration can lead to higher degradation or permeation of individual compounds through the membrane [33]. Further, each compound reacts differently with the membrane surface that depends on the membrane and compounds' chemical structure, hydrophobic, or hydrophilic interactions [44]. Cai et al. [38] studied the influence of membrane characteristics and six different phenolic compounds on membrane fouling. The analyzed phenolic compounds did not affect membrane fouling the same way, and it depended on their chemical properties, acidity coefficient, or molecular refractive index, etc. Besides operating conditions, membrane chemical composition played a significant role in membrane fouling, compounds adsorption, and retention.

3.4. Influence of Processing Parameters on Antioxidant Activity in Retentates

Phenolic compounds in wine affect the taste, feel, and color of wine, and they are mostly known as natural antioxidants [45]. Tables 6 and 7 present antioxidant activity of Cabernet Sauvignon wine, RO, and NF retentates, determined by four different assays: DPPH, ABTS, FRAP, and CUPRAC. DPPH and ABTS are decolorization assays, while

FRAP and CUPRAC are characterized by an absorbance increase at a certain wavelength as the antioxidants react with chromogenic reagent [46]. All assays differ in terms of principles and reaction conditions, and one was not sufficient to present the total antioxidant capacity of wine [47].

Table 6. Antioxidant activity (2,2-diphenyl-1-picrylhydrazil DPPH, Trolox, 2,2′-azinobis(3-ethylbenzothiazoline sulfonic acid) (ABTS), ferric reducing/antioxidant power assay (FRAP), and cupric reducing antioxidant capacity (CUPRAC)) of the initial Cabernet Sauvignon wine variety and retentates obtained by reverse osmosis at 25, 35, 45, and 55 bar with cooling (C) and without cooling (WC).

Sample	DPPH (µmol TE/100 mL)	ABTS (µmol TE/100 mL)	FRAP (µmol TE/100 mL)	CUPRAC (µmol TE/100 mL)
Wine	10.34 ± 0.53 [a]	12.17 ± 0.07 [a]	1.86 ± 0.04 [a]	69.46 ± 3.45 [a]
25C	15.73 ± 0.19 [c]	22.49 ± 0.83 [c]	2.74 ± 0.01 [bc]	109.51 ± 0.15 [d]
35C	16.27 ± 0.28 [c]	25.59 ± 0.97 [d]	2.99 ± 0.16 [cd]	109.23 ± 0.13 [d]
45C	18.02 ± 0.16 [d]	26.59 ± 0.97 [de]	3.08 ± 0.27 [d]	112.29 ± 1.42 [e]
55C	18.40 ± 0.10 [d]	27.82 ± 0.93 [e]	3.82 ± 0.29 [e]	159.47 ± 2.59 [f]
25WC	14.59 ± 0.65 [b]	20.82 ± 0.27 [b]	2.51 ± 0.01 [b]	99.07 ± 3.54 [b]
35WC	14.79 ± 0.49 [b]	20.89 ± 0.40 [b]	2.63 ± 0.12 [b]	102.85 ± 2.06 [b]
45WC	15.05 ± 0.82 [bc]	21.55 ± 0.43 [bc]	2.72 ± 0.32 [bc]	107.25 ± 1.12 [c]
55WC	15.21 ± 0.54 [bc]	21.81 ± 0.18 [c]	2.79 ± 0.11 [bc]	112.51 ± 1.80 [e]

Within column, different superscript letters indicate significant differences among samples ($p < 0.05$; ANOVA, Fisher's LSD test).

Table 7. Antioxidant capacity determined by four methods of the initial Cabernet Sauvignon wine variety and retentates obtained by nanofiltration at 25, 35, 45, and 55 bar with cooling (C) and without cooling (WC).

Sample	DPPH (µmol TE/100 mL)	ABTS (µmol TE/100 mL)	FRAP (µmol TE/100 mL)	CUPRAC (µmol TE/100 mL)
Wine	10.34 ± 0.53 [a]	12.17 ± 0.07 [a]	1.86 ± 0.04 [a]	69.46 ± 3.45 [a]
25C	15.65 ± 0.23 [b]	23.62 ± 1.84 [b]	2.61 ± 0.22 [b]	108.52 ± 0.82 [d]
35C	16.56 ± 0.08 [cd]	26.14 ± 1.63 [cd]	2.79 ± 0.18 [bc]	106.88 ± 1.57 [cd]
45C	16.66 ± 0.03 [cd]	26.31 ± 0.23 [cd]	2.94 ± 0.10 [c]	115.05 ± 3.40 [e]
55C	17.03 ± 0.23 [d]	27.21 ± 0.23 [d]	3.32 ± 0.12 [d]	149.99 ± 1.61 [f]
25WC	16.27 ± 0.15 [c]	23.31 ± 0.37 [b]	2.53 ± 0.01 [b]	99.43 ± 1.98 [b]
35WC	16.58 ± 0.01 [cd]	24.31 ± 0.18 [b]	2.56 ± 0.07 [b]	103.81 ± 1.60 [c]
45WC	16.23 ± 0.02 [c]	25.48 ± 0.45 [c]	2.54 ± 0.04 [b]	109.31 ± 0.20 [d]
55WC	16.96 ± 0.64 [d]	26.55 ± 1.27 [cd]	2.84 ± 0.18 [c]	113.82 ± 0.52 [e]

Within the column, different superscript letters indicate significant differences among samples ($p < 0.05$; ANOVA, Fisher's LSD test).

The antioxidant activity of the initial wine measured by DPPH, ABTS, FRAP, and CUPRAC assay was 10.34, 12.17, 1.86, and 69.46 µmol TE/100 mL, respectively. After the reverse osmosis process, antioxidant activity in all retentates increased. At higher pressures (45 and 55 bar) and when cooling was applied, higher antioxidant activity was measured. Higher temperature (without cooling regime) resulted in lower antioxidant activity of RO retentates compared to the ones obtained with cooling at the same pressures. There were no significant differences ($p > 0.05$) between values obtained at 25, 35, 45, and 55 bar without cooling, except for CUPRAC, where an increase in antioxidant activity was observed with pressure increment. This means that the pressure had a lower influence on antioxidant activity than temperature when cooling was not applied during the reverse osmosis process.

Table 7 presents the antioxidant activity of Cabernet Sauvignon red wine and retentates obtained by nanofiltration at 25, 35, 45, and 55 bar with and without cooling. The results showed that nanofiltration processes resulted in an increase in total antioxidant activity of all retentates comparing to the initial wine. Pressure increase had a low influence on the antioxidant activity of NF retentates. Slightly higher antioxidant activity was measured in retentates obtained at 55 bar at both temperature regimes. The CUPRAC assay was again an exception: higher pressure and temperature had a significant effect on the antioxidant activity of all retentates. This means that the highest antioxidant activity was measured at the highest pressure (55 bar) with cooling (149.99 µmol/100 mL). Compared to that, notable lower antioxidant activity was obtained when cooling was not applied, 113.82 µmol/100 mL at 55 bar. Compared to the RO process, the antioxidant activity of NF retentates was slightly higher when cooling was not applied.

It was visible that there was some difference between concentrations of phenolic compounds in RO and NF retentates, meaning that the type of membrane did not affect the retention of each compound equally. However, all obtained retentates contained higher concentrations of analyzed compounds and antioxidant activity than the initial wine. This means that both membranes, RO98pHt and NF M20, can be used for wine concentration and phenolic compounds retention. The findings in this study have been consistent with previous studies where it has been shown that membrane filtration can be used for chemical composition correction of must or wine or even wine industry waste [14,18,48–51]. Arboleda Mejia et al. [7] stated that nanofiltration membranes (three cellulose acetate and one commercial) are suitable for the recovery of phenolic compounds from red grape pomace extract. Further, Bánvölgyi et al. [20] used nanofiltration membranes at 30, 40, and 50 °C for the production of red wine concentrates with enriched valuable components (anthocyanins, resveratrol, etc.). They concluded that all concentrates had higher concentrations of analyzed compounds than the initial wine. At higher temperatures, retention of those compounds decreased, and loss occurred.

3.5. Influence of Processing Parameters on the Color of Obtained Retentates

Color parameters L^*, a^*, b^*, C^*, and $°h$ were measured in the initial Cabernet Sauvignon wine and retentates obtained by reverse osmosis (Table 8) and nanofiltration (Table 9).

Table 8. Color parameters (L^*, a^*, b^*, $°h$, and C^*) in the initial Cabernet Sauvignon wine and retentates obtained by reverse osmosis at 25, 35, 45, and 55 bar, with cooling (C) and without cooling (WC).

Sample	L^*	a^*	b^*	$°h$	C^*	ΔE^*
Wine	19.54 ± 0.02 [b]	0.59 ± 0.03 [c]	0.64 ± 0.01 [c]	31.99 ± 0.11 [c]	0.74 ± 0.02 [a]	-
25C	19.36 ± 0.03 [a]	0.54 ± 0.04 [c]	0.49 ± 0.01 [a]	26.93 ± 0.29 [a]	0.88 ± 0.01 [b]	0.24 ± 0.02 [a]
35C	19.34 ± 0.04 [a]	0.56 ± 0.02 [c]	0.47 ± 0.02 [a]	26.91 ± 0.18 [a]	0.87 ± 0.01 [b]	0.26 ± 0.01 [a]
45C	19.32 ± 0.01 [a]	0.54 ± 0.03 [c]	0.47 ± 0.01 [a]	28.83 ± 0.44 [b]	0.87 ± 0.02 [b]	0.28 ± 0.02 [ab]
55C	19.34 ± 0.02 [a]	0.54 ± 0.01 [c]	0.55 ± 0.01 [b]	29.50 ± 0.50 [b]	0.91 ± 0.01 [bc]	0.22 ± 0.03 [a]
25WC	19.36 ± 0.03 [a]	0.45 ± 0.03 [b]	0.47 ± 0.02 [a]	25.96 ± 0.76 [a]	0.94 ± 0.01 [c]	0.28 ± 0.03 [ab]
35WC	19.32 ± 0.06 [a]	0.48 ± 0.00 [b]	0.46 ± 0.01 [a]	27.18 ± 0.13 [a]	0.97 ± 0.02 [c]	0.31 ± 0.01 [b]
45WC	19.39 ± 0.03 [a]	0.38 ± 0.04 [a]	0.46 ± 0.02 [a]	28.42 ± 0.64 [b]	0.96 ± 0.04 [c]	0.31 ± 0.02 [b]
55WC	19.35 ± 0.05 [a]	0.35 ± 0.04 [a]	0.57 ± 0.05 [bc]	29.18 ± 0.63 [b]	0.93 ± 0.02 [c]	0.31 ± 0.02 [b]

Significant differences ($p < 0.05$) between samples are indicated by different superscript letters within the column (ANOVA, Fisher's LSD test).

The results showed that the L^* value in the initial wine (19.54) slightly decreased during RO and NF processes, meaning that those processes lowered the wine lightness. There was no significant change in the a^* value in all retentates when cooling was applied, compared to the initial wine. A slight decrease was observed in samples without the cooling regime. The b^* values were lower in RO and NF retentates than in the initial wine, with no significant difference ($p > 0.05$) among retentates obtained at 25, 35, and 45 bar at both temperature regimes. The hue angle ($°h$) in the initial wine was 31.99°, and this value decreased in RO and NF retentates. A slightly higher $°h$ parameter was measured in retentates obtained at 45 and 55 bar in both temperature regimes than in the ones obtained at lower pressures. The C^* value increased during both processes, especially at higher temperatures, meaning that membrane filtration processes resulted in more saturated color than the initial wine. However, colour changes measured by the Lab system in analyzed samples were not large enough to be distinguished by the human eye. This is proved by the ΔE* value that represents total color differences between the initial wine and obtained retentates. The human eye can distinguish color change when the ΔE* value is higher than 1, or 5 when the wine is observed through a glass [52]. In this study, results showed that RO and NF processes did not significantly change the colour of the initial wine (all ΔE* values were lower than 1).

Table 9. Color parameters (L*, a*, b*, °h and C*) in the initial Cabernet Sauvignon wine and retentates obtained by nanofiltration at 25, 35, 45, and 55 bar, with cooling (C) and without cooling (WC).

Sample	L*	a*	b*	°h	C*	ΔE*
Wine	19.54 ± 0.02 [b]	0.59 ± 0.03 [b]	0.64 ± 0.01 [b]	31.99 ± 0.11 [c]	0.74 ± 0.02 [a]	-
25C	19.39 ± 0.03 [a]	0.52 ± 0.02 [b]	0.53 ± 0.02 [a]	28.70 ± 0.48 [a]	0.86 ± 0.03 [b]	0.21 ± 0.03 [ab]
35C	19.37 ± 0.06 [a]	0.54 ± 0.00 [b]	0.53 ± 0.00 [a]	28.36 ± 0.76 [a]	0.87 ± 0.01 [b]	0.21 ± 0.02 [ab]
45C	19.39 ± 0.04 [a]	0.55 ± 0.02 [b]	0.56 ± 0.03 [ab]	30.91 ± 0.61 [b]	0.88 ± 0.01 [b]	0.23 ± 0.04 [ab]
55C	19.40 ± 0.03 [a]	0.53 ± 0.01 [b]	0.60 ± 0.03 [b]	30.08 ± 0.93 [b]	0.84 ± 0.03 [b]	0.16 ± 0.04 [a]
25WC	19.35 ± 0.04 [a]	0.47 ± 0.01 [a]	0.55 ± 0.02 [a]	27.44 ± 0.39 [a]	0.83 ± 0.02 [b]	0.24 ± 0.01 [b]
35WC	19.37 ± 0.01 [a]	0.44 ± 0.01 [a]	0.53 ± 0.03 [a]	27.98 ± 0.63 [a]	0.85 ± 0.01 [b]	0.25 ± 0.02 [b]
45WC	19.37 ± 0.02 [a]	0.47 ± 0.02 [a]	0.54 ± 0.02 [a]	30.73 ± 0.47 [b]	0.94 ± 0.00 [c]	0.23 ± 0.02 [b]
55WC	19.34 ± 0.02 [a]	0.44 ± 0.01 [a]	0.61 ± 0.02 [b]	30.56 ± 0.30 [b]	0.94 ± 0.02 [c]	0.25 ± 0.00 [b]

Significant differences ($p < 0.05$) between samples are indicated by different superscript letters within the column (ANOVA. Fisher's LSD test).

4. Conclusions

This study showed that reverse osmosis and nanofiltration processes are suitable for fast red wine phenolic content correction. Both membrane filtration processes resulted in higher phenolic content than in the initial wine. Comparing the two types of membranes, RO98pHt M20 membranes retained slightly higher concentrations of most phenolic compounds than NF M20 due to smaller pore size, mostly when cooling was applied. The nanofiltration process resulted in a lower retentate temperature, shorter process duration, lower fouling index than the RO process. Four applied pressures had different effects on phenolics retention that were greater if the pressure was higher. Retentate temperature increased with the pressure, which had a small or no effect if cooling was applied. During reverse osmosis and nanofiltration processes without cooling, retentate temperature was higher, and it resulted in the loss of most compounds due to higher membrane permeability or thermal degradation. However, during both processes, no visible change was observed in the wine color determined by the Lab system. In conclusion, optimal operating parameters should be adjusted to achieve the desirable phenolic content and properties of red wine concentrates.

Author Contributions: Conceptualization, A.P., V.J. and J.M.; methodology, I.I., L.J., A.P. and M.K.; formal analysis, I.I., L.J., S.K. and B.M.; investigation, I.I., A.P. and M.K.; data curation, I.I., L.J. and A.P.; writing—original draft preparation, I.I., J.M.; writing—review and editing, A.P., V.J. and M.K.; supervision, A.P., L.J. and M.K.; project administration, A.P.; funding acquisition, A.P. All authors have read and agreed to the published version of the manuscript.

Funding: This research was funded by the Josip Juraj Strossmayer University in Osijek; Membrane processes: Influence of concentration on aroma and colour compounds in red wine, grant number ZUP2018-08.

Institutional Review Board Statement: Not applicable.

Informed Consent Statement: Not applicable.

Data Availability Statement: Not available.

Conflicts of Interest: The authors declare no conflict of interest.

References

1. Garrido, J.; Borges, F. Wine and grape polyphenols—A chemical perspective. *Food Res. Int.* **2013**, *54*, 1844–1858. [CrossRef]
2. Giovinazzo, G.; Grieco, F. Functional Properties of Grape and Wine Polyphenols. *Plant Foods Hum. Nutr.* **2015**, *70*, 454–462. [CrossRef] [PubMed]
3. Meral, R. Antioxidant effects of wine polyphenols. *Trakia J. Sci.* **2008**, *6*, 57–62.
4. Giovinazzo, G.; Carluccio, M.A.; Grieco, F. Wine Polyphenols and Health. In *Bioactive Molecules in Food. Reference Series in Phytochemistry*; Mérillon, J., Ramawat, K., Eds.; Springer Nature: Cham, Switzerland, 2019; pp. 1135–1155. ISBN 9783319780306.
5. Fang, F.; Li, J.-M.; Zhang, P.; Tang, K.; Wang, W.; Pan, Q.-H.; Huang, W.-D. Effects of grape variety, harvest date, fermentation vessel and wine ageing on flavonoid concentration in red wines. *Food Res. Int.* **2008**, *41*, 53–60. [CrossRef]
6. Balík, J.; Kyseláková, M.; Tříska, J.; Vrchotová, N.; Veverka, J.; Híc, P.; Totušek, J.; Lefnerová, D. The changes of selected phenolic substances in wine technology. *Czech J. Food Sci.* **2009**, *26*, S3–S12. [CrossRef]
7. Arboleda Mejia, J.A.; Ricci, A.; Figueiredo, A.S.; Versari, A.; Cassano, A.; Parpinello, G.P.; De Pinho, M.N. Recovery of Phenolic Compounds from Red Grape Pomace Extract through Nanofiltration Membranes. *Foods* **2020**, *9*, 1649. [CrossRef] [PubMed]
8. Ganorkar, P.; Nandane, A.; Tapre, A. Reverse Osmosis for Fruit Juice Concentration—A Review. *Res. Rev. A J. Food Sci. Technol.* **2012**, *1*, 23–36.
9. Saha, B.; Torley, P.; Blackman, J.W.; Schmidtke, L.M. Review of processing technology to reduce alcohol levels in wines. In Proceedings of the 1st International Symposium Alcohol level reduction in wine-Oenoviti International Network, Bordeauxq, France, 6 September 2013; pp. 78–86.
10. Ozturk, B.; Anli, E. Different techniques for reducing alcohol levels in wine: A review. *BIO Web Conf.* **2014**, *3*, 02012. [CrossRef]
11. Gil, M.; Estévez, S.; Kontoudakis, N.; Fort, F.; Canals, J.M.; Zamora, F. Influence of partial dealcoholization by reverse osmosis on red wine composition and sensory characteristics. *Eur. Food Res. Technol.* **2013**, *237*, 481–488. [CrossRef]
12. Pham, D.-T.; Stockdale, V.J.; Wollan, D.; Jeffery, D.W.; Wilkinson, K.L. Compositional Consequences of Partial Dealcoholization of Red Wine by Reverse Osmosis-Evaporative Perstraction. *Molecules* **2019**, *24*, 1404. [CrossRef] [PubMed]
13. Longo, R.; Blackman, J.W.; Torley, P.J.; Rogiers, S.Y.; Schmidtke, L.M. Changes in volatile composition and sensory attributes of wines during alcohol content reduction. *J. Sci. Food Agric.* **2016**, *97*, 8–16. [CrossRef] [PubMed]
14. Banvolgyi, S.; Savaş Bahçeci, K.; Vatai, G.; Bekassy, S.; Bekassy-Molnar, E. Partial dealcoholization of red wine by nanofiltration and its effect on anthocyanin and resveratrol levels. *Food Sci. Technol. Int.* **2016**, *22*, 677–687. [CrossRef] [PubMed]
15. Bellona, C. Nanofiltration—Theory and Application. In *Desalination*; Kucera, J., Ed.; Scrivener Publishing LLC: Salem, MA, USA; Clarkson University: Potsdam, NY, USA, 2019; pp. 163–207.
16. Massot, A.; Mietton-Peuchot, M.; Peuchot, C.; Milisic, V. Nanofiltration and reverse osmosis in winemaking. *Desalination* **2008**, *231*, 283–289. [CrossRef]
17. Chakraborty, S.; Bag, B.C.; DasGupta, S.; Basu, J.K.; De, S. Prediction of permeate flux and permeate concentration in nanofiltration of dye solution. *Sep. Purif. Technol.* **2004**, *35*, 141–152. [CrossRef]
18. Cassano, A. Recovery of Polyphenols from Wine Wastewaters by Membrane Operations. In *Encyclopedia of Membranes*; Springer: Berlin, Heidelberg, 2016; pp. 1717–1718.
19. Yammine, S.; Rabagliato, R.; Vitrac, X.; Mietton-Peuchot, M.; Ghidossi, R. The use of nanofiltration membranes for the fractionation of polyphenols from grape pomace extracts. *Oeno One* **2019**, *53*, 11–26. [CrossRef]
20. Banvolgyi, S.; Kiss, I.; Bekassy-Molnar, E.; Vatai, G. Concentration of red wine by nanofiltration. *Desalination* **2006**, *198*, 8–15. [CrossRef]
21. Di Giacomo, G.; Taglieri, L. Production of Red Wine Polyphenols as Ingredient for the Food and Pharmaceutical Industry. *Int. J. Food Sci. Nutr. Eng.* **2012**, *2*, 12–15. [CrossRef]
22. Ough, C.S.; Amerine, M.A. *Methods Analysis of Musts and Wines*; John Wiley & Sons Inc.: New York, NY, USA, 1988.
23. Kim, D.O.; Jeong, S.W.; Lee, C.Y. Antioxidant capacity of phenolic phytochemicals from various cultivars of plums. *Food Chem.* **2003**, *81*, 321–326. [CrossRef]
24. Giusti, M.M.; Wrolstad, R.E. Characterization and measurement of anthocyanins by UV–Visible spectroscopy. In *Current Protocols in Food Analytical Chemistry*; Wrolstad, R.E., Schwartz, S.J., Eds.; John Wiley & Sons Inc.: New York, NY, USA, 2001; pp. 5–69.
25. Brand-Williams, W.; Cuvelier, M.E.; Berset, C. Use of a free radical method to evaluate antioxidant activity. *LWT Food Sci. Technol.* **1995**, *28*, 25–30. [CrossRef]
26. Re, R.; Pellegrini, N.; Proteggente, A.; Pannala, A.; Yang, M.; Rice-Evans, C. Antioxidant activity applying an improved ABTS radical cation decolorization assay. *Free Radic. Biol. Med.* **1999**, *26*, 1231–1237. [CrossRef]
27. Benzie, I.F.F.; Strain, J.J. Ferric reducing/antioxidant power assay: Direct measure of total antioxidant activity of biological fluids and modified version for simultaneous measurement of total antioxidant power and ascorbic acid concentration. *Methods Enzymol.* **1999**, *299*, 15–27. [CrossRef] [PubMed]
28. Özyürek, M.; Güçlü, K.; Tütem, E.; Bakan, K.S.; Erçağ, E.; Esin Çelik, S.; Baki, S.; Yildiz, L.; Karaman, Ş.; Apak, R. A comprehensive review of CUPRAC methodology. *Anal. Methods* **2011**, *3*, 2439–2453. [CrossRef]
29. Vukoja, J.; Pichler, A.; Kopjar, M. Stability of Anthocyanins, Phenolics and Color of Tart Cherry Jams. *Foods* **2019**, *8*, 255. [CrossRef]
30. Siddiqui, M.U.; Arif, A.F.M.; Bashmal, S. Permeability-selectivity analysis of microfiltration and ultrafiltration membranes: Effect of pore size and shape distribution and membrane stretching. *Membranes* **2016**, *6*, 40. [CrossRef]

31. Popović, K.; Pozderović, A.; Jakobek, L.; Rukavina, J.; Pichler, A. Concentration of chokeberry (Aronia melanocarpa) juice by nanofiltration. *J. Food Nutr. Res.* **2016**, *55*, 159–170.
32. Díaz-Reinoso, B.; Moure, A.; Domínguez, H.; Parajó, J.C. Ultra- and nanofiltration of aqueous extracts from distilled fermented grape pomace. *J. Food Eng.* **2009**, *91*, 587–593. [CrossRef]
33. Pozderovic, A.; Popovic, K.; Pichler, A.; Jakobek, L. Influence of processing parameters on permeate flow and retention of aroma and phenolic compounds in chokeberry juice concentrated by reverse osmosis. *Cyta J. Food* **2016**, *14*, 382–390. [CrossRef]
34. Gurak, P.D.; Cabral, L.M.C.; Rocha-Leão, M.H.M.; Matta, V.M.; Freitas, S.P. Quality evaluation of grape juice concentrated by reverse osmosis. *J. Food Eng.* **2010**, *96*, 421–426. [CrossRef]
35. Koo, C.H.; Mohammad, A.W.; Suja', F.; Meor Talib, M.Z. Use and development of fouling index in predicting membrane fouling. *Sep. Purif. Rev.* **2013**, *42*, 296–339. [CrossRef]
36. El Rayess, Y.; Albasi, C.; Bacchin, P.; Taillandier, P.; Mietton-Peuchot, M.; Devatine, A. Analysis of membrane fouling during cross-flow microfiltration of wine. *Innov. Food Sci. Emerg. Technol.* **2012**, *16*, 398–408. [CrossRef]
37. Koo, C.H.; Mohammad, A.W.; Suja', F.; Meor Talib, M.Z. Review of the effect of selected physicochemical factors on membrane fouling propensity based on fouling indices. *Desalination* **2012**, *287*, 167–177. [CrossRef]
38. Cai, M.; Hou, W.; Li, Z.; Lv, Y.; Sun, P. Understanding Nanofiltration Fouling of Phenolic Compounds in Model Juice Solution with Two Membranes. *Food Bioprocess Technol.* **2017**, *10*, 2123–2131. [CrossRef]
39. Arsuaga, J.M.; López-Muñoz, M.J.; Sotto, A. Correlation between retention and adsorption of phenolic compounds in nanofiltration membranes. *Desalination* **2010**, *250*, 829–832. [CrossRef]
40. Burin, V.M.; Arcari, S.G.; Costa, L.L.F.; Bordignon-Luiz, M.T. Determination of some phenolic compounds in red wine by RP-HPLC: Method development and validation. *J. Chromatogr. Sci.* **2011**, *49*, 647–651. [CrossRef] [PubMed]
41. Jiang, B.; Zhang, Z.W. Comparison on phenolic compounds and antioxidant properties of cabernet sauvignon and merlot wines from four wine grape-growing regions in China. *Molecules* **2012**, *17*, 8804–8821. [CrossRef]
42. Šeruga, M.; Novak, I.; Jakobek, L. Determination of polyphenols content and antioxidant activity of some red wines by differential pulse voltammetry, HPLC and spectrophotometric methods. *Food Chem.* **2011**, *124*, 1208–1216. [CrossRef]
43. López-Muñoz, M.J.; Sotto, A.; Arsuaga, J.M.; Van der Bruggen, B. Influence of membrane, solute and solution properties on the retention of phenolic compounds in aqueous solution by nanofiltration membranes. *Sep. Purif. Technol.* **2009**, *66*, 194–201. [CrossRef]
44. Conidi, C.; Cassano, A. Recovery of phenolic compounds from bergamot juice by nanofiltration membranes. *Desalin. Water Treat.* **2015**, *56*, 3510–3518. [CrossRef]
45. López-Vélez, M.; Martínez-Martínez, F.; Valle-Ribes, C. Del The Study of Phenolic Compounds as Natural Antioxidants in Wine. *Crit. Rev. Food Sci. Nutr.* **2003**, *43*, 233–244. [CrossRef]
46. Apak, R.; Güçlü, K.; Birsen, D.; Özyürek, M.; Esin Çelik, S.; Bektaşoğlu, B.; Berker, K.I.; Özyurt, D. Comparative evaluation of various total antioxidant capacity assays applied to phenolic compounds with the CUPRAC assay. *Molecules* **2007**, *12*, 1496–1547. [CrossRef] [PubMed]
47. Büyüktuncel, E.; Porgalı, E.; Çolak, C. Comparison of total phenolic content and total antioxidant activity in local red wines determined by spectrophotometric methods. *Food Nutr. Sci.* **2014**, *5*, 1660–1667. [CrossRef]
48. Kiss, I.; Vatai, G.; Bekassy-Molnar, E. Must concentrate using membrane technology. *Desalination* **2004**, *162*, 295–300. [CrossRef]
49. Versari, A.; Ferrarini, R.; Parpinello, G.P.; Galassi, S. Concentration of grape must by nanofiltration membranes. *Food Bioprod. Process. Trans. Inst. Chem. Eng. Part C* **2003**, *81*, 275–278. [CrossRef]
50. Pati, S.; La Notte, D.; Clodoveo, M.L.; Cicco, G.; Esti, M. Reverse osmosis and nanofiltration membranes for the improvement of must quality. *Eur. Food Res. Technol.* **2014**, *239*, 595–602. [CrossRef]
51. Bui, K.; Dick, R.; Moulin, G.; Galzy, P. Partial Concentration of Red Wine by Reverse Osmosis. *J. Food Sci.* **1988**, *53*, 647–648. [CrossRef]
52. Pérez-Magariño, S.; González-Sanjosé, M.L. Application of absorbance values used in wineries for estimating CIELAB parameters in red wines. *Food Chem.* **2003**, *81*, 301–306. [CrossRef]

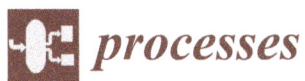

Article

Evaluation of Direct Ultrasound-Assisted Extraction of Phenolic Compounds from Potato Peels

Shusheng Wang [1,2], Amy Hui-Mei Lin [3,†], Qingyou Han [4] and Qin Xu [2,*]

1. College of Life Science, Jilin Agricultural University, Changchun 130118, China; wangshusheng@jlau.edu.cn
2. Department of Food Science, Purdue University, W. Lafayette, IN 47907, USA
3. Bi-State School of Food Science, University of Idaho, Moscow, ID 83844, USA; amy_lin@sifbi.a-star.edu.sg
4. School of Engineering Technology, Purdue University, W. Lafayette, IN 47907, USA; hanq@purdue.edu
* Correspondence: xuq@purdue.edu; Tel.: +1-765-494-4183
† Present address: Clinical Nutrition Research Center, Singapore Institute of Food and Biotechnology Innovation, Agency for Science, Research and Technology, Singapore 117609, Singapore.

Received: 16 November 2020; Accepted: 15 December 2020; Published: 17 December 2020

Abstract: Potato peels (PPs) are generally considered as agriculture waste. The United States alone generates over one million tons of PPs a year. However, PPs contain valuable phenolic compounds with antioxidant activities. In this study, we evaluated the efficiency of ultrasound-assisted extraction techniques in recovering antioxidants from PPs. These techniques included a direct ultrasound-assisted extraction (DUAE), an indirect ultrasound-assisted extraction (IUAE), and a conventional shaking extraction (CSE). Results of this study showed that DUAE was more effective in extracting phenolic compounds than IUAE and CSE. We also evaluated the factors affecting the yield of total phenolic compounds (TPC) in DUAE, including the temperature, time, acoustic power, ratio of solvent to solids, and size of PPs particles. TPC yield of DUAE was higher, and the extraction rate was faster than IUAE and CSE. Furthermore, TPC yield was strongly correlated to the temperature of the mixture of PPs suspension. SEM images revealed that the irradiation of ultrasound energy from DUAE caused micro-fractures and the opening of PPs cells. The extract obtained from DUAE was found to have antioxidant activity comparable to commercial synthetic antioxidants. Results of this preliminary study suggest that DUAE has the potential to transform PPs from agricultural waste to a valuable ingredient. A future systematic research study is proposed to advance the knowledge of the impact of processing parameters in the kinetics of phenolic compounds extraction from potato peels using various extraction methods.

Keywords: potato peel; ultrasound; phenolic compound; antioxidant

1. Introduction

Potatoes (*Solanum tuberosum* L.), along with corn, rice, and wheat, are a staple food source [1], and its processed foods are popular globally. As most potatoes are peeled before processing, the United States alone generates over one million tons of potato peels yearly, creating disposal, sanitation, and environmental problems [2,3]. However, potato peels contain valuable substances such as phenolic compounds, which are natural antioxidants. On average, potato tubers contain 25–125 mg of phenolic compounds per 100 g fresh weight, and approximately 50% of the phenolic compounds are in peels and adjoining tissues [4,5]. The primary phenolic compounds found in potatoes are chlorogenic acid, caffeic acid, p-coumaric acid, and ferulic acid [6,7]. Phenolic compounds in plants are involved in many physiological processes, such as cell growth, root formation, seed germination, and fruit ripening. Moreover, phenolic compounds can act as reducing agents, hydrogen donors, and scavengers of reactive oxygen species [8]. In addition to antioxidant activity, phenolic compounds have antidiabetic, anti-microbial, anti-allergy, vasodilation, and cardio-protective activities [9]. The food industry relies on synthetic antioxidants, such as butylated hydroxytoluene (BHT), butylated hydroxyanisole (BHA), and tert-butylhydroquinone (TBHQ) for preventing lipid oxidation [10]. However, synthetic antioxidants are associated with some health risks, such as hepatic damage and the development of cancers [11]. Therefore, there is a demand for natural antioxidants, for which potato peel extract is an ideal source.

Methods for the extraction of phenolic compounds can be categorized into conventional and novel methods. The conventional method requires a high quantity of organic solvents during solid–liquid interaction and a long extraction time with low yields [12–14]. Novel methods are more effective in extracting phenolic compounds. Novel methods include subcritical water extraction, microwave-assisted extraction, high-pressure homogenization extraction, pressured liquid extraction, and ultrasound-assisted extraction [15–17]. The ultrasound-assisted extraction methods have received considerable attention due to their high capability and efficiency of extraction [18]. In addition, the ultrasound-assisted extraction methods are simple, flexible, versatile, and economic [19].

The ultrasound-assisted extraction method can be further categorized into indirect ultrasound-assisted extraction (IUAE) using an ultrasound bath and direct ultrasound-assisted extraction (DUAE) using an ultrasound probe. IUAE has been tested for extracting phenolic compounds from potato peels; however, DUAE, which has much higher ultrasonic power density than that of IUAE, has not yet been examined for extracting phenolic compounds from potato peels. The high level of ultrasonic irradiation in DUAE can accelerate the extraction, but its impact on the production and antioxidant activity have not been investigated either. This study examined the extraction efficacy of the DUAE and compared it with that of both IUAE and CSE. The study also examined the antioxidant activity of the extract produced by DUAE and compared it with that of popular synthetic antioxidants. The long-term goal of this investigation was to efficiently process a large number of potato peels, which are otherwise wasted, and turn this waste product into a valuable commodity.

2. Materials and Methods

2.1. Materials

Potato peels were from Basic American Foods (Blackfoot, ID, USA). Peels were dried in a convection oven at 45 °C for 48 h. The dehydrated potato peels were ground into powders using a spice grinder (Waring spice grinder, model-WSG 30, Waring Products, Torrington, CT, USA). The powders were sieved through 45- and 100-mesh screens that allowed particles with a diameter smaller than 0.354 and 0.150 mm, respectively, to pass through. Potato peel samples were then divided into four fractions according to their sizes: original (without grind), particles retained on the 45-mesh screen (referred to as >45 mesh), particles that passed through the 45-mesh screen but retained on the 100-mesh screen (referred to as 45–100 mesh), and particles that passed through the 100-mesh screen (referred to as <100 mesh). Potato peel powders were sealed in Ziploc® bags (S.C. Johnson & Son, Inc., Racine, WI, USA) and stored at −18 °C until used.

All chemicals were reagent grade, obtained from Sigma-Aldrich Co. (St. Louis, MO, USA) or Fisher Scientific (Pittsburgh, PA, USA), and used without further purifications or treatments.

2.2. Conventional Shaking Extraction (CSE)

Potato peel powders (0.25 g) were extracted with 5 mL of methanol (50%, v/v) in a glass cylinder, and then put in an incubator shaker (Environmental incubator shaker, G24, New Brunswick Co., Inc., Edison, NJ, USA) in triplicate. The incubator shaker was controlled at 25 °C and 150 rpm, and the extraction time was 1, 2, 5, 10, 15, 30, 45, and 60 min. The mixture was centrifuged at 1500× g for 15 min after extraction. Two samples were taken per extraction, and the total phenolic compounds (TPC) in the supernatant was quantified in triplicates.

2.3. Indirect Ultrasound-Assisted Extraction (IUAE)

Ground peel powders (0.25 g) were suspended in 5 mL of methanol (50%, v/v) and transferred into a glass cylinder, which was placed in an ultrasound water bath (SharperTek®, Pontiac, MI, USA) set at a frequency of 40 kHz (500 W) at 25 °C for 1, 2, 5, 10, 15, 30, 45, and 60 min. The mixture was centrifuged at 1500× g for 15 min after extraction, and the extraction under each condition was performed three times. The TPC in the supernatant was quantified in triplicates.

2.4. Direct Ultrasound-Assisted Extraction (DUAE) and Temperature Measurement

Potato peel powders were mixed with methanol and transferred to a glass cylinder, which was set in a water bath (Figure 1). An ultrasound probe was submerged 5 mm below the surface of the potato peel suspension in the glass cylinder. A thermocouple (E-Type Thermocouple Extension Wire, National Instruments, Roscoe, IL, USA) was inserted into the glass cylinder to monitor the temperature of potato peel suspension. The mixture temperature was automatically recorded by PicoLog recorder (PicoLog software version 5.25.3, Picolog Technology, TX, USA), and the peak temperature was reported. The setup of DUAE also consisted of a waveform generator (Agilent Technologies, model 33120A, Santa Clara, CA, USA), an amplifier (Amplifier Research, model 150A-100B, Pleasanton, CA, USA), an air-cooled piezoelectric converter (Sonics & Materials, model CV-154, Newtown, CT, USA), and a probe (Sonotrode, model 1102, a diameter of 12.7 mm, Sonics & Materials, Newtown, CT, USA).

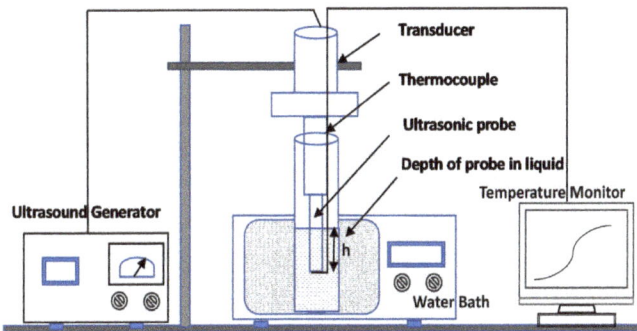

Figure 1. Schematic of the setup of direct ultrasound-assisted extraction (DUAE) method.

In order to understand the impact of ultrasound parameters on extraction efficiency, several parameters were examined in this study. The solvent-to-solid ratios were controlled at 10:1, 20:1, 40:1, and 60:1 by suspending 25 mg (dry wt.) of potato peel powders with various amounts (2.5, 5, 10, or 15 mL) of methanol (50%, v/v). The temperature of the water bath was controlled at −2, 25, 45, and 60 °C. The ultrasonic probe was oscillated at a frequency of 22.95 kHz with an output power of 120 W for 1, 2, 5, 10, 15, 30, 45, and 60 min. The extractions were performed with various amplitudes, 200, 400, 600, and 900 millivolts peak-to-peak (mVpp) of the input sine waveform. After the extraction, the mixture was centrifuged at 1500× g for 15 min, and the TPC in each extract was quantified. Each extraction condition was performed in triplicates.

2.5. Quantification of Total Phenolic Compounds (TPC) in Potato Peel Extracts

Phenolic compounds in potato peel extracts were quantified using the Folin–Ciocalteu method of Mohdaly et al. [10] with modifications. The potato peel extract (1 mL) was mixed with 2 mL of 10-fold diluted Folin-Ciocalteu reagent in a tube, followed by adding 2 mL of sodium bicarbonate solution (5%, w/v) to the mixture. The mixture was vortexed and then incubated at 25 °C for 30 min. The absorbance of each mixture was measured at 765 nm using a UV-VIS spectrophotometer (Genesys-10S, Thermo Fisher Scientific, Waltham, MA, USA). Methanol (50%, v/v) was used as the blank of the spectrophotometer measurement. Gallic acid solutions, 10–500 μg/mL, were used to construct a calibration curve with absorbance against various concentrations. The yields of extraction were expressed as milligrams of gallic acid equivalents per gram dry weight of potato peel powders (mg GAE/g dry wt.).

2.6. Examination of Potato Peel Powders with Scanning Electron Microscope (SEM)

Potato peel powders, before and after extractions, were sputter-coated with a thin layer of gold-palladium for 60 s at 25 °C and examined using a field-emission scanning electron microscope (Quanta 3D FEG, FEI Co., Hillsboro, OR, USA) at 10 kV.

2.7. Determination of DPPH Radical Scavenging Activity of Extracted Phenolic Compounds

The free radical scavenging activity of potato peel extracts on 2,2-diphenyl-1-picrylhydrazyl (DPPH) radicals was measured as described previously [5]. An aliquot (50 μL) of potato peel extracts was added to DPPH (1.5 mL, 3.94 mg/100 mL methanol). As free electrons in DPPH are paired off in the presence of antioxidants, the absorption decreases as the result of the extinction of the purple color of DPPH. Decolorization was determined by measuring the absorbance at 517 nm with a UV-VIS spectrophotometer after 20 min of reaction. The measurement was performed three times. The scavenging activity on DPPH radicals was calculated as percentage (%) inhibition using the following equation [10]:

$$\text{DPPH radical scavenging activity (\%)} = [(\text{Abs}_{control} - \text{Abs}_{sample})/\text{Abs}_{control}] \times 100 \quad (1)$$

2.8. Statistical Analysis

Analysis of variance was conducted using SPSS, Version 23.0 (SPSS Inc., Chicago, IL, USA). The Pearson correlation coefficient (r) was calculated to demonstrate the linear correlations between variables. All results are presented as the mean (M) of triplicate measurements. The level of significance was set at $p < 0.05$.

3. Results and Discussion

3.1. Comparison of Three Extraction Methods

Figure 2 shows a significant difference of extraction efficiencies of the three methods by using TPC as a function of extraction times.

When comparing DUAE with CSE in Figure 2, the maximum yield of TPC from DUAE (9.3 mg GAE/g dry wt.) was about 48% higher than that of CSE (6.26 mg GAE/g dry wt.) with an extraction time of 60 min. In addition, there was a significant difference in extraction rate between DUAE and CSE. Within 1 min of extraction, CSE generated 3.35 mg GAE/g dry wt. of TPC, while DUAE generated 7.6 mg GAE/g dry wt. of TPC, an amount that was about two times higher. In order to achieve this amount of TPC using the CSE, it would require more than 60 min. The high efficiency of DUAE was associated with the phenomenon of ultrasound-induced cavitation. The collapse of cavitation bubbles produced ultrasonic jets. The ultrasonic jets further improved the infusion of the solvent to the solid particles, disrupted the potato peel cells, and enhanced the extraction of phenolic compounds from the potato peels [20,21]. The CSE was less efficient than DUAE. A prolonged extraction time could increase the TPC yield of CSE and decrease the difference in TPC yield between CSE and DUAE. The ultrasound probe in DUAE immersed in the potato peel suspension transferred higher ultrasonic energy to potato peels.

Data shown in Figure 2 also indicate that DUAE was more efficient than IUAE. The maximum yield of TPC using DUAE (9.33 mg GAE/g dry wt.) was about 2.6% higher than that of IUAE (9.09 mg GAE/g dry wt.) with an extraction time of 30 min. To achieve a TPC yield of 7.6 mg GAE/g dry wt., 1 min was needed for DUAE compared to 5 min. of extraction time necessary when using IUAE. Thus, it can be noted that when extracting phenolic compounds from potato peels, the extraction efficiency of DUAE is about five times faster than IUAE. These experimental results agree with those of other researchers using similar methods for extracting phenolic compounds from various materials [22,23]. Compared to an ultrasound bath, the ultrasound probe delivers a higher power to promote mass transfer. Capelo-Martinez et al. [24] explain that the ultrasound probe, which is immersed directly in the extraction mixture, transferred higher ultrasonic energy to the samples, as the ultrasonic waves do not need to cross both the water in the bath and the cylinder wall before reaching the sample to be treated. However, there was little significant difference in TPC yield between these two ultrasound treatment methods after a prolonged extraction time (30 min.), which differs from the results attained from our previous work with walnut shells [25].

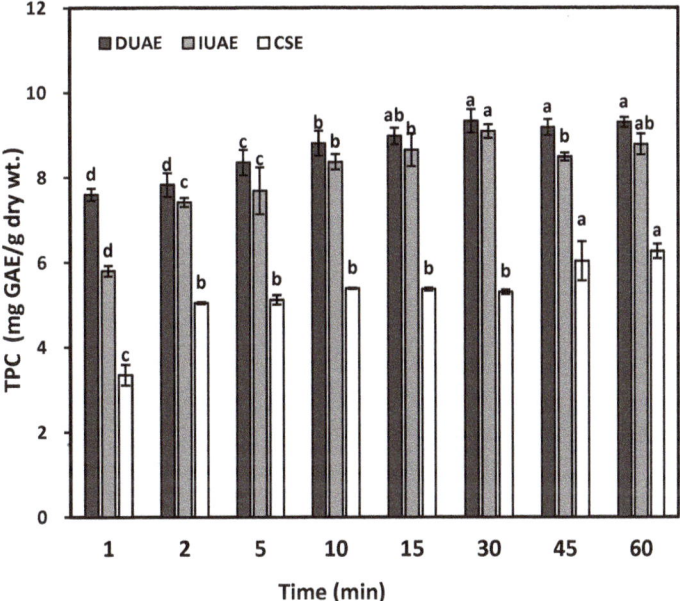

Figure 2. Yields of total phenolic compounds (TPC) from potato peels extracts obtained using the conventional shaking extraction (CSE), direct ultrasound-assisted extraction (DUAE), and indirect ultrasound-assisted extraction (IUAE) methods. Data are means of three measurements, and the error bars indicate standard deviations. Data denoted with the same letter (a, b, c, or d) were not significantly different from the same extraction method at different timings ($p > 0.05$). Setting for the two ultrasound methods, DUAE and IUAE, were 23 kHz, 25 °C water bath temperature, 600 mVpp, solvent-to-solid ratio 40:1, and particle size smaller than 0.354 mm.

The morphology of potato peel cells was examined by SEM. The untreated potato peels had closed cells with rough surfaces (Figure 3a). All three methods caused a significant expansion in cell volume. In the CSE method, the surface of potato peel cells became smooth with cracks in some cells (Figure 3b). Both ultrasound-assisted methods produced some ruptured cells with large perforations (Figure 3c,d), and these phenomena were caused by cavitation. DUAE caused more damage to cells with hollow openings (Figure 3d) than IUAE and CES. The disrupting of potato peel cells allowed the solvent to penetrate into cells and accelerated the release of phenolic compounds from potato peels.

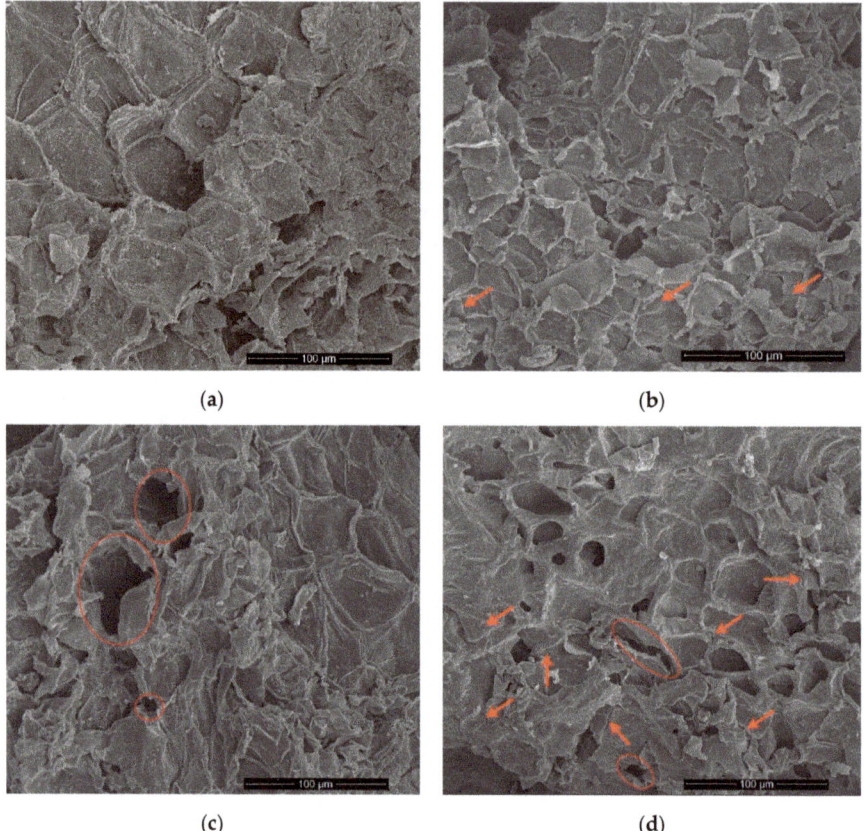

Figure 3. SEM images of cells in potato peels before extraction (**a**), after extraction by the CSE method (**b**), after extraction by the IUAE method (**c**), and after extraction by the DUAE method (**d**). All three methods were conducted with a solvent-to-solid ratio of 40:1 in a water bath controlled at 25 °C for 30 min.

3.2. Parameters Affecting the Yield of TPC Using the DUAE Method

3.2.1. Effects of Extraction Time on TPC Yield

Prolonged extraction time produced a higher yield of TPC. The yield was 7.60 mg GAE/g dry wt. at 1 min and 9.30 mg GAE/g dry wt. at 60 min of extraction (Figure 4). Because the extraction of phenolic compounds is a diffusion-controlled process, the yield was time dependent. These results also agree with those of researchers who attribute the effect of ultrasound on the extraction yield to acoustic-induced effects, such as cavitation, streaming, and shock waves [26,27]. During the extraction, both the TPC yield and temperature of the potato peel suspensions were at or near the peak values after 45 min in a constant water bath temperature of 25 °C. Increasing the extraction time to 60 min did not further increase TPC yield, and the mixture temperature decreased from 50.5 °C to 48 °C. Results showed that TPC yield correlated more with mixture temperature ($r = 0.974$, $p < 0.01$) than with extraction time ($r = 0.795$, $p = 0.11$). Findings in this study suggest a need to balance the temperature and reaction time during extraction.

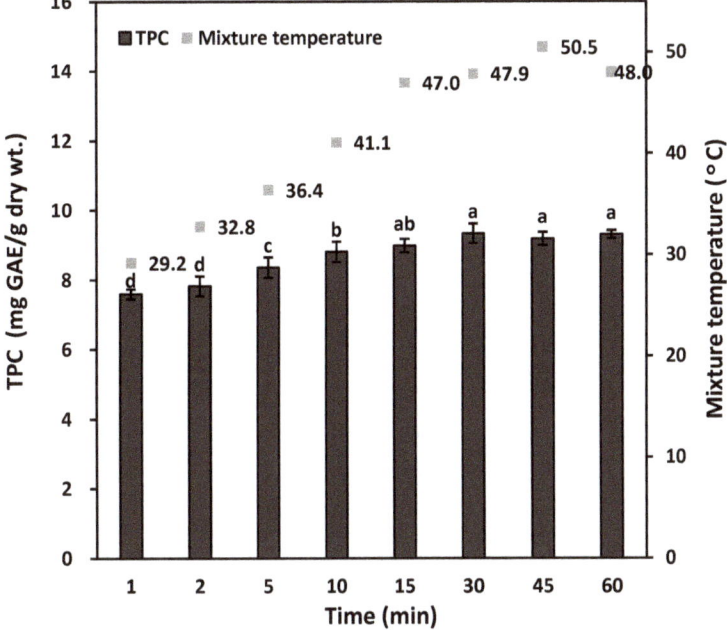

Figure 4. The relationship among the yield of total phenolic compounds (TPC), extraction time (min), and the temperature of potato peels suspension in DUAE. Numbers indicated in the graph denote the temperature of the potato peels suspension. Data are means of three measurements, and error bars indicate standard deviations. Data denoted with the same letter (a, b, c, or d) were not significantly different ($p > 0.05$). Ultrasound extraction parameters were 23 kHz, 600 mVpp, water bath temperature 25 °C, solvent-to-solid ratio 40:1, and particle size smaller than 0.354 mm.

The ultrasonic energy injected into the glass container heated up the mixture directly, and the heat exchange between the glass container and the water bath was not enough to overcome the temperature increase in the container. As a result, in our experiments, the temperature in the mixture was higher than the bath temperature during the DUAE of phenolic compounds from potato peels. Further research is required to confirm if the mixture temperature affects the solubility of phenolic compounds in the solvent.

3.2.2. Effects of Extraction Temperature on TPC Yield

Temperature greatly affects extraction efficiency. However, the actual reaction temperature of potato peels suspension almost always deviated from the water bath temperature. The ultrasonic energy injected into the glass cylinder, where it holds the potato peel suspension, heat up the mixture quickly. However, the heat transfer between the glass cylinder and water bath was not quick enough to offset the temperature difference. In this study, the water bath temperature was controlled at −2, 25, 45, and 60 °C, but the mixture temperature was found to be 13.8, 47.9, 53.0, and 69.5 °C, respectively (Figure 5). Results showed that both water bath temperature and mixture temperature positively correlated with TPC yield. It has been shown that high temperature reduces the surface extension of solvents [25], increases solvent solubility, enhances the infusion of solvent into potato cells, and promotes the disruption of cells [28]. Results of this study showed that both mixture temperature ($r = 0.993$, $p = 0.02$) and water bath temperature ($r = 0.967$, $p = 0.08$) were correlated with TPC yields.

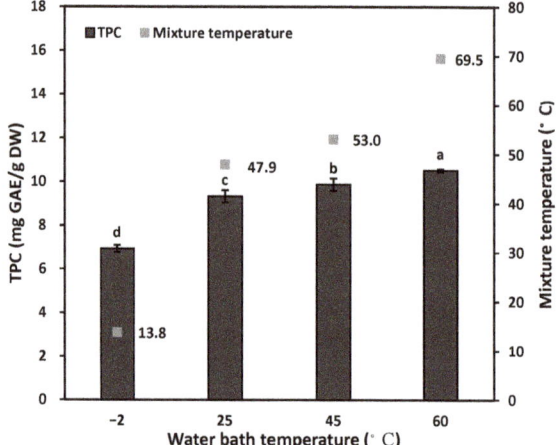

Figure 5. The relationship among the yield of total phenolic compounds (TPC), water bath temperature, and mixture temperature in DUAE. Numbers indicated in the graph denote the mixture temperature. Data are means of three measurements, and error bars are standard deviations. Data denoted with the same letter (a, b, c, or d) were not significantly different ($p > 0.05$). The ultrasound extraction parameters were 23 kHz, 600 mVpp, solvent-to-solid ratio 40:1, 30-min extraction, and particle size smaller than 0.354 mm.

3.2.3. Effects of Amplitude of Ultrasonic Vibration on TPC Yield

The amplitude of the input sine waveform also had a positive impact on the extraction yield. When the amplitude was increased from 200 mVpp to 400 mVpp and 600 mVpp, the TPC yield increased from 7.67 GAE/g to 9.12 GAE/g and 9.33 GAE/g dry wt., respectively (see Figure 6). While the amplitude was 200, 400, 600, and 900 mVpp, the mixture temperature was 32.1, 41.8, 47.9, and 50.2 °C, respectively, despite the water bath temperature being at 25 °C. It has been shown that high ultrasound amplitude delivers more power to the mixture of potato peels suspension, increases mixture temperature, enhances solvent penetration, and induces more cavitation damage to cell walls [27,28]. Results showed that TPC yield strongly correlated with both temperature ($r = 0.962$, $p < 0.01$) and ultrasound amplitude ($r = 0.800$, $p = 0.05$).

There was no significant improvement in TPC yield when the amplitude was increased from 600 to 900 mVpp. Capelo-Martinez [24] reported that high amplitude could degrade extracts. When the amplitude reached a level at which extraction and degradation offset each other, no further increase in yield would be observed. Rakita and Han [29] reported that stable cavitation could be obtained between 200 and 300 mVpp in pure water. Results from this study indicated that the balance was at 600 mVpp. The higher amplitude shortened the time to achieve the maximum TPC yield, but did not further increase the yield.

3.2.4. Effects of Solvent-to-Solid Ratio on TPC Yield

The extraction yields were 7.16, 9.44, 9.33, and 10.02 mg GAE/g dry wt. when the solvent-to-solid ratios were 10:1, 20:1, 40:1, and 60:1, respectively (Figure 7). Increasing the ratio of solvent-to-solid from 10:1 to 20:1 improved the yield, but a further increase in the ratio had no additional effect. The mass transfer from solid to solvent is concentration-dependent. Therefore, an increase in the solvent resulted in a better defection rate. An increase in the solvent-to-solid ratio was found to enlarge the difference between the temperature of the water bath and the mixture of potato peels suspension. It has been observed that a large amount of cavitation bubbles was formed when a high solvent-to-solid ratio was applied to the extraction. Results showed that TPC yield had a strong relationship with both mixture temperature ($r = 0.816$, $p = 0.01$) and solvent-to-solid ratio ($r = 0.796$, $p = 0.11$).

3.2.5. Effects of the Particle Size of Potato Peels on TPC Yield

Results in this study showed that the extraction yields were 2.54, 7.48, 9.26, and 10.29 mg GAE/g dry weight when the particle sizes of potato peel powders were original (20–30 mm), >45 mesh (>0.354 mm), 45–100 mesh (0.354–0.150 mm), and <100 mesh (0.150 mm), respectively (Figure 8). Finer particles were found to generate much higher yield, as small particles have a bigger total surface area and shorter solvent diffusion path. The mixture temperature of finer particles was higher than that of bigger particles. The mixture temperature of particles 2–3 mm and smaller than 0.15 mm were 39.1 °C and 52.4 °C, respectively. It was claimed that the ultrasound energy is absorbed more in the mixture having a greater area of particle/liquid interface. Such solid–liquid interface with the ultrasound-induced shear flow dissipates ultrasonic energy into heat in the solvent, resulting in an increased temperature in the mixture.

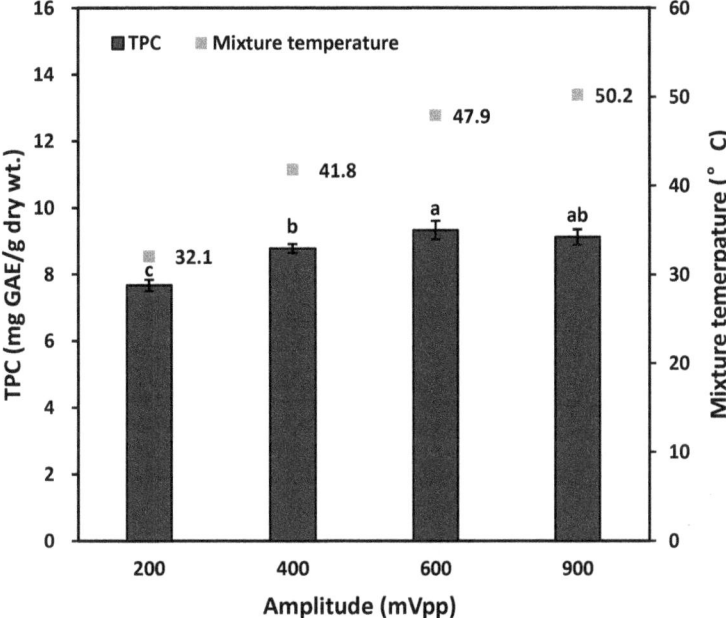

Figure 6. Relationships among the yield of total phenolic compounds (TPC), extraction amplitude, and mixture temperature in DUAE. Numbers indicated in the graph denote the temperature of the potato peels suspension. Data are means of three measurements, and error bars indicate standard deviations. Data denoted with the same letter (a, b, c, or d) were not significantly different ($p > 0.05$). Ultrasound extraction parameters were 23 kHz, 600 mVpp, water bath temperature 25 °C, solvent-to-solid ratio 40:1, and particle size smaller than 0.354 mm.

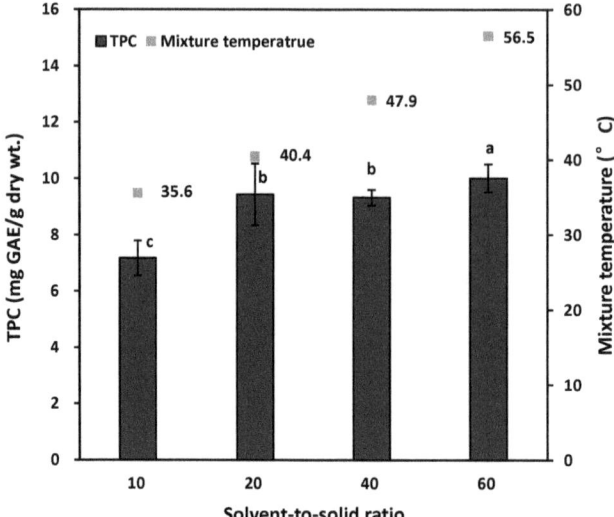

Figure 7. The relationship among the yield of total phenolic compounds (TPC), solvent-to-solid ratio, and mixture temperature in DUAE. Numbers indicated in the graph denote the temperature of the potato peels suspension. Data are means of three measurements, and error bars indicate standard deviations. Data denoted with the same letter (a, b, c, or d) were not significantly different ($p > 0.05$). Ultrasound extraction parameters were 23 kHz, 600 mVpp, water bath temperature 25 °C, solvent-to-solid ratio 40:1, and particle size smaller than 0.354 mm.

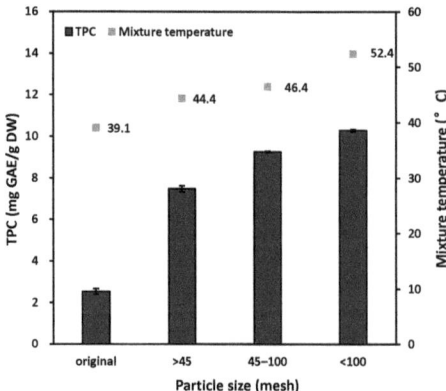

Figure 8. The relationship among the yield of total phenolic compounds (TPC), particle size, and mixture temperature during the DUAE extraction. Numbers indicated in the graph denote the temperature of the potato peels suspension. Data are means of three measurements, and error bars indicate standard deviations. Data denoted with the same letter (a, b, c, or d) were not significantly different ($p > 0.05$). Ultrasound extraction parameters were 23 kHz, 600 mVpp, water bath temperature 25 °C, and solvent-to-solid ratio 40:1. Particle sizes: 20–30 mm (original); >45 mesh (>0.354 mm); 45–100 mesh (0.354–0.150 mm); and <100 mesh (<0.150 mm).

3.3. Scavenging Activity of Phenolic Compounds Extracted from Potato Peels

Plant phenolic compounds are natural antioxidants for delaying the oxidation of oils and fats in food during storage. With the concern of their negative impact on health, synthetic antioxidants, such as tert-butylhydroquinone (TBHQ), butylated hydroxytoluene (BHT), and butylated hydroxyanisole

(BHA), are less desired [27]. To confirm the antioxidant activity of potato peel extracts generated by the DUAE method, their free radical scavenging activity on 2,2-diphenyl-1-picrylhydrazyl (DPPH) was determined. Results showed that the antioxidant activities of the potato peel extract correlated with the quantity of TPC in the potato peel extracts ($p < 0.05$; Figure 9). Our findings suggest that the antioxidant activity in potato peel extracts was primarily influenced by the quantity of phenolic compounds, results that agree with the findings of other researchers [30]. As detailed by many reports, the phenolic compounds in potato peels contain higher amounts of phenolic acids and flavonoids [1,2]. These components have great antioxidant activity. Therefore, potato peels have the potential to be used as a natural source of antioxidants in the food and agriculture industry [31].

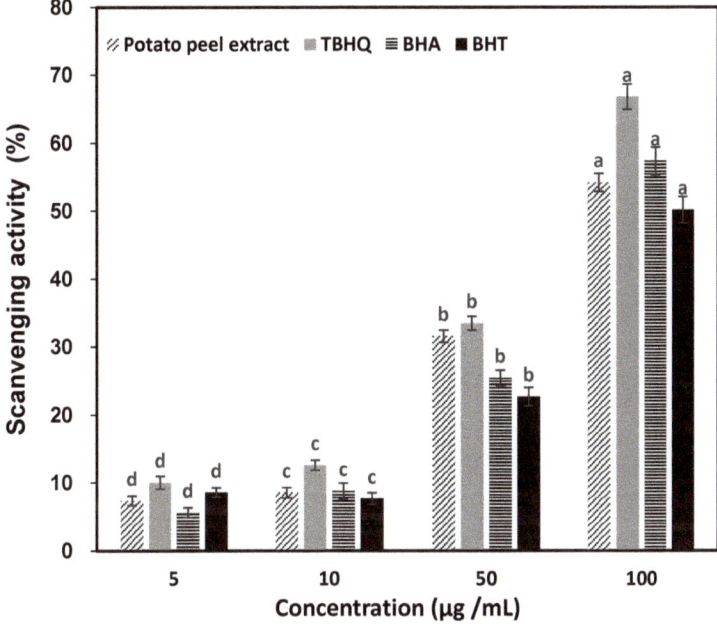

Figure 9. Scavenging activity of potato peel extract compared with that of tert-butylhydroquinone (TBHQ), butylated hydroxyanisole (BHA), and butylated hydroxytoluene (BHT). Data are means of three measurements, and error bars indicate standard deviations. Data denoted with the same letter (a, b, c, or d) were not significantly different ($p > 0.05$). DUAE parameters were 23 kHz, 600 mVpp, water bath temperature 25 °C, solvent-to-solid ratio 40:1, 30-min extraction, and particle size smaller than 0.354 mm.

The antioxidant activity of potato peel extracts was further compared with TBHQ, BHA, and BHT. The comparison was normalized to the quantity of total phenolic compounds (Section 2.5). At the concentration of 50 µg/mL, the scavenging activities of the potato peel extracts and TBHQ were higher than that of BHA and BHT. At a higher concentration of 100 µg/mL, TBHQ had the highest antioxidant activity (66.8%), followed by BHA (57.4%) and the potato peel extracts (54.2%), while BHT had the lowest antioxidant activity (50.2%). These results suggest that DUAE-extracted potato peels extract is comparable to that of these synthetic antioxidant products.

4. Conclusions

This study demonstrates the effectiveness of the DUAE of valuable antioxidants from potato peels. The direct contact of an ultrasound probe with potato peel suspension greatly enhanced the extraction efficiency. The extraction yield of TPC using DUAE was about two times higher than that of CBS at one minute, and the maximum yield of TPC was 48% higher than that of CSE. To achieve a TPC of 7.6 mg GAE/g dry wt., it took 1 min using DUAE, 5 min using IUAE, and more than 60 min using CSE. The setup of DUAE in this study allowed the reaction temperature to be measured, and it was discovered that a balance of reaction time and temperature was needed for obtaining the maximum yield of total phenolic compounds. The high efficiency of DUAE was associated with the transfer of high ultrasound energy and temperature to potato peel suspension. DUAE generated more disruption of potato cells, but did not diminish the antioxidant activity. DUAE-extracted potato peel extract had comparable antioxidant activity to popular synthetic antioxidants. Findings of this study suggest that DUAE has the potential to transform a large number of potato peels to valuable ingredients, and, thus, promote sustainability. Further research for pre-treatment of potato peels, such as cleaning, and removal of undesired compounds, such as alkaloids, is recommended. Moreover, to further investigate the mechanism of the antioxidant activity of phenolic extracts from potato peels, additional purification steps and determination of phenolic profiles by HPLC are required. In summary, this preliminary study proved the concept of using a simplified ultrasound extraction to increase profitability for the potato industry by producing antioxidants from potato peels.

Author Contributions: Investigation: Q.X. and S.W.; resources: Q.X., Q.H., and A.H.-M.L.; writing—original draft preparation: S.W.; writing—review and editing: Q.X., Q.H., and A.H.-M.L.; supervision: Q.X. and A.H.-M.L. All authors have read and agreed to the published version of the manuscript.

Funding: This research was funded by John & Emma Tse, Li-Fu Chen Memorial Laboratory Fund and the Center for Materials Processing Research at Purdue University (W. Lafayette, IN, USA); Science and Technology Department of Jilin Province (No. 20170101108JC, Jilin, China); Idaho State Department of Agriculture Specialty Crop Block Grant Program-Farm Bill 2015 (15-SCBGP-ID-0015); and the Potato Research Endowment (FY 2014) sponsored by Basic American Foods (Blackfoot, ID, USA) at University of Idaho (Moscow, ID, USA).

Acknowledgments: We thank Xingtao Liu for assistance with SEM examinations, and Wilson Xu and Milan Rakita (Purdue University, W. Lafayette, IN, USA) for operating the ultrasound equipment and participating in the discussion. We appreciate Basic American Foods for providing potato peels. We acknowledge Laurie L Van Keppel (Purdue University, W. Lafayette, IN, USA) and Hannah Han (University of California, Los Angeles, USA) for editing the manuscript.

Conflicts of Interest: The authors declare no conflict of interest.

References

1. Singh, B.; Singh, J.; Singh, J.P.; Kaur, A.; Singh, N. Phenolic compounds in potato (*Solanum tuberosum* L.) peel and their health-promoting activities. *Int. J. Food Sci. Technol.* **2020**, *55*, 2273–2281. [CrossRef]
2. Akyol, H.; Riciputi, Y.; Capanoglu, E.; Caboni, M.F.; Verardo, V. Phenolic Compounds in the Potato and Its Byproducts: An Overview. *Int. J. Mol. Sci.* **2016**, *17*, 835. [CrossRef] [PubMed]
3. Kumari, B.; Tiwari, B.K.; Hossain, M.B.; Rai, D.K.; Brunton, N.P. Ultrasound-assisted extraction of polyphenols from potato peels: Profiling and kinetic modelling. *Int. J. Food Sci. Technol.* **2017**, *52*, 1432–1439. [CrossRef]
4. Al-Weshahy, A.; Rao, A.V. Isolation and characterization of functional components from peel samples of six potatoes varieties growing in Ontario. *Food Res. Int.* **2009**, *42*, 1062–1066. [CrossRef]
5. Singh, A.; Sabally, K.; Kubow, S.; Donnelly, D.J.; Gariepy, Y.; Orsat, V.; Raghavan, G.S. Microwave-assisted extraction of phenolic antioxidants from potato peels. *Molecules* **2011**, *16*, 2218–22132. [CrossRef] [PubMed]
6. Albishi, T.; John, J.A.; Al-Khalifa, A.S.; Shahidi, F. Phenolic content and antioxidant activities of selected potato varieties and their processing by-products. *J. Funct. Foods* **2013**, *5*, 590–600. [CrossRef]
7. Arun, K.B.; Chandran, J.; Dhanya, R.; Krishna, P.; Jayamurthy, P.; Nisha, P. A comparative evaluation of antioxidant and antidiabetic potential of peel from young and matured potato. *Food Biosci.* **2015**, *9*, 36–46. [CrossRef]
8. Pereira, D.M.; Valentão, P.; Pereira, J.A.; Andrade, P.B. Phenolics: From chemistry to biology. *Molecules* **2009**, *14*, 2202–2211. [CrossRef]
9. Balasundram, N.; Sundram, K.; Samman, S. Phenolic compounds in plants and agri-industrial by-products: Antioxidant activity, occurrence, and potential uses. *Food Chem.* **2006**, *99*, 191–203. [CrossRef]
10. Mohdaly, A.A.A.; Sarhan, M.A.; Smetanska, I.; Mahmoud, A. Antioxidant properties of various solvent extracts of potato peel, sugar beet pulp and sesame cake. *J. Sci. Food Agric.* **2010**, *90*, 218–226. [CrossRef]

11. van Esch, G.J. Toxicology of tert-butylhydroquinone (TBHQ). *Food Chem. Toxicol.* **1986**, *24*, 1063–1065. [CrossRef]
12. Borah, P.P.; Das, P.; Badwaik, L.S. Ultrasound treated potato peel and sweet lime pomace based biopolymer film development. *Ultrason. Sonochem.* **2017**, *36*, 11–19. [CrossRef] [PubMed]
13. Sánchez Maldonado, A.F.; Mudge, E.; Gänzle, M.G.; Schieber, A. Extraction and fractionation of phenolic acids and glycoalkaloids from potato peels using acidified water/ethanol-based solvents. *Food Res. Int.* **2014**, *65*, 27–34. [CrossRef]
14. Wu, Z.G.; Xu, H.Y.; Ma, Q.; Cao, Y.; Ma, J.N.; Ma, C.M. Isolation, identification and quantification of unsaturated fatty acids, amides, phenolic compounds and glycoalkaloids from potato peel. *Food Chem.* **2012**, *135*, 2425–2429. [CrossRef] [PubMed]
15. Jacotet-Navarro, M.; Rombaut, N.; Fabiano-Tixier, A.S.; Danguien, M.; Bily, A.; Chemat, F. Ultrasound versus microwave as green processes for extraction of rosmarinic, carnosic and ursolic acids from rosemary. *Ultrason. Sonochem.* **2015**, *27*, 102–109. [CrossRef] [PubMed]
16. Galhano dos Santos, R.; Ventura, P.; Bordado, J.C.; Mateus, M.M. Valorizing potato peel waste: An overview of the latest publications. *Rev. Environ. Sci. Bio/Technol.* **2016**, *15*, 585–592. [CrossRef]
17. Kumari, B.; Tiwari, B.K.; Hossain, M.B.; Brunton, N.P.; Rai, D.K. Recent advances on application of ultrasound and pulsed electric field technologies in the extraction of bioactives from agro-industrial by-products. *Food Bioprocess Technol.* **2018**, *11*, 223–241. [CrossRef]
18. Garcia-Salas, P.; Morales-Soto, A.; Segura-Carretero, A.; Fernandez-Gutierrez, A. Phenolic-compound-extraction systems for fruit and vegetable samples. *Molecules* **2010**, *15*, 8813–8826. [CrossRef]
19. Patist, A.; Bates, D. Ultrasonic innovations in the food industry: From the laboratory to commercial production. *Innov. Food Sci. Emerg. Technol.* **2008**, *9*, 147–154. [CrossRef]
20. Friedman, M.; Kozukue, N.; Kim, H.J.; Choi, S.H.; Mizuno, M. Glycoalkaloid, phenolic, and flavonoid content and antioxidative activities of conventional nonorganic and organic potato peel powders from commercial gold, red, and Russet potatoes. *J. Food Compos. Anal.* **2017**, *62*, 69–75. [CrossRef]
21. Esclapez, M.D.; García-Pérez, J.V.; Mulet, A.; Cárcel, J.A. Ultrasound-Assisted Extraction of Natural Products. *Food Eng. Rev.* **2011**, *3*, 108–120. [CrossRef]
22. Hossain, M.B.; Brunton, N.P.; Patras, A.; Tiwari, B.; O'Donnell, C.P.; Martin-Diana, A.B.; Barry-Ryan, C. Optimization of ultrasound assisted extraction of antioxidant compounds from marjoram (*Origanum majorana* L.) using response surface methodology. *Ultrason. Sonochem.* **2012**, *19*, 582–590. [CrossRef] [PubMed]
23. Ghafoor, K.; Choi, Y.H.; Jeon, J.Y.; Jo, I.H. Optimization of ultrasound-assisted extraction of phenolic compounds, antioxidants, and anthocyanins from grape (*Vitis vinifera*) seeds. *J. Agric. Food Chem.* **2009**, *57*, 4988–4994. [CrossRef] [PubMed]
24. Capelo-Martínez, J.-L. *Ultrasound in Chemistry: Analytical and Applications*; Wiley-VCH: Weinheim, Germany, 2009; pp. 55–76.
25. Han, H.; Wang, S.; Rakita, M.; Wang, Y.; Han, Q.; Xu, Q. Effect of ultrasound-assisted extraction of phenolic compounds on the characteristics of walnut shells. *Food Nutr. Sci.* **2018**, *9*, 1034–1045. [CrossRef]
26. Riciputi, Y.; Diaz-de-Cerio, E.; Akyol, H.; Capanoglu, E.; Cerretani, L.; Caboni, M.F.; Verardo, V. Establishment of ultrasound-assisted extraction of phenolic compounds from industrial potato by-products using response surface methodology. *Food Chem.* **2018**, *269*, 258–263. [CrossRef]
27. Samarin, A.M.; Poorazarang, H.; Hematyar, N.; Elhamirad, A. Phenolics in potato peels: Extraction and utilization as natural antioxidants. *World Appl. Sci.* **2012**, *18*, 191–195.
28. Chemat, F.; Rombaut, N.; Sicaire, A.-G.; Meullemiestre, A.; Fabiano-Tixier, A.-S.; Abert-Vian, M. Ultrasound assisted extraction of food and natural products: Mechanisms, techniques, combinations, protocols and applications. A review. *Ultrason. Sonochem.* **2017**, *34*, 540–560. [CrossRef]
29. Rakita, M.; Han, Q. Influence of pressure field in melts on the primary nucleation in solidification processing. *Metall. Mater. Trans. B* **2017**, *48*, 2232–2244. [CrossRef]
30. Singh, N.; Kamath, V.; Narasimhamurthy, K.; Rajini, P.S. Protective effect of potato peel extract against carbon tetrachloride-induced liver injury in rats. *Environ. Toxicol. Pharmacol.* **2008**, *26*, 241–246. [CrossRef]
31. Javed, A.; Ahmad, A.; Tahir, A.; Shabbir, U.; Nouman, M.; Hameed, A. Potato peel waste—Its nutraceutical, industrial and biotechnological applications. *AIMS Agric. and Food* **2019**, *4*, 807–823.

Publisher's Note: MDPI stays neutral with regard to jurisdictional claims in published maps and institutional affiliations.

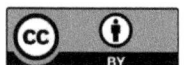 © 2020 by the authors. Licensee MDPI, Basel, Switzerland. This article is an open access article distributed under the terms and conditions of the Creative Commons Attribution (CC BY) license (http://creativecommons.org/licenses/by/4.0/).

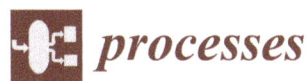

Article

Phenolics Dynamics and Infrared Fingerprints during the Storage of Pumpkin Seed Oil and Thereof Oleogel

Andreea Pușcaș [1], Andruța Mureșan [1,*], Floricuța Ranga [2], Florinela Fetea [2], Sevastița Muste [1], Carmen Socaciu [2] and Vlad Mureșan [1,*]

[1] Department of Food Engineering, Faculty of Food Science and Technology, University of Agricultural Sciences and Veterinary Medicine Cluj-Napoca, 400372 Cluj-Napoca, Romania; andreea.puscas@usamvcluj.ro (A.P.); sevastita.muste@usamvcluj.ro (S.M.)
[2] Department of Food Science, Faculty of Food Science and Technology, University of Agricultural Sciences and Veterinary Medicine Cluj-Napoca, 400372 Cluj-Napoca, Romania; floricutza_ro@yahoo.com (F.R.); florinelafetea@yahoo.com (F.F.); carmen.socaciu@usamvcluj.ro (C.S.)
* Correspondence: andruta.muresan@usamvcluj.ro (A.M.); vlad.muresan@usamvcluj.ro (V.M.); Tel.: +40-264-596-384

Received: 4 October 2020; Accepted: 3 November 2020; Published: 5 November 2020

Abstract: Cold-pressed pumpkin seed oil is a valuable source of bioactive molecules, including phenolic compounds. Oleogels are designed for trans and saturated fats substitution in foods, but also demonstrate protection and delivery of bioactive compounds. Consequently, the present work aimed to assess individual phenolic compounds dynamics and infrared fingerprints during the ambient storage of pumpkin seed oil and thereof oleogel. For oleogels production, a 5% ternary mixture of waxes, composed by 3% beewax, 1% sunflower wax and 1% rice bran wax, was used. Phenolic compounds were extracted by traditional liquid–liquid extraction, followed by HPLC-MS quantification. FTIR (400–4000 cm^{-1}) was used for characterizing and monitoring the oxidative stability of all samples and for the evaluation of intermolecular forces between oleogelator mixtures and oil. Specific wavenumbers indicated oxidative processes in stored sample sets; storage time and sample clustering patterns were revealed by chemometrics. Isolariciresinol, vanillin, caffeic and syringic acids were quantified. The main changes were determined for isolariciresinol, which decreased in liquid pumpkin seed oil samples from 0.77 (T1) to 0.13 mg/100 g (T4), while for oleogel samples it decreased from 0.64 (T1) to 0.12 mg/100 g (T4). However, during the storage at room temperature, it was concluded that oleogelation technique might show potential protection of specific phenolic compounds such as syringic acid and vanillin after 8 months of storage. For isolariciresinol, higher amounts are registered in the oleogel (0.411 mg/100 g oil) than in the oil (0.37 mg/100 g oil) after 5 months of ambient temperature storage (T3). Oxidation processes occurred after 5 months storage for both oil and oleogel samples.

Keywords: pumpkin seed oil; oleogels; polyphenols; HPLC-MS; Fourier transform infrared spectroscopy; chemometrics; storage follow-up

1. Introduction

Cold-pressed pumpkin seed oil is a dichromatic, viscous oil, abundant in valuable compounds such as unsaturated fatty acids (mostly linoleic and oleic), tocopherols, sterols, β-carotene, and lutein, the content of the bioactive compounds differing among the species and varieties, or due to climate and cultivation conditions [1,2]. The oil preserves its nutritional profile because, in general, the temperature during pressing does not exceed 50 °C. However, other studies also revealed considerable contents of polyphenols in pumpkin seed oil obtained under different extraction temperatures or solvents, imparting overall antioxidant activity to this oil [3–5]. The numerous nutritive-pharmacological properties such as cancer prevention, anti-inflammation, anti-diabetic and lowering of cholesterol levels, are the main reasons for promoting the increase in the consumption of pumpkin seed oil [6,7]. Few previous studies regarding the oxidative stability of pumpkin seed oil have been conducted, especially for the cold-pressed type [4]. At this moment, it is mostly consumed as a salad dressing or encapsulated, despite its physicochemical properties which make it suitable for industrial applications too [2].

Oleogelation, a structuring technique which transforms vegetable oils into solid-like materials with the use of oleogelators, will soon be adopted as a current practice by processors and the food industry, increasing their consumption possibilities. This would be mainly due to consumers' awareness regarding healthier food and recent legislation regarding trans and saturated fat-containing products, which will be replaced by oleogels containing healthy mono or polyunsaturated oils. There are numerous possibilities of developing an oleogel, but the direct method, implying the dispersion of the structuring agents in the heated oil, followed by cooling and crystallization, is usually chosen because it is a method which is easy to up-scale. The indirect method based on an emulsion template is currently being intensively exploited and improved by researchers, but implies supplementary equipment such as spray or freeze-driers [8,9]. Oleogels can be formed from a wide range of structuring agents which can be classified as non-triacylglycerol gelators, more specifically crystalline particles or self-assembling structures, self-assembled fibrillar networks, polymers and inorganic compounds, or lipid-based gelators such as waxes, ceramides, phytosterols, fatty acids, fatty alcohols, and monoglycerides, etc. [10]. Recently, novel structuring agents were synthesized by enzyme catalysis [11–13]. Among them, natural waxes are cost-effective food-grade substances that demonstrated structuring capacity even at a low concentration and improved functionality when they were forming mixtures [14,15]. Waxes were also used to structure fish oil, in the study of oxidation of fish oil oleogel in comparison to bulk oil [16].

The versatility of oleogel process design permits the inclusion of certain fatty acids in foods, but also different liposoluble molecules and bioactive compounds, originating from the oil, from the structuring agents or added purposefully, to increase the nutritional value of the products [17–19]. β-carotene or curcumin have been included in the composition of different oleogels to exploit their health-promoting implications and to assess if model hydrophobic compounds can be protected against processing conditions and storage through oleogelation [20–23]. The usage of solely lipophilic structuring molecules can result in a negative digestibility response towards the system, and implicitly lowers the bioavailability [24]. β-sitosterol and δ-oryzanol organogelators used as a mixture are an example of structuring agents which facilitate the reduction in the controversial fats through oleogelation and also provide prophylactic effects on heart diseases through cholesterol levels management, which they are able to control as phytosterols [25,26]. In addition, ceramides are a class of oleogelators demonstrating tumor suppressing capacity [27]. The delivery of hydrophilic bioactive compounds through oleogel was also possible, by designing functional emulsion gels containing condensed tannins, capsaicin or inulin [28–30]. Polyphenols are able to form stable crystals which stabilize emulsion template oleogels and transform the oleogel into a functional matrix due to their biological activity [8,31].

Polyunsaturated vegetable oils, such as pumpkin seed oil, which are already abundant in polyphenols or other biologically active compounds, are more desirable for oleogel formulation and inclusion in food products such as meats, diary, pastry, and confectionary, to improve their nutritional profile. Moreover, oil blends should be developed, since the addition of only 1% cold-pressed pumpkin seed oil to sunflower oil demonstrated an antioxidant effect [32].

Most of the research focuses on evaluating if the oleogel can mimic the rheological, textural, and sensory properties of the fat and their inclusion in foods [33,34]. The present study follows the impact of oleogelification on the biologically active compounds delivered by the oil, namely the specific polyphenols, which might be altered by the oleogelation processes such as mixing, heating, or during UV storage [33,34]. Regarding the chemical and nutritional characterization of different pumpkin seed oils, it has been reported repeatedly that the fatty acid composition of the oil consists of mono-

and poly-unsaturated fats, the double bonds inside the alkyl chains of the fatty acids making the pumpkin seed oil prone to oxidation [35,36]. Additionally, a decrease in the total polyphenols of the pumpkin seed oil stored up to 120 days was reported [37]. Consequently, the present work aimed to assess individual phenolic compounds dynamics in fresh state (T1) and during the ambient storage of pumpkin seed oil and thereof oleogel, after one month (T2), five months (T3) and eight months (T4), but also the infrared fingerprints and chemometrics, in order to study oxidation and the implication of the oloegel in retarding the phenomenon or the polyphenols' antioxidant effect.

2. Materials and Methods

2.1. Materials

Cold-pressed pumpkin seed oil was purchased from Luna Solai, a Romanian producer. The waxes are natural and were kindly provided by Kahlwax (Trittau, Germany). HPLC filters, Chromafil, with a pore size of 0.45 µm and filter diameter of 13 mm, were also used for extractions. Hexane and MeOH were purchased from Merck (Darmstadt, Germany). Acetonitrile and acetic acid used for HPLC-MS analysis were purchased from Merck (Darmstadt, Germany). All other chemicals were of analytical grade.

2.2. Oleogel Production

For oleogel production, a 5% wax ternary mixture was used to gel cold-pressed pumpkin seed oil. As a structuring agent, a ternary mixture of waxes was chosen since it was previously found that it leads to the formation of oleogels with excellent physical properties. The mixture was formed by 3% beeswax, 1% sunflower wax and 1% rice bran wax. The wax and the oil were heated above the highest melting point of the waxes (80 °C) on a magnetic hot stirrer plate. The melted mixture was poured in aliquots of 30 g (OD), and these were closed and stored at room temperature under light exposure along with the liquid oil (UD), with different transparent polypropylene vessels (50 mL volume) being used for sampling each storage time (fresh—T1, one month—T2, five months—T3 and eight months—T4).

2.3. Phenolic Compounds Extraction

Phenolic compounds extraction consisted of a traditional liquid–liquid extraction as mentioned Ricciutelli et al. [38]. A volume of 3 mL of the oil or oleogel sample and 3 mL hexane were transferred into a 15 mL centrifuge tube which was vortexed (MX-S, Dlab Scientific Co., Beijing, China) for 30 s, until the mixture was homogenized. A volume of 5 mL of methanolic solution (3:2) was added, then it was subjected to sonication (Bandelin SONOREX, Sigma Aldrich, Berlin, Germany) for 15 min and centrifuged (DM0412 Dlab Scientific Co., Beijing, China) for 10 min with 3000 rot/min. The supernatant was disposed and 3 mL hexane was re added to the methanolic pellet in order to dilute the remaining lipidic compounds and the vortex, sonication and centrifugation steps were repeated for 2–3 times, until the supernatant was clear. Furthermore, a concentration step at 35 °C under reduced pressure was conducted (Rotavapor Heidolph). The evaporated samples were solubilized in 1 mL of methanol, filtered through 0.45 µm Millipore nylon filter and used for HPLC-MS analysis.

2.4. HPLC-MS Quantification of Specific Phenolic Compounds

High-performance liquid chromatography (HPLC) remains one of the most important analytical tools for fingerprinting and quantifying bioactive compounds. HPLC analysis was performed on Agilent 1200 system equipped with a quaternary pump, a degasser DGU-20 A3 (Prominence), an autosampler, an UV–VIS detector with photodiode (DAD), coupled with a single-quadrupole Mass Detector Agilent model 6110 (Agilent Technologies, Santa Clara, CA, USA). The compound separation was conducted on Eclipse XDB C18 column (5 µm, 4.6 × 150 mm). The mobile phase consisted of two solvents, A and B, injected at 25 °C for 30 min, at a flow rate of 0.5 mL/min and a gradient which is described in the following, together with the solvents. The mobile phase composition: solvent A—bi-distilled water and 0.1% acetic acid/acetonitrile (99/1) v/v, B—acetonitrile and acetic acid 0.1%. The solvent gradient applied was as follows: 0 min, 5% B; 0–2 min, 5% B; 2–18 min, 5–40% B; 18–20 min, 40–90% B; 20–24 min, 90% B; 24–25 min, 90–5% B; 25–30 min, 5% B. The chromatograms were monitored at 280 and 340 nm, respectively. The mass spectrometric data were obtained using a single-quadrupole 6110 mass spectrometer (Agilent Technologies, Chelmsford, MA, USA) equipped with an ESI probe. The measurements were performed in the positive mode with an ion-spray capillary voltage of 3000 V, and a temperature of 300 °C. The nitrogen flow rate was 7 L/min. Data were collected in full scan mode within the range 100 to 1200 m/z. The data reading and acquiring was done using Agilent ChemStation software.

2.5. Fourier Transform Infrared Spectroscopy

The FTIR spectra were acquired with Shimadzu IR Prestige-21 equipment (Shimadzu Corporation, Kyoto, Japan) in order to evaluate the oxidative stability of oleogel and reference oil, but also to analyze the intermolecular forces between the wax ternary mixture and the oil. The oil and the oleogel samples were placed directly on the sampling device equipped with a single reflection attenuated total reflectance (ATR). Spectra were scanned in the 600–4000 cm^{-1} wave number range with a resolution of 4 cm^{-1} and 64 scans. The spectral data were processed with Origin PRO8. To remove noise and eliminate background effects, the acquired spectral values were processed with standard normal variate (SNV) and the scatter effects were removed by centering and scaling each individual spectrum.

2.6. Chemometrics

By principal component analysis (PCA), using the Unscrambler 10.1 Software, version 10.1 (Camo Software AS, Oslo, Norway), the variability and similarities between samples registered during FTIR analysis were depicted. The PLS analysis (partial least squares) was also performed in order to reveal the possible relations existing between the presence of the polyphenols in the sample and the resulting FTIR spectra during the 8 months of storage, both for the oils and oleogels.

2.7. Statistical Analysis

Two-way analysis of variance (ANOVA) using Minitab Statistical Software v.19 (Minitab Inc., State College, PA, USA) was performed in order to assess the influence of pumpkin seed oil's physical state (oil vs. oleogel) and storage time on individual phenolic concentrations; for each compound, Tukey's comparison tests were performed at a 95% confidence level.

3. Results and Discussion

3.1. Phenolic Compounds Extraction and Individual Characterization

The samples were subjected to a traditional liquid–liquid extraction, with hexane and methanolic solution as solvents with no further acid hydrolysis. Then, compound identification and peak assignments, or the total polyphenolic content, were assessed based on the retention times, UV-VIS spectra and also comparing with LDI MS results. The HPLC-MS analysis allowed the identification and quantification of individual polyphenolic components and revealed the presence of isolariciresinol, vanillin, caffeic and syringic acids, based on the parameters described in Table 1, both in the oil and oleogel samples.

The extraction method proved efficiency, since in another study, where the phenolic compounds extracted with the solid phase method (SPE) from a sample consisting of cold-pressed pumpkin seed oil produced for commercial purpose could not be individually identified [5]. The original method of solid phase extraction (SPE) of the phenolic compounds is not suitable for pumpkin seed oil and needs adaptation, but is preferred, because is a premise of good separation of the interest compounds, according to a research which investigates different extraction methods and protocols [4]. The lack of accuracy of the Folin–Ciocalteu method for the calculation of total polyphenolic content of pumpkin seed oil was also discussed and seems to be due to the influence of the carotenoids on the SPE extraction and on the method, the bleaching of oil before this measurement not being indicated because it affects specific polyphenolic compounds and would not solve the inconvenience [4].

Table 1. Phenolic compounds identification in cold-pressed pumpkin seed oil by HPLC-MS.

Retention Time (min)	UV Max	[M + H]+ (m/z)	Identification
12.12	320	181	Caffeic acid
15.05	280	198	Syringic acid
16.31	265, 320	153	Vanillin
26.27	280	360	Isolariciresinol

In the present study, the total phenolic contents of the cold-pressed pumpkin seed oils and their correspondent oleogels were also assessed by HPLC-MS and the results were 1.087 mg/100 g for the oil at fresh state and 0.999 mg/100 g for the oleogel (T1), a similar content being reported by the literature for the oil [39]. From our knowledge, this is the first time when the total polyphenols are analyzed for a pumpkin seed oil oleogel. The content of the individual and total polyphenols in the cold-pressed pumpkin seed oil and oleogel during storage, expressed as mg/100 g oil, is represented in Figure 1. For all individual phenolics (caffeic acid, syringic acid, vanillin, isolariciresinol, as well as total phenolics), the two-way ANOVA revealed high significant differences ($p < 0.05$) for both factors (oil physical state and storage time) as well as their interaction. Consequently, the oil state–storage time interactions were analyzed by several one-way ANOVA tests and compared by Tukey's method. Thus, the influence of oleogelation and storage duration over the phenolics dynamics is depicted by Figure 1, including the statistical significance.

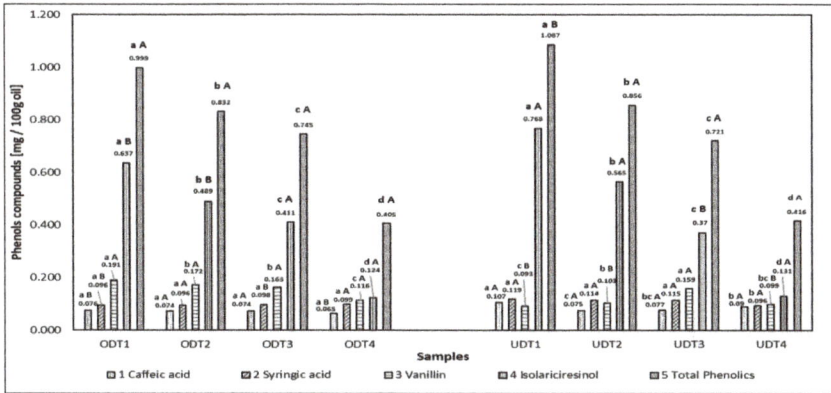

Figure 1. Individual and total phenolic compounds detected by HPLC-MS in cold-pressed pumpkin seed oil (UD) and oleogel (OD) fresh (T1) but also stored for one (T2), five (T3) and eight months (T4) at room temperature. For the same compound, lower-case letters within each sample group (oleogel or oil) indicate no significant difference ($p > 0.05$); for the same compound and storage time, upper-case letters between each sample type (oleogel vs. oil) indicate no significant difference ($p > 0.05$).

For caffeic acid, syringic acid and isolariciresinol lower amounts were detected in the oleogel samples in comparison with the oil. Isolariciresinol is a lignan commonly identified in the pumpkin seed, but which is present in lower amounts in the oil too. In addition, it might be thermolabile, since in oleogel it is present in slightly lower amounts than in the oil at fresh state. For the cold-pressed pumpkin seed oil investigated in our research, isolariciresinol was the most abundant polyphenolic compound detected (0.768 mg/100 g in the fresh oil). The content of another oligomer of this lignan, the secoisolariciresinol, it is reported to be lowered both in seed and oil, because of the roasting process [4]. From the class of hydroxycinnamic acids, the caffeic acid was identified (0.107 mg/100 g oil in the fresh state) and from the class of hydroxybenzoic acids, the syringic acid was present in an amount of 0.119 mg/100 g oil. In the oleogel samples, caffeic and syringic acids showed no statistically significant differences during storage ($p > 0.05$), while in the oil samples, a varying trend was noticed, as depicted in Figure 1. An overall statistically significant higher content of vanillin ($p < 0.05$), a compound of the class of hydroxy benzaldehydes, is present in the oleogel samples, in each moment of storage, in comparison to the oil samples. In the oleogel, 0.191 mg/100 g was detected, while in the fresh oil it was 0.093 mg/100 g, thus the thermal treatment might promote the release of this compound. The amount of vanillin in the oleogel samples decreased during storage and a statistically significant difference between samples was revealed; in the oil samples, the vanillin concentrations were varying during the eight months storage (Figure 1).

The content of the total polyphenols decreased during storage to less than half, both for the oil and the oleogel samples, the main changes being determined for isolariciresinol, which statistically significant decreased ($p < 0.05$) in liquid pumpkin seed oil samples from 0.77 (T1) to 0.13 mg/100 g (T4), while for oleogel samples from 0.64 (T1) to 0.12 mg/100 g (T4). Therefore, during the storage at room temperature, it can be observed that oleogelation technique might show potential protection of overall phenolic compounds, especially for the syringic acid and vanillin, higher content being registered in the oleogel sample in comparison to the oil, in samples stored at room temperature for 8 months (T4). For isolariciresinol, statistically significant higher amounts ($p < 0.05$) are registered in the oleogel (0.411 mg/100 g oil) than in the oil (0.37 mg/100 g oil) after 5 months of ambient temperature storage (T3).

3.2. Fourier Transform Infrared Spectroscopy

FTIR spectroscopy coupled with the chemometrics techniques is a recently intensively exploited method in the fast, simple and non-invasive analysis of edible oils. It is suitable for determining both the composition and the quality of oils. The FTIR spectra, scanned using attenuated total reflectance mode, displayed both for the oil and oleogel samples, raw and SNV-treated, peaks characteristic for vegetable oils. For instance, the peak at 3007 cm^{-1} is denoting the poly unsaturation of the oil, sharp peaks also being registered in the 2924, 2852, and 1745 cm^{-1} region, to reveal the abundance of triglycerides in the samples (Figure 2). At the lower frequencies, the band near 720 cm^{-1} is assigned to the rocking vibration of the CH$_2$ group which build up the long-chain mono and polyunsaturated fatty acids of the pumpkin seed oil. The broad peak at 1160 cm^{-1} might be due to C-O stretching of a tertiary alcohol or even due to the presence of the phenolic compounds. Other studies describing the FTIR spectra of pumpkin seed oil also registered smaller intensity peaks in the region of 1695, 1460, 1378, 1237, 1160, 1110, 1097, 950 and 850 cm^{-1}, some small shifts in the peaks to left or right being registered due to the particularity of the oils composition [40–42].

During the oleogel formation, the cold-pressed pumpkin seed oil was subjected to a thermal treatment of 80 °C for up to 5 min and to shearing, and even if oleogelation does not affect the chemical properties of oil, different molecular arrangements occur due to the crystallization of the ternary mixture of waxes and the oil, during cooling, affecting the appearance of the spectra, depending on the oil and the oleogelation technique. Beside changes in intensities, it can be affirmed that there was no variability in the peak appearance or shifts for the oleogels in comparison to the oils (Figure 2), which indicates that physical interactions, and not changes in the chemical structure, are the reason for oleogel formation. Usually in the study of oleogels, medium intensity bands in the 3550–3450 cm^{-1} range indicate intermolecular bounding and 3570–3540 cm^{-1} range bands indicate the presence of some intramolecular hydrogen bonds in the FTIR spectra [43]. The spectra of the wax based oleogels usually lack a well-resolved band in this region [44]; also, other authors evaluate the bands at 2924 cm^{-1} specific for the lipid acyl-chains, which in our study for the cold-pressed pumpkin seed the oleogel sample displays lower intensity, and thus a slightly higher conformational ordering than the oil [45].

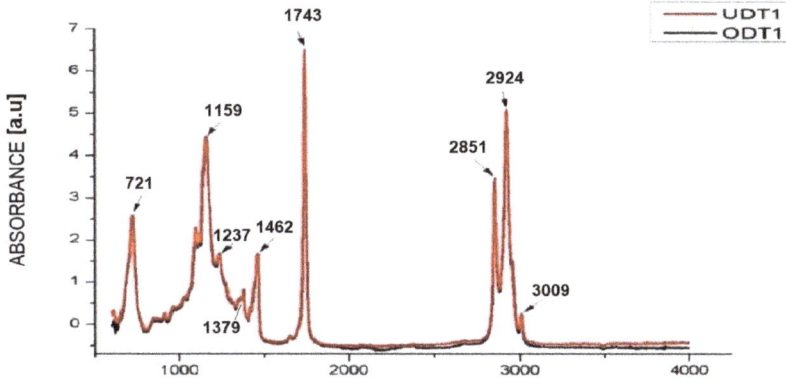

Figure 2. FTIR raw spectra of pumpkin seed oil (UDT1) and oleogel (ODT1) in fresh state (T1).

It is already concluded that oxidation processes during heating occur more slowly in oils extracted from 4–12 min microwave roasted pumpkin seeds in comparison to oils from unroasted seeds [46]. In the present study, the effect of thermal treatment on the oxidative stress of the oleogel samples is evaluated, by comparing the different intensities of several key absorbances for the oil and oleogel samples at T1, in fresh state (Figure 2). The heat-induced oxidation can be monitored at the 3050–2800 cm^{-1} or 1743–1465 cm^{-1} spectral region, where slight differences in the values of the intensities were registered for the oil and oleogel samples in fresh state [46]. In the 1500–1300 cm^{-1} region, the bending vibration of methyl and methylen groups can be analyzed. For the oleogel samples in fresh state, higher intensities were registered and this might be due to the waxes' contribution, which are derived from mixtures of long-chain hydrocarbons.

Oil oxidation is a set of natural phenomena governed by intrinsic and extrinsic factors, determining the shelf life, nutritional and sensorial properties of edible oils. This is a multidimensional result of the fatty acid composition of oil, and the presence of antioxidant components such as phenolic compounds, concurring with oxygen, light or heat [47]. The samples analysed by HPLC-MS for the quantification of total polyphenolic compounds displayed a decrease of almost 50% during the 8 months of storage; therefore, higher oxidation of the oils and oleogels is expected to be registered as the storage time increases. Both the oil and oleogel samples stored for 5 months display peaks overlaid with the peaks of the rest of the samples (at fresh state and stored for 1 months) and, in conclusion, at that moment, oxidation processes were not advanced. In the raw spectra, the intensity of the peaks displayed for the oleogel sample stored for 8 months (ODT4) are lower than the rest of the samples in the following regions: 2924, 2850, 1743, and 1157 cm^{-1}, but did not decreased for 3008, 1465, and 715 cm^{-1}.

The raw and SNV-treated FTIR spectra were registered for both the oil (Figure 3a,b) and oleogel samples (Figure 3c,d) in different moments of the storage period: fresh (T0), 1 month (T1), 5 months (T3) and 8 months (T4) in order to follow the oxidation during the 8 months of storage and to reveal the influence of the total polyphenols. The spectra started to reveal significant differences in terms of the intensity and position of the relevant bands (the shifts were not large but visible). For the SNV-treated spectra, the increase in a peak can be seen in regions of 1743 cm^{-1} for the oleogel in comparison to the oil, which is due to the formation of carbonylic compounds and cis allylic during oxidation. For the raw spectra of the oleogel, the peak at 3008 cm^{-1} was decreased because of the decrease in cis allylic (C=CH) bonds and is slightly shifted to the right, in comparison to the peak registered for the oil samples.

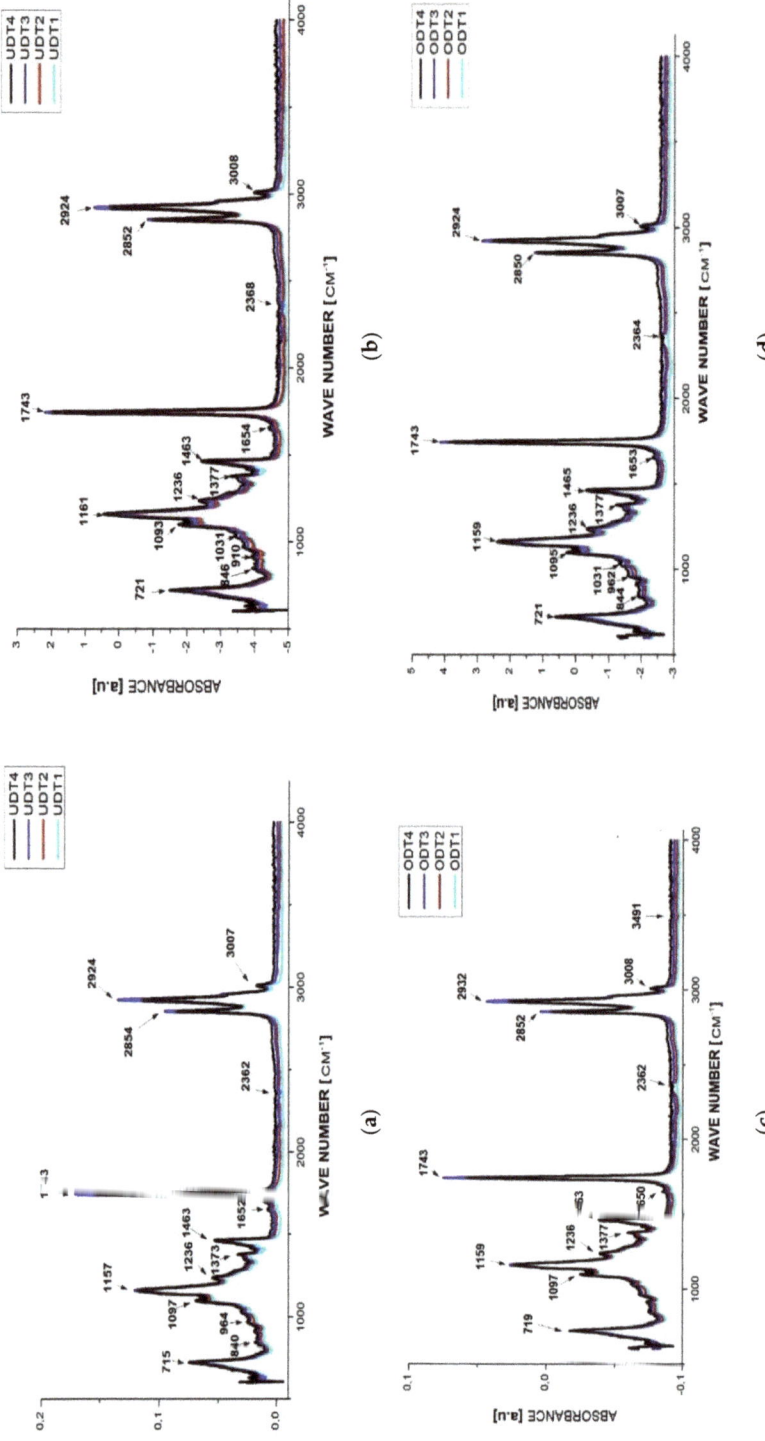

Figure 3. FTIR spectra of pumpkin seed oil (UD) and oleogel (OD) at fresh (T1), and stored one month (T1), five (T2) and eight months (T4) at room temperature: (a) oil raw spectra; (b) standard normal variate (SNV)-treated oil spectra; (c) oleogel raw spectra; (d) SNV-treated oleogel spectra.

During oxidation, double bonds will be converted in single bonds, as a first step to hydroperoxide formation, and this can be confirmed by an increase in the ratio of intensities 2850/3008 cm^{-1}. Figure 4 depicts the ratio of intensities 2850/3008 cm^{-1} during the storage of oil and oleogel samples. It was established in order to inspect the effect of the oleogelation related to storage and its potential protection against oxidation or loss of bio-active compounds, by comparing the 8 months stored oleogel and oil samples. Figure 4 indicates a more intense oxidation for the oleogel sample after 5 months of storage in comparison to the oil. The current study hypothesis that oleogelation protects the cold-pressed pumpkin seed oil from oxidation or from the loss of polyphenols is thus invalidated for samples stored longer than 5 months.

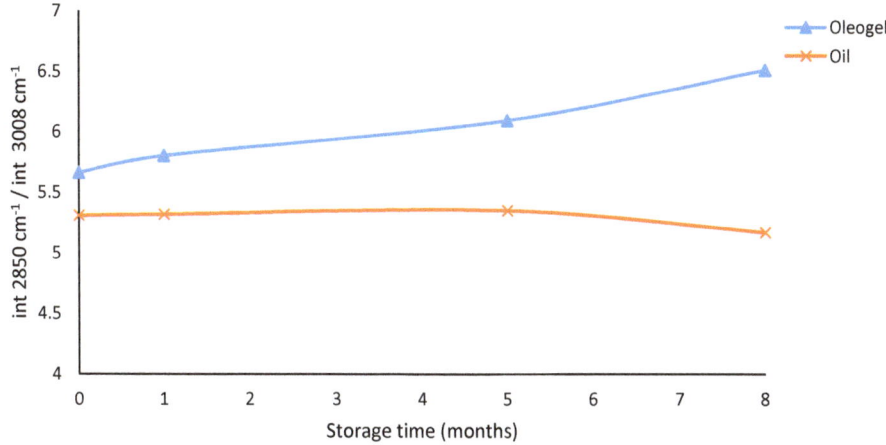

Figure 4. Ratio of intensities 2850 cm^{-1}/3008 cm^{-1} of the oil and oleogel samples during storage.

3.3. Principal Component Analysis

Due to the similarities in terms of chemical composition, the visual comparison of the spectra of pumpkin seed oil and oleogels during storage can lead to inaccurate perceptions and the principal component analysis could better aid in the classification of the samples. PCA was performed in order to group the samples based on their similarities and differences registered in the FTIR analysis. PCA was projected by its principal components (PCs) using raw and SNV-treated FTIR spectral data from 600 to 4000 cm^{-1}. For the raw spectra, PC1 and PC2 accounted, respectively, for 62% and 25% of the total data variance. In PCA, the first principle component (PC1) accounts for the most variation, meanwhile the second principle component (PC2) accounts for the samples which fall out of the trend. In the projections of PC1 and PC2, it can be observed that oil samples are well separated from the oleogel samples. As shown in Figure 5a, there is a high similarity between the principal component scores of the raw FTIR spectrum of the oleogel sample in fresh state (ODT1) and those of the oil sample after 1 month of storage (UDT2).

The oil samples of UDT1, UDT2, UDT3 do, however, form a cluster in the upper right side of the plot, while the oil sample stored for 8 months (UDT4) is in the upper left side. A similar trend is also observed for the oleogel samples, leading to the formation another separate cluster. The SNV pre-treated FTIR spectra PC1 horizontal axis explains 60% of the total variance, while the PC2 vertical axis explains 20%. The principal component analysis (PCA) scores and loadings, for standard normal variate (SNV) pre-treated FTIR spectra 600–4000 cm^{-1} also allow the visualization of both oil and oleogel samples stored for 8 months falling out of the trend established by the rest of the sample. The rest of the samples are, however, disseminated closely in the upper and lower right side of the plot, while for the raw FTIR spectra, all the oil samples are in the upper right side and all the oleogel samples are in the lower right side.

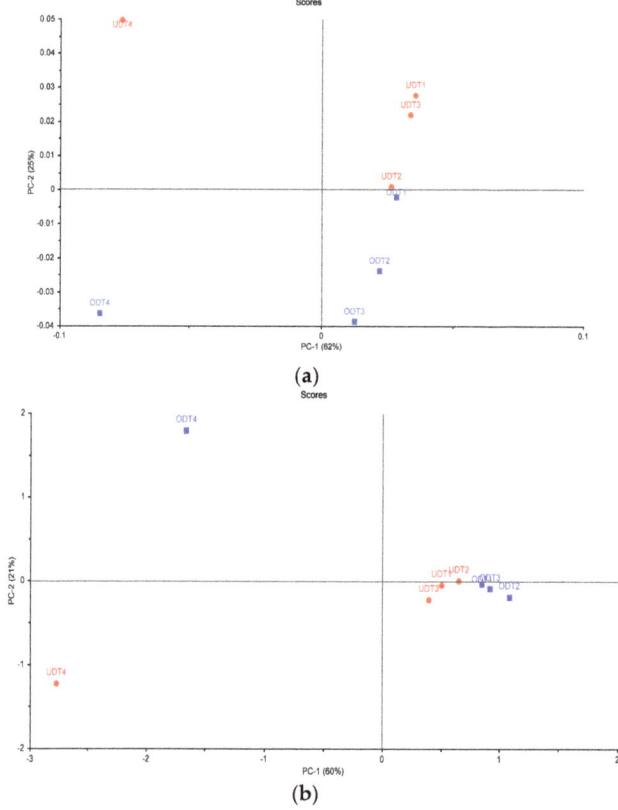

Figure 5. Principal component analysis (PCA) scores, for raw (**a**) and SNV-treated (**b**) FTIR spectra of oils and oleogels in the wave range of 600–4000 cm^{-1}.

3.4. Partial Least Square Analysis

A prefeasibility study was conducted with the four samples of the pumpkin seed oil and the four samples of the ternary wax mixture oleogels in different storage moments for predicting the content of the total phenols during the storage of pumpkin oil or oleogels, based on FTIR coupled with partial least square (PLS) calibration and cross-validation models. The leave-one-out cross-validation procedure was performed. The partial least square (PLS) calibration and full cross-validation models for total phenolic prediction by using raw (Figure 6a,b) or SNV (Figure 6c,d) FTIR spectra 600–4000 cm^{-1} were computed. The PLS calibration and cross-validation models showed encouraging coefficients of determination R^2 for raw spectra (0.89 for calibration and 0.73 for cross-validation) and SNV-treated spectra (0.9 for calibration and 0.86 for cross-validation). The attempt to optimize the spectral region of the PLS model (956–2961 cm^{-1} optimized region based on regression coefficients), revealed R^2 increased to 0.93, indicating a good modelling of the data the calibration model (Figure 7); however, the PLS cross-validation model presented an unsatisfactory coefficient of determination R^2 of 0.57. Consequently, for this prefeasibility study conducted, it was concluded that the best PLS calibration and cross-validation models are obtained when full SNV treated spectra are used (Figure 6c,d), with a standard error of calibration (SEC) of 0.07 and a standard error of cross-validation (SECV) of 0.1 being obtained.

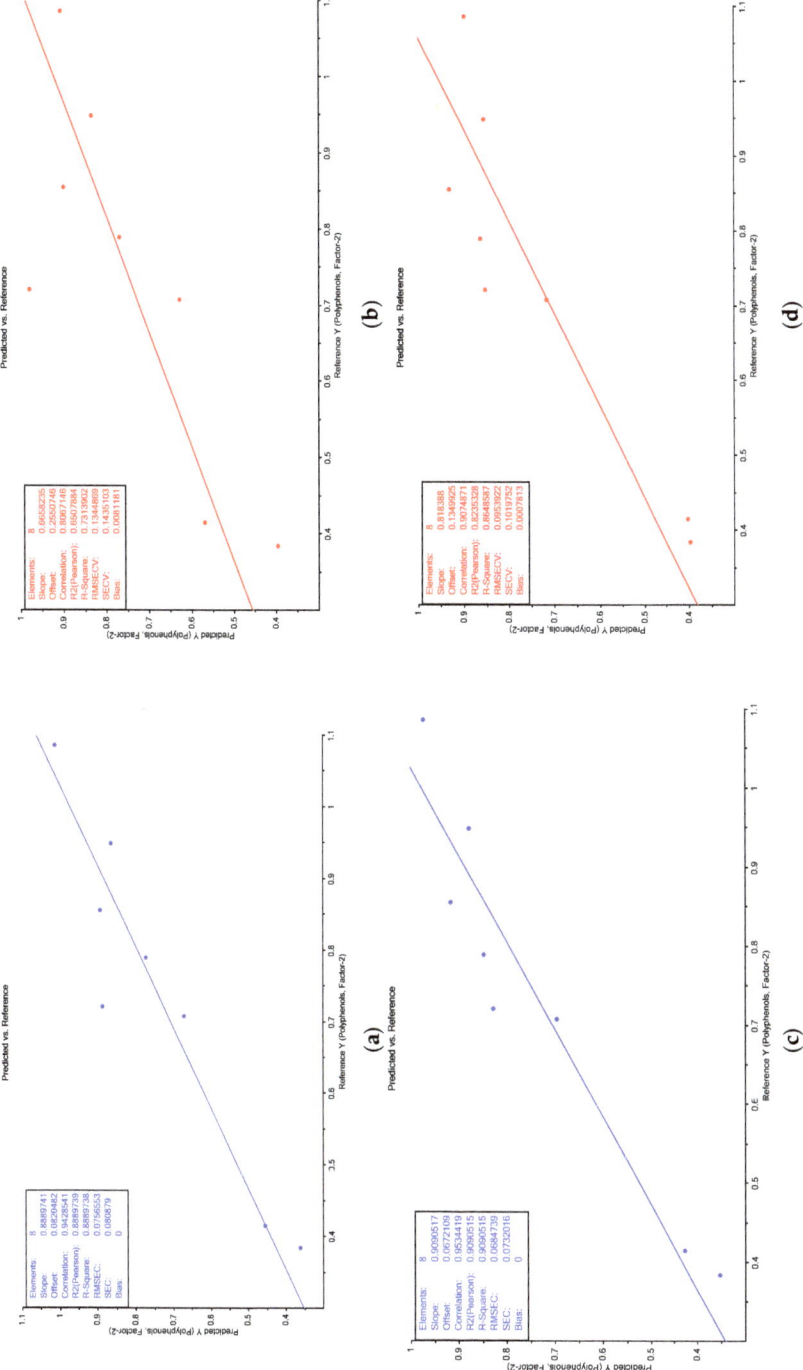

Figure 6. Partial least square (PLS) calibration (**a**,**c**) and full cross-validation (**b**,**d**) models for total phenolic prediction by using raw (**a**,**b**) or pre-treated standard normal variate (**c**,**d**) FTIR spectra 600–4000 cm^{-1}.

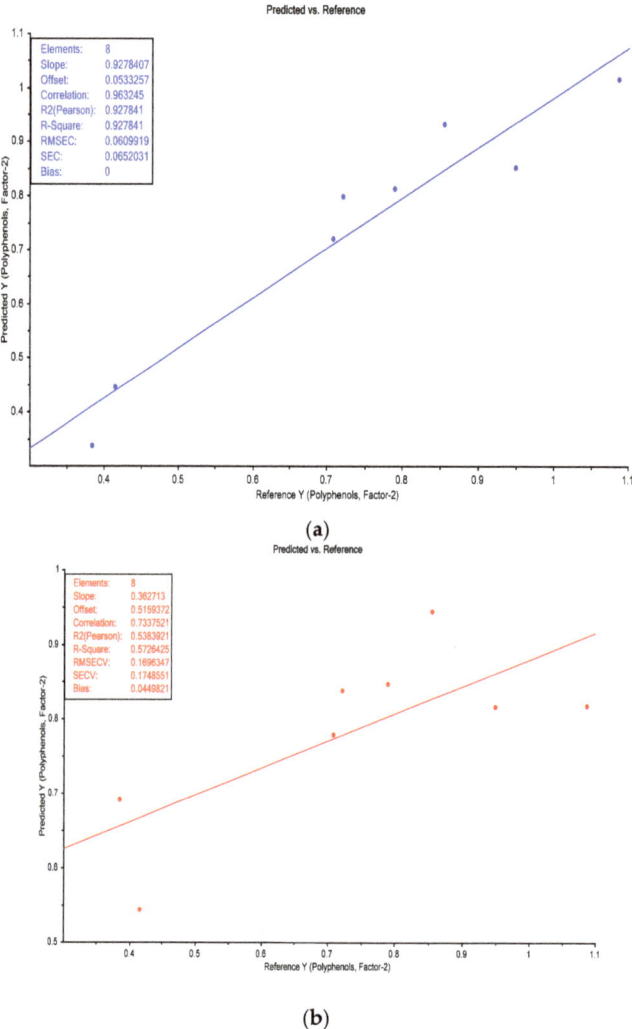

Figure 7. Partial least square (PLS) calibration (**a**) and full cross-validation (**b**) models for total phenolic prediction by using pre-treated standard normal variate (SNV) FTIR spectra—optimum spectral regions selected.

4. Conclusions

Liquid–liquid extraction of polyphenols from cold pressed pumpkin seed oil and oleogel, and their total and individual quantification by HPLC-MS, were performed during ambient storage. Isolariciresinol was the most abundant phenolic compound, but vanillin, caffeic and syringic acids were also identified.

The influence of oleogelation and storage duration on the phenolics dynamics was examined for 8 months. The content of the total polyphenolic compounds was decreased to almost half of the initial content. It is concluded that specific phenolic compounds, such as syringic acid and vanillin, might have been better protected during storage due to oleogelation for 8 months and also isolariciresinol for 5 months.

FTIR spectroscopy revealed similar trends for the oxidation process in oil and oleogel samples, but after 5 months storage, the oleogel samples became more degraded. The ratio of intensities at 2850/3008 cm^{-1} and the PCA analysis also confirm this. For the raw data, PCA revealed high similarities between the sample of oleogel in fresh state (ODT1) and the oil sample after 1 month of storage (UDT2).

On a pioneered level, due to the low number of samples, the contents of the total phenols during storage of pumpkin oil or oleogels, based on FTIR coupled with partial least square (PLS) calibration and cross-validation models, were studied. It was concluded that the best PLS calibration and cross-validation models were obtained when full SNV-treated spectra were used, with a standard error of calibration (SEC) of 0.07 and a standard error of cross-validation (SECV) of 0.1 being obtained.

Author Contributions: Conceptualization, V.M.; Formal analysis, A.P., A.M., F.R. and F.F.; Funding acquisition, V.M.; Methodology, A.M., F.R. and F.F.; Supervision, S.M., C.S. and V.M.; Writing—original draft, A.P.; Writing—review and editing, V.M. All authors have read and agreed to the published version of the manuscript.

Funding: This work was supported by a grant of Ministry of Research and Innovation, CNCS—UEFISCDI, project number PN-III-P1-1.1-PD-2016-0113, within PNCDI III. The publication fee was supported by funds from the National Research Development Projects to finance excellence (PFE)-37/2018–2020 granted by the Romanian Ministry of Research and Innovation.

Acknowledgments: The authors would like to thank Iasmina Blidar for technical assistance for oleogel sample preparation.

Conflicts of Interest: The authors declare no conflict of interest. The funders had no role in the design of the study; in the collection, analyses, or interpretation of data; in the writing of the manuscript, or in the decision to publish the results.

References

1. Rezig, L.; Chouaibi, M.; Ojeda-Amador, R.M.; Gomez-Alonso, S.; Salvador, M.D.; Fregapane, G.; Hamdi, S. Cucurbita maxima pumpkin seed oil: From the chemical properties to the different extracting techniques. *Not. Bot. Horti Agrobot. Cluj-Napoca* **2018**, *46*, 663–669. [CrossRef]
2. Stevenson, D.G.; Eller, F.J.; Wang, L.; Jane, J.-L.; Wang, T.; Inglett, G.E. Oil and tocopherol content and composition of pumpkin seed oil in 12 cultivars. *J. Agric. Food Chem.* **2007**, *55*, 4005–4013. [CrossRef] [PubMed]
3. Parry, J.; Hao, Z.; Luther, M.; Su, L.; Zhou, K.; Yu, L.L. Characterization of cold-pressed onion, parsley, cardamom, mullein, roasted pumpkin, and milk thistle seed oils. *J. Am. Oil Chem. Soc.* **2006**, *83*, 847–854. [CrossRef]
4. Andjelkovic, M.; Van Camp, J.; Trawka, A.; Verhé, R. Phenolic compounds and some quality parameters of pumpkin seed oil. *Eur. J. Lipid Sci. Technol.* **2010**, *112*, 208–217. [CrossRef]
5. Van Hoed, V.; Sampaio, K.A.; Felkner, B.; Bavec, F.; Scippo, M.L.; Brose, F.; Bavec, M.; Verhé, R. Tocopherols and polyphenols in pumpkin seed oil are moderately affected by industrially relevant roasting conditions. *Eur. J. Lipid Sci. Technol.* **2017**, *119*, 1700110. [CrossRef]
6. Yadav, M.; Jain, S.; Tomar, R.; Prasad, G.; Yadav, H. Medicinal and biological potential of pumpkin: An updated review. *Nutr. Res. Rev.* **2010**, *23*, 184–190. [CrossRef]
7. Bora, N.S. Beneficial properties of pumpkin seed oil as an antioxidant nutraceutical. *EC Pharmacol. Toxicol.* **2018**, *6*, 498–499.
8. Luo, S.-Z.; Hu, X.-F.; Jia, Y.-J.; Pan, L.-H.; Zheng, Z.; Zhao, Y.-Y.; Mu, D.-D.; Zhong, X.-Y.; Jiang, S.-T. Camellia oil-based oleogels structuring with tea polyphenol-palmitate particles and citrus pectin by emulsion-templated method: Preparation, characterization and potential application. *Food Hydrocoll.* **2019**, *95*, 76–87. [CrossRef]
9. Jiang, Y.; Liu, L.; Wang, B.; Sui, X.; Zhong, Y.; Zhang, L.; Mao, Z.; Xu, H. Cellulose-rich oleogels prepared with an emulsion-templated approach. *Food Hydrocoll.* **2018**, *77*, 460–464. [CrossRef]
10. Co, E.D.; Marangoni, A.G. Chapter 1—Oleogels: An Introduction. In *Edible Oleogels*, 2nd ed.; Marangoni, A.G., Garti, N., Eds.; AOCS Press: San Diego, CA, USA, 2018; pp. 1–29. [CrossRef]

11. Samateh, M.; Sagiri, S.S.; Sanni, R.; Chee, C.; Satapathy, S.; John, G. Tuning aesthetic and mechanical properties of oleogels via formulation of enzyme-enabled stereoisomeric molecular gelators. *J. Agric. Food Chem.* **2019**. [CrossRef]
12. Ghosh, M.; Begg, F.; Bhattacharyya, D.K.; Bandyopadhya, N.; Ghosh, M. Nutritional evaluation of oleogel made from micronutrient rich edible oils. *J. Oleo Sci.* **2017**, *66*, 217–226. [CrossRef]
13. Nicholson, R.A.; Marangoni, A.G. Enzymatic glycerolysis converts vegetable oils into structural fats with the potential to replace palm oil in food products. *Nat. Food* **2020**, 1–9. [CrossRef]
14. Tavernier, I.; Doan, C.D.; Van de Walle, D.; Danthine, S.; Rimaux, T.; Dewettinck, K. Sequential crystallization of high and low melting waxes to improve oil structuring in wax-based oleogels. *RSC Adv.* **2017**, *7*, 12113–12125. [CrossRef]
15. Winkler-Moser, J.K.; Anderson, J.; Felker, F.C.; Hwang, H.S. Physical properties of beeswax, sunflower wax, and candelilla wax mixtures and oleogels. *J. Am. Oil Chem. Soc.* **2019**, *96*, 1125–1142. [CrossRef]
16. Hwang, H.S.; Fhaner, M.; Winkler-Moser, J.K.; Liu, S.X. Oxidation of fish oil oleogels formed by natural waxes in comparison with bulk oil. *Eur. J. Lipid Sci. Technol.* **2018**, *120*, 1700378. [CrossRef]
17. Wang, X.; Wang, S.-J.; Nan, Y.; Liu, G. The effects of oil type and crystallization temperature on the physical properties of vitamin C-loaded oleogels prepared by an emulsion-templated approach. *Food Funct.* **2020**, *11*, 8028–8037. [CrossRef]
18. Martins, A.J.; Cerqueira, M.A.; Cunha, R.L.; Vicente, A. Fortified beeswax oleogels: Effect of β-carotene on the gel structure and oxidative stability. *Food Funct.* **2017**, *8*, 4241–4250. [CrossRef]
19. Masotta, N.E.; Martinefski, M.R.; Lucangioli, S.; Rojas, A.M.; Tripodi, V.P. High-dose coenzyme Q10-loaded oleogels for oral therapeutic supplementation. *Int. J. Pharm.* **2019**, *556*, 9–20. [CrossRef]
20. Mao, L.; Wang, D.; Liu, F.; Gao, Y. Emulsion design for the delivery of β-carotene in complex food systems. *Crit. Rev. Food Sci. Nutr.* **2016**, *58*, 770–784. [CrossRef] [PubMed]
21. Hughes, N.E.; Marangoni, A.G.; Wright, A.J.; Rogers, M.A.; Rush, J.W.E. Potential food applications of edible oil organogels. *Trends Food Sci. Technol.* **2009**, *20*, 470–480. [CrossRef]
22. Li, L.; Wan, W.; Cheng, W.; Liu, G.; Han, L. Oxidatively stable curcumin-loaded oleogels structured by β-sitosterol and lecithin: Physical characteristics and release behaviour in vitro. *Int. J. Food Sci. Technol.* **2019**, *54*, 2502–2510. [CrossRef]
23. Perez, J.A.V.; Remacho, C.R.; Rodriguez, J.R.; Pulido, J.M.O.; De La Fuente, E.B.; Martinez-Ferez, A. Optimization of Oleogel Formulation for Curcumin Vehiculization and Lipid Oxidation Stability by Multi-response Surface Methodology. *Chem. Eng. Trans.* **2019**, *75*, 427–432.
24. Martins, A.J.; Vicente, A.A.; Pastrana, L.M.; Cerqueira, M.A. Oleogels for development of health-promoting food products. *Food Sci. Hum. Wellness* **2020**, *9*, 31–39. [CrossRef]
25. Bot, A.; Agterof, W.G.M. Structuring of edible oils by mixtures of γ-oryzanol with β-sitosterol or related phytosterols. *J. Am. Oil Chem. Soc.* **2006**, *83*, 513–521. [CrossRef]
26. Calligaris, S.; Mirolo, G.; Da Pieve, S.; Arrighetti, G.; Nicoli, M.C. Effect of oil type on formation, structure and thermal properties of γ-oryzanol and β-sitosterol-based organogels. *Food Biophys.* **2013**, *9*, 69–75. [CrossRef]
27. Rogers, M.A.; Spagnuolo, P.A.; Wang, T.M.; Angka, L. A potential bioactive hard-stock fat replacer comprised of a molecular gel. *Food Sci. Nutr.* **2017**, *5*, 579–587. [CrossRef]
28. Li, F. Inulin-Monoglycerides Emulsion Gel as Potential Fat Replacer and Effect of Inulin to Delay Lipid Oxidation. Master's Thesis, Carleton University, Ottawa, ON, Canada, 2019.
29. Freire, M.; Cofrades, S.; Pérez-Jiménez, J.; Gómez-Estaca, J.; Jiménez-Colmenero, F.; Bou, R. Emulsion gels containing n-3 fatty acids and condensed tannins designed as functional fat replacers. *Food Res. Int.* **2018**, *113*, 465–473. [CrossRef] [PubMed]
30. Lu, M.; Cao, Y.; Ho, C.-T.; Huang, Q. Development of organogel-derived capsaicin nanoemulsion with improved bioaccessibility and reduced gastric mucosa irritation. *J. Agric. Food Chem.* **2016**, *64*, 4735–4741. [CrossRef]
31. Qiu, C.; Huang, Y.; Li, A.; Ma, D.; Wang, Y. Fabrication and characterization of oleogel stabilized by gelatin-polyphenol-polysaccharides nanocomplexes. *J. Agric. Food Chem.* **2018**, *66*, 13243–13252. [CrossRef]
32. Rexhepi, F. Antioxidant activity of pumpkin seed oil and its effect on oxidative stability of sunflower oil monitored by FTIR spectroscopy technique. *Eur. J. Mater. Sci. Eng.* **2020**, *5*, 51–57. [CrossRef]
33. Pușcaș, A.; Mureșan, V.; Socaciu, C.; Muste, S. Oleogels in food: A review of current and potential applications. *Foods* **2020**, *9*, 70. [CrossRef] [PubMed]

34. Martins, A.J.; Vicente, A.A.; Cunha, R.L.; Cerqueira, M.A. Edible oleogels: An opportunity for fat replacement in foods. *Food Funct.* **2018**, *9*, 758–773. [CrossRef]
35. Rezig, L.; Chouaibi, M.; Meddeb, W.; Msaada, K.; Hamdi, S. Chemical composition and bioactive compounds of Cucurbitaceae seeds: Potential sources for new trends of plant oils. *Process. Saf. Environ. Prot.* **2019**, *127*, 73–81. [CrossRef]
36. Montesano, D.; Blasi, F.; Simonetti, M.S.; Santini, A.; Cossignani, L. Chemical and nutritional characterization of seed oil from *Cucurbita maxima* L (var. Berrettina) pumpkin. *Foods* **2018**, *7*, 30. [CrossRef]
37. Poiana, M.-A.; Alexa, E.; Moigradean, D.; Popa, M. The influence of the storage conditions on the oxidative stability and antioxidant properties of sunflower and pumpkin oil. In Proceedings of the 44th Croatian & 4th International Symposium of Agriculture, Opatija, Croatia, 16–20 February 2009; pp. 449–453.
38. Ricciutelli, M.; Marconi, S.; Boarelli, M.C.; Caprioli, G.; Sagratini, G.; Ballini, R.; Fiorini, D. Olive oil polyphenols: A quantitative method by high-performance liquid-chromatography-diode-array detection for their determination and the assessment of the related health claim. *J. Chromatogr. A* **2017**, *1481*, 53–63. [CrossRef] [PubMed]
39. Gorjanović, S.Ž.; Rabrenović, B.B.; Novaković, M.M.; Dimić, E.B.; Basić, Z.N.; Sužnjević, D.Ž. Cold-pressed pumpkin seed oil antioxidant activity as determined by a DC polarographic assay based on hydrogen peroxide scavenge. *J. Am. Oil Chem. Soc.* **2011**, *88*, 1875–1882. [CrossRef]
40. Irnawati, I.; Riyanto, S.; Martono, S.; Rohman, A. The employment of FTIR spectroscopy and chemometrics for authentication of pumpkin seed oil from sesame oil. *Food Res.* **2019**, *4*, 42–48. [CrossRef]
41. Rohman, A.; Man, Y.C.; Nurrulhidayah, A. Fourier-transform infrared spectra combined with chemometrics and fatty acid composition for analysis of pumpkin seed oil blended into olive oil. *Int. J. Food Prop.* **2015**, *18*, 1086–1096. [CrossRef]
42. Irnawati, I.; Riyanto, S.; Martono, S.; Rohman, A. Determination of sesame oil, rice bran oil and pumpkin seed oil in ternary mixtures using FTIR spectroscopy and multivariate calibrations. *J. Food Sci.* **2019**, *4*, 135–142. [CrossRef]
43. Öğütcü, M.; Arifoğlu, N.; Yılmaz, E. Preparation and characterization of virgin olive oil-beeswax oleogel emulsion products. *J. Am. Oil Chem. Soc.* **2015**, *92*, 459–471. [CrossRef]
44. Yılmaz, E.; Öğütcü, M. Oleogels of virgin olive oil with carnauba wax and monoglyceride as spreadable products. *Grasas Y Aceites* **2014**, *65*, e040. [CrossRef]
45. Gómez-Estaca, J.; Herrero, A.M.; Herranz, B.; Álvarez, M.D.; Jiménez-Colmenero, F.; Cofrades, S. Characterization of ethyl cellulose and beeswax oleogels and their suitability as fat replacers in healthier lipid pâtés development. *Food Hydrocoll.* **2019**, *87*, 960–969. [CrossRef]
46. Ali, M.A.; Nargis, A.; Othman, N.H.; Noor, A.F.; Sadik, G.; Hossen, J. Oxidation stability and compositional characteristics of oils from microwave roasted pumpkin seeds during thermal oxidation. *Int. J. Food Prop.* **2017**, *20*, 2569–2580. [CrossRef]
47. Rohman, A.; Man, Y.C. Application of FTIR spectroscopy for monitoring the stabilities of selected vegetable oils during thermal oxidation. *Int. J. Food Prop.* **2013**, *16*, 1594–1603. [CrossRef]

Publisher's Note: MDPI stays neutral with regard to jurisdictional claims in published maps and institutional affiliations.

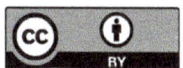

© 2020 by the authors. Licensee MDPI, Basel, Switzerland. This article is an open access article distributed under the terms and conditions of the Creative Commons Attribution (CC BY) license (http://creativecommons.org/licenses/by/4.0/).

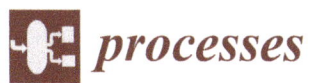

Article

Polyphenolic Profiling of Forestry Waste by UPLC-HDMS[E]

Colin M. Potter [1,*] and David L. Jones [1,2]

[1] Centre for Environmental Biotechnology, School of Natural Sciences, Bangor University, Gwynedd, Bangor LL57 2UW, UK; d.jones@bangor.ac.uk
[2] UWA School of Agriculture and Environment, The University of Western Australia, Perth, WA 6009, Australia
* Correspondence: colin.potter@bangor.ac.uk

Received: 22 October 2020; Accepted: 1 November 2020; Published: 4 November 2020

Abstract: Polyphenols constitute a diverse array of naturally occurring secondary metabolites found in plants which, when consumed, have been shown to promote human health. Greater consumption may therefore aid in the fight against diseases such as obesity, diabetes, heart disease, cancer, etc. Tree bark is polyphenol-rich and has potential to be used in food supplements. However, it is important to gain insight into the polyphenol profile of different barks to select the material with greatest concentration and diversity. Ultra-performance liquid chromatography (UPLC) was coupled with an ion mobility time-of-flight high-definition/high-resolution mass spectrometer (UPLC-HDMS[E]) to profile ethanol extracts of three common tree barks (*Pinus contorta, Pinus sylvestris, Quercus robur*) alongside a commercial reference (Pycnogenol® extracted from *Pinus pinaster*). Through the use of Progenesis QI informatics software, 35 high scoring components with reported significance to health were tentatively identified across the three bark extracts following broadly the profile of Pycnogenol®. Scots Pine had generally higher compound abundances than in the other two extracts. Oak bark extract showed the lowest abundances but exhibited higher amounts of naringenin and 3-*O*-methylrosmarinic acid. We conclude that forestry bark waste provides a rich source of extractable polyphenols suitable for use in food supplements and so can valorise this forestry waste stream.

Keywords: polyphenolic; Phenol-Explorer; I-Class; Synapt G2-Si; phenolomics

1. Introduction

Polyphenols encompass a very broad range of compounds (e.g., flavonoids, phenolic acids, polyphenolic amides) which can be present in some foods in high concentrations [1]. Consumption of polyphenols can provide significant benefits to human health [2,3]. Most of these positive effects are attributed to their antioxidant and antimicrobial properties which may help prevent a range of diseases, such as cancer and bacterial infections [4,5]. There is also evidence that polyphenols can cross the blood–brain barrier and participate in the regulation of neuropeptides involved in mental wellbeing [6,7]. In relation to the current obesity crisis, polyphenols have also been shown to promote satiety and reduce food intake [8,9]. Specifically, dietary polyphenols have been shown to reduce the proliferation of adipocytes, suppress triglyceride accumulation, stimulate lipolysis, and reduce inflammation [10]. Polyphenols have also been shown to positively alter the gut microbiome [11]. The wide range of perceived benefits associated with polyphenols has led to calls from health agencies to both increase the consumption of polyphenol-rich foods, to breed crops with higher polyphenol contents and to potentially supplement food with polyphenols to promote human wellbeing [12]. A range of controlled trials have subsequently confirmed the benefits of these approaches [13].

One of the major challenges faced by the food industry is that over 8000 polyphenols have thus far been identified in food; however, the evidence base for the short- and long-term health effects for most of these polyphenols remains poorly understood or absent [14]. In addition, the interactive effects of polyphenol mixtures on human health remains virtually unknown [15]. Further, some polyphenols have been shown to be detrimental to human health, particularly when consumed in large quantities [16]. Greater knowledge is therefore needed about the diversity, concentration, and bioavailability of polyphenols in foods and natural products used as food supplements.

The bark, wood, seeds, and leaves of trees frequently contain large quantities of polyphenols which can be readily extracted on an industrial scale [17–19]. Trials have also indicated that wood-derived polyphenols may be useful in the treatment of Type II diabetes and heart disease amongst other ailments [20–22]. This supports historical reports of their use for treating a range of human diseases [23]. The relative abundance of forestry products, therefore, makes them a suitable target for bulk extraction of polyphenols for use in the food and beverage industry and in pharmaceutical and nutraceutical production [24–26]. The concentration and types of polyphenols, however, is known to vary widely between tree species [27,28]. This variation is due to intrinsic differences in secondary metabolism between species, ontological stage, and also the influence of external factors such as climate, herbivory, and soil type [29,30].

Although many approaches are available for the extraction and characterisation of phenolics in tree tissues, many of these lack sensitivity or are designed for targeted analysis of specific phenolic groups with proven bioactive properties. Advances in analytical capability, however, now allow the untargeted analysis and mass profiling of low molecular weight phenolics [31,32]. For example, a UPLC-ESI-QTOF-MS (separation achieved with ultra-performance liquid chromatography (UPLC) followed by electrospray ionization and detection via a quadrupole time-of-flight mass spectrometer) approach was used to putatively annotate 262 phenolic compounds from *Moringa oleifera* leaves [33] and 187 from tea leaves [34]. These approaches, however, have not been widely applied to the bioprospecting of forestry waste. The development of UPLC with ion mobility time-of-flight high definition MS (UPLC-HDMS^E) provides multiple degrees of orthogonal separation and unprecedented peak capacity through the added dimension of ion mobility separation [35,36]. This approach provides increased confidence in interpreting phenolomic datasets and identifying individual compounds. The primary aim of this study was to demonstrate the use of UPLC-HDMS^E for characterising the main polyphenols present in three common bark wastes which can be obtained commercially. Our second aim was to broadly compare our findings to an existing nutraceutical product.

2. Materials and Methods

2.1. Forestry Waste Samples

Representative bulk samples of bark waste were provided by a commercial forestry contractor (B.R. Warner Ltd., Amlwch, Anglesey, UK). The samples were from mature Lodgepole pine (LPP; *Pinus contorta*), Scots pine (SP; *Pinus sylvestris*), and Oak (O; *Quercus robur*). The commercial bark-derived dietary supplement, Pycnogenol® extracted from Maritime pine (*Pinus pinaster*) was used as a reference material. Reviews on the use of Pycnogenol® and its impacts on human health are presented elsewhere [37–39].

2.2. Sample Preparation

Changes in sample preparation methods will alter the polyphenol profile obtained in the subsequent extract. Ethanol was chosen here to provide the highest abundance of polyphenols [40] and also to comply with the EU directive for Good Manufacturing Practice (GMP) for food stuffs [41]. Briefly, each bark sample was ground to a fine powder and then 10 g placed in a glass beaker containing 100 mL of ethanol. After covering with Parafilm®, the mixture was sonicated in an ultrasonic bath for 30 min. Ethanol was chosen as a solvent due to its legislative approval for use in the food industry [41]. The mixture was then left for 24 h at 4 °C before re-sonicating for 30 min. Once the solid material had settled, the liquid layer was placed in polypropylene tubes and centrifuged (10,000 rev min^{-1}, 30 min).

The resultant supernatant was concentrated to 10 mL by gentle heating to 60 °C in a fume cupboard (i.e., 1 mL extract g^{-1} bark). The resultant extract was kept at −20 °C until required. The method described was repeated for each bark type in quadruplicate.

2.3. Analytical Instrumentation

An untargeted, discovery method was developed in negative ion mode using an I-class UPLC with a Synapt G2-Si in $HDMS^E$ mode (Waters UK Ltd., Wilmslow, UK). HD refers to ion mobility while MS^E is a data-independent terminology for an acquisition that gathers mass spectrometer (MS) data, within a specified mass range, on all ions formed in the gas phase. These parent ions are subsequently fragmented to create product ions. The Synapt G2-Si is a quadrupole time-of-flight MS (Q-ToF) with incorporated ion mobility. A Z-Spray™ source was used in which chromatographically separated analytes arrive via one probe and the lock mass is infused via another. A metal baffle was set to switch periodically to allow either the analytes or the lock mass to enter the MS. Data were acquired and stored as continuum spectral data. Leucine enkephalin (Tyr-Gly-Gly-Phe-Leu) was the lock mass chosen for mass axis correction.

2.4. UPLC Conditions

The UPLC used was a Waters I-class instrument equipped with a Waters Cortecs UPLC C18+ 2.7 μm × 2.1 mm × 100 mm superficially porous column. This stationary phase has a positive charge present on the surface which provides better selectivity and peak shape for negatively charged analytes such as polyphenols. The use of 0.1% acetic acid as the mobile phase modifier was found to be the combination of modifier and concentration that gave the highest signal-to-noise ratio for polyphenolic compounds. Briefly, the mobile phase consisted of water modified with 0.1% acetic acid in A and MeOH modified with 0.1% acetic acid in B. The flow rate was 0.5 mL min^{-1}, the column temperature 40 °C and the injection volume 1.0 μL. The mobile phase composition was initially 90% A with 10% B, changing linearly to 1% A with 99% B over 4 min, and finally back to the initial conditions over 0.2 min.

2.5. Synapt G2-Si Conditions

Data were acquired and stored as continuum in a mass range of 50 to 1200 Da in negative ion resolution mode. The cone voltage was set to 40 V and the scan time was set to 0.2 s using an average of 3 scans and a mass window of ± 0.5 Da. The leucine enkephalin lock mass (554.2615 Da) was acquired every 30 s throughout the run but was not used for on-the-fly correction; this mass reference was acquired and stored for later use in data processing.

2.6. Data Processing

$HDMS^E$ data were processed using Progenesis QI software (NonLinear Dynamics Ltd., Newcastle upon Tyne, UK). Firstly, the acquired data were imported, then aligned to compensate for the small drifts in retention time between runs. A between-subjects experimental design was chosen creating 3 groups for the bark extracts, 1 for the reference (Pycnogenol®), and 1 group for blank extracts. Peaks were picked to locate the analytes in the samples and then ions were deconvoluted. These ions were then compared to the ChemSpider Polyphenols database [42] with a 5 ppm precursor tolerance. Theoretical fragmentation (in silico) was also performed with a fragment tolerance of 5 ppm. Only isotope similarity scores above 90% were used and also a filter for elemental composition was set to take into account compounds with elemental composition of H, C, and O. As a result of collecting ion mobility data as well as MS^E data ($HDMS^E$ mode), Progenesis QI was more able to distinguish co-eluting components due to differences in drift times of the parent ions.

Identifications made through comparison to external databases should always be treated as tentative. In Progenesis QI, data were filtered so that only the best quality data were selected for further investigation. Filters were setup to show only compounds that had ANOVA p values ≤ 0.01 and blanks were the lowest mean. All compound abundances lower than 100, with no fragmentation and showing blanks as the highest mean, were removed from the dataset. Of a maximum possible score of 60 for this experimental setup only scores above 40 were chosen for further evaluation. Metrics for retention time similarity and collision cross-section (CCS) similarity were zero.

After processing through Progenesis QI, data were then exported to EZInfo (Umetrics, Umeå, Sweden) which provided a multivariate analysis (MVA) approach to this discovery data. Multivariate data analysis was achieved by undertaking Principal Component Analysis (PCA) in EZInfo giving an overview of the sample data via a scores plot. This plot shows the observations that are likely to be most similar (close together) and also the ones that are most dissimilar (far away) allowing for the visualisation of atypical observations, trends and other patterns within the data. The heat map was produced in Matlab (MatWorks Inc., Natlick, MA, USA).

3. Results and Discussion

3.1. Bioactive Phenolic Compounds in Tree Bark Extracts

A summary of the results obtained from the analysis of the three bark extracts is presented in the detailed Excel file in Supplementary Materials (XL-SM). Tentative identifications for compounds are ordered with the highest scoring results from top to bottom. In summary, a total of 35 components were tentatively identified across the three bark extracts with scores of 40 or above. Accurate mass values are given for parent and main product ions plus retention time (min.), drift time (ms) and normalised abundances for all sample injections. All components showed very low ANOVA-p and q values, indicating a false discovery rate (FDR) approaching zero in many cases with a maximum FDR of 0.5%. Isotope similarity scores above 90 and mass errors of ≤ 5 ppm can also be seen. Pycnogenol®, which was used as a reference material, generally exhibited higher abundances of polyphenols than the bark extracts, which was probably due to the extraction and concentration resulting from its proprietary production process. Additional references are given for each identified polyphenol component which have been shown to have bioactive significance in terms of human health benefits. Three components which could not be distinguished from their isobaric species have their various possibilities listed, which is felt to be better than exclusion. Total ion chromatograms and ion intensity graphs to illustrate the alignment and vector editing processes, are available in supplementary materials (Figures S1–S8). Molecular structures of the 35 identified components can be found in Figure S9.

As an aid to visualisation, a heat map has been created using averaged abundances for each sample type across the 35 identified polyphenols (Figure 1). From this overview of the identifications it can be seen that the 2 *Pinus sp.* more closely represent the general trend of Pycnogenol® (*Pinus pinaster*) than does oak.

It is also noted that compound abundances are generally higher in the Scots Pine extract than in the other two bark extracts with the Oak sample showing the lowest abundances. Oak, on the other hand, does exhibit higher amounts of naringenin and 3-O-methylrosmarinic acid than the other samples. Several biological activities have been ascribed to naringenin, including antioxidant, antitumor, antiviral, antibacterial, anti-inflammatory, antiadipogenic, and cardioprotective effects. The most promising activity being related to cardiovascular disease protection, in pure form and in complex polyphenolic mixtures, and also naringenin's ability to improve endothelial function [43]. The 3-O-methylrosmarinic acid is thought to contribute to the properties of the *Cistus* genus which is a plant used in traditional folk medicine for wound healing and its anti-inflammatory properties [44].

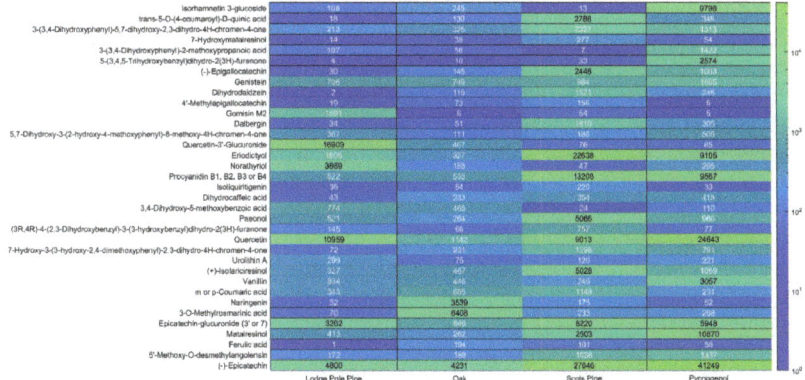

Figure 1. Heat map created using averaged abundances for each sample type across the 35 tentatively identified polyphenols.

As an overview of the data, a scores plot, using principal component analysis (PCA) with Pareto scaling, was created which showed tight clustering of the bark extracts sample replicates and a general separation between bark types (Figure 2). This figure includes an expanded area view of the more closely situated clusters. This shows tight clustering within each group of replicates and clear differences between the sample types. Furthermore, also available in the supplementary material is a loadings bi-plot (Figure S11) which illustrates how the components relate to the samples i.e., the closer an ion is to a sample cluster the more this describes the sample's composition and therefore also highlights the differences between the bark extracts.

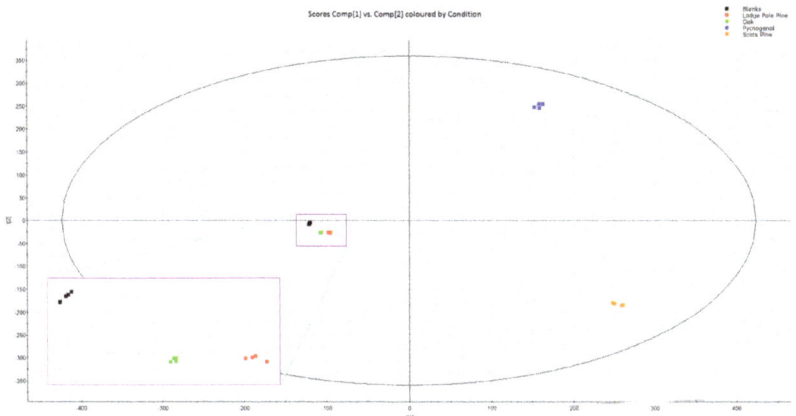

Figure 2. Scores plot with Pareto scaling showing tight clustering of the bark extract sample replicates and separation between bark types including an expanded area view of the more closely situated clusters.

To continue to point out the highlights of this discovery work (additional references for each compound are available in supplementary information) it can be seen in XL-SM and Figure 1 that quercetin, eriodictyol and (−)-epicatechin are compounds with significant abundance. Dietary supplementation with quercetin or plant extracts containing quercetin has been shown to attenuate high fat diet induced obesity and insulin resistance [45] and also decreases inflammation [46]. Quercetin is seen to be abundant across all 4 extracts. Eriodictyol, which is particularly prominent in Scots Pine, has been shown to stimulate insulin secretion in mice islets, improving glucose tolerance and increasing plasma insulin in non-diabetic and diabetic rats [47]. Furthermore, research shows that neuro-inflammatory response to experimental stroke is inhibited by eriodictyol [48] as is inflammation in osteoarthritis [49]. Epicatechin's benefits have been discussed prolifically in literature with a primary focus on anti-oxidant, anti-microbial, anti-inflammatory, and anti-cancer effects [50] plus, more specifically, cardiovascular and neuropsychological health [51].

Quercetin, which is seen in all samples analysed here, and quercetin-3'-glucuronide, which is abundant in lodgepole pine bark, have both been shown to be active against human breast cancer [52]. Furthermore, also abundant in lodgepole pine is norathyriol which is noted for its potential towards suppression of skin cancers induced by UV radiation [53], as a new candidate for the treatment of hypouricaemic [54] and also its regulatory effect on lipid metabolism making it useful for protection against hepatic lipid metabolic disorders and the treatment of non-alcoholic fatty liver disease [55].

The diverse array of higher abundance components is most evident in Scots Pine; some of these components have already been mentioned. In addition, procyanidin (B1, B2, B3 or B4), is observed in Scots Pine bark in very high abundance and is also evident in the other extracts to a lesser extent. These molecules are the pigments often associated with apples, grapes, and berries and their related health benefits. Procyanidins have been reported to target diverse molecular switches in carcinogen metabolism including inflammation, cell proliferation, cell cycle, apoptosis, and the development of new blood vessels (angiogenesis) and consequently studies on Procyanidins have shown that they inhibit the proliferation of various cancer cells in vitro and in vivo [56].

3.2. Tentative Identification of Polyphenols

It is often the case that databases do not contain fragmentation data so in silico theoretical predictions are relied upon here. This can be quite effective in the context of polyphenolic compounds as their mechanisms of fragmentation are well documented. They are generally in the category referred to as Retro-Diels–Alder (RDA) reactions [57]. Furthermore, the sugar moiety, which is present in many polyphenols, may also fragment by RDA. Often, a water loss precedes the RDA fragmentation by remote hydrogen rearrangement, forming an unsaturated sugar moiety, which facilitates the RDA process. All mass spectra are available in the supplementary material (Figure S10).

The parent ion identified at 1.38 min. was m/z 477.1036 which related to [M-H]$^-$ for $C_{22}H_{22}O_{12}$ with a mass error of −0.4 ppm. This gave rise to the product ion m/z 462.0796 which indicates a further loss of CH_3. This was identified as isorhamnetin-3-glucoside which has a ChemSpider ID of CSID4477169 and has the highest score of all components identified in this study. Parent ion, m/z 355.1192, was also observed at 1.38 min which corresponds to [M-H$_2$O-H]$^-$ for 7-hydroxymatairesinol but was separated from m/z 477.1036 by drift time. The former being 4.3400 ms and the latter being 3.2550 ms. The main fragment for 7-Hydroxymatairesinol produced by MS/MS was m/z 340.0948 which also indicates a loss of CH_3 i.e., [M-H$_2$O- CH$_3$-H]$^-$.

At retention time 1.04 min m/z 337.0929 [M-H]$^-$ was observed which gave rise to m/z 163.0389 as the main MS/MS product ion. This indicates the loss of coumaric acid and therefore leads to the identification of trans-5-O-(4-coumaroyl)-D-quinic acid (CSID4945466). Next, 3-(3,4-dihydroxyphenyl)-5,7-dihydroxy-2,3-dihydro-4H-chromen-4-one (CSID35015212) which was present as [2M-H]$^-$. [2M 11 110.001.70] was observed as the main product ion which was probably due to a fission of the C-ring.

The 3-(3,4-dihydroxyphenyl)-2-methoxypropanoic acid (CSID35015213) was identified at 0.93 min by its [M-H$_2$O-H]$^-$ ion at m/z 193.0499 which was further validated by its main product ion m/z 109.0285 which relates to $C_6H_5O_2$. At 2.57 min the [2M-H]$^-$ ion relating to 5-(3,4,5-trihydroxybenzyl)dihydro-2(3H)-furanone is found (m/z 447.1289) with m/z 413.1239 [$C_{11}H_9O_3$+e+M]$^-$ and m/z 343.0811 [$C_7H_5O_2$-H+M]$^-$ being the major product ions resulting from the loss of 34.0050 Da and 104.0478 Da, respectively. An isotope similarity score of 95.4% and a mass accuracy of −1.6 ppm gave credibility to the empirical formula $C_{11}H_{12}O_5$.

The identification of (-)-epigallocatechin was achieved via observation of the [M-H$_2$O-H]$^-$ adduct at m/z 287.0557 eluting at 1.23 min and the main MS/MS fragment of m/z 259.0605 [C$_{14}$H$_{12}$O$_5$-H]$^-$. Next on the table of highest scoring identifications is genistein which is apparent as the [M-H]$^-$ adduct (m/z 269.0448) at 3.85 min. The main MS/MS product ions of m/z 241.0487 [C$_{14}$H$_{10}$O$_4$-H]$^-$ and m/z 225.0542 [C$_{14}$H$_8$O$_3$+e]$^-$ strengthen this identification.

Dihydrodaidzein (CSID154076), was elucidated via its [M-H]$^-$ adduct (m/z 255.0663) at 1.95 min. Major fragments of m/z 223.0749 [C$_{15}$H$_{10}$O$_2$+e]$^-$ and m/z 211.0750 [C$_{14}$H$_{10}$O$_2$+e]$^-$ were observed in the high energy MS/MS signal although other product ions were apparent. It is noted that its drift time of 2.3870 ms differs from that of the co-eluter identified as ferulic acid ([2M-H]$^-$, m/z 387.1071) whose drift time was 3.2008 ms. This illustrates the benefit of the orthogonality of ion mobility spectrometry (IMS) in separating co-eluting components. Ferulic acid also gave the main product ions m/z 326.1159 [C$_9$H$_7$O+e+M]$^-$ and m/z 311.0921 [C$_8$H$_6$O-H+M]$^-$ which agreed with in silico fragmentation. On top of this, further complexity is added by the co-elution of 2 more compounds at 1.95 min. These are (+)-isolariciresinol ([M-H$_2$O-H, M-H]$^-$, 360.1577Da) and dalbergin ([M-H]$^-$ m/z 267.0665) which have drift times of 3.4720 ms and 2.4955 ms, respectively. Good IMS separation can be seen across all four co-eluters in this cluster at 1.95 min which would have otherwise been difficult to transform into tentative identifications. This indicates four parent ions of different size and shape and therefore different CCS values. Portable CCS values are not yet available in databases, to our knowledge, but the future potential here for assisting identification is clear. For completeness the main MS/MS product ions for (+)-isolariciresinol were m/z 341.1394 [C$_{20}$H$_{22}$O$_5$-H]$^-$, m/z 326.1159 [C$_{19}$H$_{19}$O$_5$-H]$^-$, and m/z 283.0971 [C$_{17}$H$_{18}$O$_5$ -H$_2$O-H]$^-$ and for dalbergin m/z 255.0645 [C$_{15}$H$_{11}$O$_4$+e]$^-$ and m/z 211.0750 [C$_{14}$H$_{11}$O$_2$+e]$^-$ were observed.

The 4'-methylepigallocatechin was identified in Progenesis QI at 2.37 min by its [2M-H]$^-$ adduct at m/z 639.1708 and main product ions of m/z 285.0759 [C$_{16}$H$_{13}$O$_5$+e]$^-$ and m/z 183.1017 [C$_9$H$_{12}$O$_4$ -H]$^-$. At 2.52 min, m/z 385.1639 was identified as the [M-H]$^-$ adduct for the allergic inflammation mediator, gomisin M2, which was found at its highest abundance in lodge pole pine. From the MS/MS data, m/z 181.0866 [C$_{10}$H$_{13}$O$_3$+e]$^-$ was observed as the base peak. The 5,7-dihydroxy-3-(2-hydroxy-4-methoxyphenyl)-8-methoxy-4H-chromen-4-one (CSID30777598) was also identified from the [M-H]$^-$ adduct when compared to Phenol-Explorer, which has an accurate mass of m/z 329.0663 at 2.49 min and a base peak product ion of m/z 301.0742 which corresponds to [C$_{16}$H$_{14}$O$_6$-H]$^-$.

The [M-H]$^-$ adduct for procyanidin can be seen at 0.99 min although which isomer this corresponds to cannot be determined by accurate mass alone. The molecule could be B1, B2, B3 or B4. m/z 577.1345 has one base peak fragment at m/z 451.1006 [C$_{24}$H$_{19}$O$_9$+e]$^-$. Comparison of retention time and drift time to analytical standards would help to clarify the correct isomer, or alternatively NMR. Close in terms of drift time to this is m/z 575.1191 which elutes at 0.66 min and is suggested to be eriodictyol as the [2M-H]$^-$ adduct. This has product ions of m/z 451.1031 [C$_{24}$H$_{19}$O$_9$+e]$^-$, m/z 407.0770 [C$_{22}$H$_{16}$O$_8$-H]$^-$ and m/z 289.0711 [C$_{15}$H$_{13}$O$_6$+e]$^-$, which is the same (−1.9 ppm) as the ChemSpider published exact mass of the (-)-epicatechin [M-H]$^-$ adduct. It is also noted that the flavan-3-ol, (-)-epicatechin is observed at 0.83 min and m/z 289.0723 [M-H]$^-$ and is confirmed by its familiar fragment m/z 245.0811 which is due to the loss of 44 Da [M-CH$_3$CHO-H]$^-$ [58]. This component is ubiquitous throughout much of the plant kingdom and can, therefore, be seen to be present in all of the extracts analysed.

Quercetin-3'-glucuronide is identified at 1.70 min and m/z 477.0686 ([M-H]$^-$) which has a mass error of 2.4 ppm compared to its theoretical mass. Product ions were found at m/z 449.0737 which relates to [C$_{20}$H$_{18}$O$_{12}$-H]$^-$ and m/z 286.0115 which is due to the loss of the glucuronide moiety. Furthermore, norathyriol was identified by its [M-H]$^-$ adduct which was visible at 1.22 min m/z 259.0243 with main product ions in MS/MS of m/z 231.0283 ([C$_{12}$H$_8$O$_5$-H]$^-$) and m/z 203.0334 ([C$_{11}$H$_8$O$_4$-H]$^-$). Isoliquiritigenin (CSID553829) was observed via its [M-H]$^-$ adduct, m/z 255.0657, at 1.53 min with its product ion m/z 163.0385 [C$_9$H$_7$O$_3$+e]$^-$ seen as a result of MS/MS. The [2M-H] adduct for dihydrocaffeic acid was identified through its accurate mass of m/z 363.1081 at 1.25 min. The main ions produced in MS/MS were m/z 331.1187 [C$_9$H$_8$O$_2$+e+M]$^-$ and m/z 316.0947 [C$_8$H$_8$O$_2$-H+M]$^-$. The mass error was −1.2 ppm and the isotope similarity scored high at 95.3 out of 100. Similarly, the [2M-H] adduct for 3,4-dihydroxy-5-methoxybenzoic acid was identified through its accurate mass of m/z 367.0654 at 1.48 min with the main product ion being m/z 333.0628 [C$_8$H$_5$O$_3$+e+M]$^-$.

Paeonol, which has a wealth of health claims in current research [59–62], was identified due to the accurate mass of its [2M-H]$^-$ adduct which had a mass error of −0.4 ppm and an isotope similarity of 93.96. This produced a base peak fragment of m/z 316.0947 [C$_8$H$_7$O$_3$-H+M]$^-$ in the high energy MS/MS spectra.

Although it is clear that there are many different arrangements of phenol groups in (3R,4R)-4-(2,3-dihydroxybenzyl)-3-(3-hydroxybenzyl)dihydro-2(3H)-furanone, a tentative identification was made for this molecule, or the five positional isomers, through the [M-H$_2$O-M]$^-$ adduct. This was found at its highest abundance in Scots Pine. The base peak product ion was m/z 269.1185 [C$_{18}$H$_{18}$O$_5$ -CO$_2$-H]$^-$ following the loss of CO$_2$ from the deprotonated parent molecule.

Quercetin, which derives its name from the oak tree, is very much a common component found in the analysis of natural plant products. From its mass spectra, the [M-H]- adduct m/z 301.0357 is seen at 1.50 min which agrees with the accurate mass expected from theory and literature (mass error 1.2 ppm). The base peak product ion m/z 125.0239 is explained by fragment [C$_6$H$_6$O$_3$ -H]$^-$. Epicatechin-3′-glucuronide was identified by its [M-H$_2$O-H]$^-$ adduct at 1.99 min. but could equally be identified as epicatechin-7-glucuronide. The product ions were used to aid with confirmation of identity with the observation of m/z 289.0712 [epicatechin -H]$^-$ and the familiar fragment m/z 245.0807 [epicatechin - CH$_3$CHO -H]$^-$. m/z 177.0535 relates to the remainder of the molecule after the separation of m/z 289.0712 i.e., glucuronic acid minus a phenol group.

The 7-hydroxy-3-(3-hydroxy-2,4-dimethoxyphenyl)-2,3-dihydro-4H-chromen-4-one was identified using its [M-H]- and [M-H$_2$O-H]- adducts at 2.02 min. The mass error was −0.86 ppm. m/z 226.0617 [C$_{11}$H$_{14}$O$_5$+e]$^-$ was seen as the base peak product ion in the MS/MS spectra and also m/z 285.0746 was observed which arose due to the loss of CH$_3$O and the formation of the [C$_{16}$H$_{13}$O$_5$+e]$^-$ ion. Urolithin A was found to be most abundant in Lodgepole Pine. It was identified by the [M-H]$^-$ adduct at 1.51 min and the product ion at m/z 183.0436 which was explained by the loss of CO$_2$, [M-CO$_2$-H]$^-$.

The identification of vanillin was made via the [3M-H] adduct at 0.41 min. and the product ion m/z 134.0361 which is thought to be [C$_8$H$_7$O$_2$ -H]$^-$ i.e., the loss of H$_2$O from the parent. Coumaric acid was also identified although whether this was para or meta could not be determined by this technique. Accurate mass of the [2M-H]$^-$ adduct was used which was present at 1.65 min plus the MS/MS fragment m/z 253.0860, [C$_7$H$_4$+e+M]$^-$ was used for confirmation. From literature, naringenin was expected to be present in oak [63] and was found in greatest abundance in the oak extract data. Naringenin was identified by the [M-H]$^-$ adduct only as the fragmentation was not conclusive and would therefore require more work to make this satisfactory.

The identification of 3-O-methylrosmarinic acid was aided by an array of fragments for identification. The [M-H$_2$O-H]$^-$ was detected at 2.21 min. From the MS/MS spectra, 3 product ions were chosen to strengthen the initial identification using accurate mass. m/z 195.0658 [C$_{10}$H$_{11}$O$_4$+e]$^-$, m/z 135.0443 [C$_8$H$_7$O$_2$+e]$^-$ and m/z 121.0284 [C$_7$H$_6$O$_2$-H]$^-$ were the qualifiers observed with m/z 135.0443 being the base peak. Matairesinol was identified at 2.17 min by its [M-H]$^-$ adduct and the MS/MS fragment m/z 342.1099 [C$_{19}$H$_{19}$O$_6$ -H]$^-$. The product ion showed a 0.44 ppm mass error compared to its theoretical mass and had an isotope similarity of 96.35. To conclude this section, 5′-methoxy-O-desmethylangolensin was identified at 1.36 min by its [M-H]$^-$ adduct and the MS/MS fragment m/z 257.0808 [C$_{15}$H$_{13}$O$_4$+e]$^-$. The [M-H]$^-$ adduct showed a −0.42 ppm mass error compared to its theoretical mass and had an isotope similarity of 91.64.

3.3. Potential Use of Bark Waste for Nutraceutical Production

The wide spectrum of polyphenols found in these bark samples illustrates the potential to produce a nutritional supplement from a range of tree species. It also raises the possibility to blend products from different tree species to obtain a more balanced bioactive phenolic profile. This may involve the use of other tree species not investigated here which may have vastly different physical structures and chemical compositions (e.g., *Betula* spp., *Salix* spp., and *Eucalyptus* spp.). In addition, an expansion of this study is necessary to provide more detail on the importance of factors which may affect the polyphenol profile, such as tree stand age, harvesting season, time, and conditions of storage prior to processing. Future work should also focus on the most efficient and cost-effective extraction techniques. One such route, would be to investigate the use of supercritical fluid extraction i.e., liquid CO_2 (and possibly modifiers such as ethanol) as a food-friendly alternative to the processes detailed here. The fast diffusion rate of liquid CO_2 may result in more rapid extraction. Furthermore, it is shown that different enzymatic pre-treatments can facilitate control of selectivity as to which components are extracted [64]. Extraction solvents may also be recycled from batch to batch. Future work should also focus on the use of the solid waste remaining after the extraction process e.g., conversion into fuel pellets [65].

4. Conclusions

Here we demonstrate the effective use of UPLC-HDMS^E for the detailed analysis of forestry waste and its application in the development of novel food nutritional supplements. In our extracts we identified 35 components with bioactive properties which have the potential to benefit human and animal health by providing a preventative measure against many life threatening conditions. Furthermore, the phenolic components can be easily extracted from low value forestry waste making the low carbon process suitable for commercialisation.

Supplementary Materials: The following are available online at http://www.mdpi.com/2227-9717/8/11/1411/s1, Figure S1: Total ion chromatogram of Lodge Pole Pine, Figure S2: Ion intensity map of Lodge Pole Pine, Figure S3: Total ion chromatogram of Oak, Figure S4: Ion intensity map of Oak, Figure S5: Total ion chromatogram of Scots Pine, Figure S6: Ion intensity map of Scots Pine, Figure S7: Total ion chromatogram of Pycnogenol®, Figure S8: Ion intensity map of Pycnogenol®, Figure S9 Molecular structures of identifications ordered from high to low score value, Figure S10 Mass spectra of identifications ordered from high to low score value, Figure S11 Loadings bi-plot of the bark extract data, XL SM is a spreadsheet of identifications, abundances and additional references.

Author Contributions: The project was conceptualized by C.M.P. who was also responsible for methodology and formal analysis. The samples were prepared and analysed by C.M.P. The first draft of the manuscript was prepared by C.M.P. and reviewed and edited by D.L.J. All authors have read and agreed to the published version of the manuscript.

Funding: This research received no external funding.

Acknowledgments: The authors are very grateful to the Welsh European Funding Office (WEFO) for funding the Centre for Environmental Technology at Bangor University. The authors also acknowledge the kind support of Brian Warner of B. R. Warner Services Ltd. and Radek Braganca at the BioComposites Centre, Bangor University. Furthermore, the kind assistance of E.S. Potter is acknowledged for her work in the creation of the heat map.

Conflicts of Interest: The authors declare that they have no known competing financial interests or personal relationships that could have appeared to influence the work reported in this paper.

References

1. El Gharras, H. Polyphenols: Food sources, properties and applications—A review. *Int. J. Food Sci. Technol.* **2009**, *44*, 2512–2518. [CrossRef]
2. De La Iglesia, R.; Milagro, F.I.; Campión, J.; Boqué, N.; Martínez, J.A. Healthy properties of proanthocyanidins. *BioFactors* **2010**, *36*, 159–168. [CrossRef] [PubMed]
3. Krikorian, R.; Kalt, W.; Mcdonald, J.E.; Shidler, M.D.; Summer, S.S.; Stein, A.L. Cognitive performance in relation to urinary anthocyanins and their flavonoid-based products following blueberry supplementation in older adults at risk for dementia. *J. Funct. Foods* **2019**, 103667. [CrossRef]
4. Watson, R.R.; Preedy, S.Z. *Polyphenols in Human Health and Disease*; Academic Press: Cambridge, MA, USA, 2014; Volume 1.
5. Lattanzio, V.; Kroon, P.A.; Ralph, J.; Harris, P.; Dixon, R.A.; Dangles, O.; Lamotte, O. *Recent Advances in Polyphenol Research*; John Wiley & Sons: Hoboken, NJ, USA, 2008; Volume 1.

6. Liu, Y.; Jia, G.; Gou, L.; Sun, L.; Fu, X.; Lan, N.; Li, S.; Yin, X. Antidepressant-like effects of tea polyphenols on mouse model of chronic unpredictable mild stress. *Pharmacol. Biochem. Behav.* **2013**, *104*, 27–32. [CrossRef] [PubMed]
7. Panickar, K.S. Effects of dietary polyphenols on neuroregulatory factors and pathways that mediate food intake and energy regulation in obesity. *Mol. Nutr. Food Res.* **2013**, *57*, 34–47. [CrossRef] [PubMed]
8. McDougall, G.J.; Stewart, D. The inhibitory effects of berry polyphenols on digestive enzymes. *BioFactors* **2005**, *23*, 189–195. [CrossRef]
9. Zhang, W.L.; Zhu, L.; Jiang, J.G. Active ingredients from natural botanicals in the treatment of obesity. *Obes. Rev.* **2014**, *15*, 957–967. [CrossRef]
10. Wang, S.; Moustaid-Moussa, N.; Chen, L.X.; Mo, H.B.; Shastri, A.; Su, R.; Bapat, P.; Kwun, I.; Shen, C.L. Novel insights of dietary polyphenols and obesity. *J. Nutr. Biochem.* **2014**, *25*, 1–18. [CrossRef]
11. Alonso, V.R.; Guarner, F. Linking the gut microbiota to human health. *Br. J. Nutr.* **2013**, *109* (Suppl. 2), S21–S26. [CrossRef]
12. Espley, R.V.; Bovy, A.; Bava, C.; Jaeger, S.R.; Tomes, S.; Norling, C.; Crawford, J.; Rowan, D.; McGhie, T.K.; Brendolise, C.; et al. Analysis of genetically modified red-fleshed apples reveals effects on growth and consumer attributes. *Plant Biotechnol. J.* **2013**, *11*, 408–419. [CrossRef]
13. Martinez-Dominguez, E.; de la Puerta, R.; Ruiz-Gutierrez, V. Protective effects upon experimental inflammation models of a polyphenol-supplemented virgin olive oil diet. *Inflamm. Res.* **2001**, *50*, 102–106.
14. Cory, H.; Passarelli, S.; Szeto, J.; Tamez, M.; Mattei, J. The role of polyphenols in human health and food systems: A mini-review. *Front. Nutr.* **2018**, *5*, 87. [CrossRef] [PubMed]
15. Vejdovszky, K.; Schmidt, V.; Warth, B.; Marko, D. Combinatory estrogenic effects between the isoflavone genistein and the mycotoxins zearalenone and alternariol in vitro. *Mol. Nutr. Food Res.* **2017**, *61*, 1600526. [CrossRef]
16. Jain, A.; Manghani, C.; Kohli, S.; Nigam, D.; Rani, V. Tea and human health: The dark shadows. *Toxicol. Lett.* **2013**, *220*, 82–87. [CrossRef]
17. Kumar, P.S.; Kumar, N.A.; Sivakumar, R.; Kaushik, C. Experimentation on solvent extraction of polyphenols from natural waste. *J. Mater. Sci.* **2009**, *44*, 5894–5899. [CrossRef]
18. Bolling, B.W.; Chen, C.-Y.O.; McKay, D.L.; Blumberg, J.B. Tree nut phytochemicals: Composition, antioxidant capacity, bioactivity, impact factors. *Nutr. Res. Rev.* **2011**, *24*, 244–275. [CrossRef] [PubMed]
19. Withouck, H.; Boeykens, A.; Broucke, M.V.; Moreira, M.M.; Delerue-Matos, C.; De Cooman, L. Evaluation of the impact of pre-treatment and extraction conditions on the polyphenolic profile and antioxidant activity of Belgium apple wood. *Eur. Food Res. Technol.* **2019**, *245*, 2565–2578. [CrossRef]
20. Feldman, E.B. The scientific evidence for a beneficial health relationship between walnuts and coronary heart disease. *J. Nutr.* **2002**, *132*, 1062S–1101S. [CrossRef] [PubMed]
21. Debeljak, J.; Ferk, P.; Čokolič, M.; Zavratnik, A.; Tavč Benković, E.; Kreft, S.; Štrukelj, B. Randomised, double blind, cross-over, placebo and active controlled human pharmacodynamic study on the influence of silver fir wood extract (Belinal) on post-prandial glycemic response. *Pharmazie* **2016**, *71*, 566–569. [CrossRef]
22. Ogawa, S.; Matsuo, Y.; Tanaka, T.; Yazaki, Y. Utilization of flavonoid compounds from bark and wood. III. Application in health foods. *Molecules* **2018**, *23*, 1860. [CrossRef]
23. Liu, J.K.; Henkel, T. Traditional Chinese medicine (TCM): Are polyphenols and saponins the key ingredients triggering biological activities? *Curr. Med. Chem.* **2002**, *9*, 1483–1485. [CrossRef]
24. Gironi, F.; Piemonte, V. Temperature and solvent effects on polyphenol extraction process from chestnut tree wood. *Chem. Eng. Res. Des.* **2011**, *89*, 857–862. [CrossRef]
25. Comandini, P.; Lerma-García, M.J.; Simó-Alfonso, E.F.; Toschi, T.G. Tannin analysis of chestnut bark samples (Castanea sativa Mill.) by HPLC-DAD-MS. *Food Chem.* **2014**, *157*, 290–295. [CrossRef]
26. Câmara, C.R.S.; Schlegel, V. A review on the potential human health benefits of the black walnut: A comparison with the english walnuts and other tree nuts. *Int. J. Food Prop.* **2016**, *19*, 2175–2189. [CrossRef]
27. Donno, D.; Boggia, R.; Zunin, P.; Cerutti, A.K.; Guido, M.; Mellano, M.G.; Prgomet, Z.; Beccaro, G.L. Phytochemical fingerprint and chemometrics for natural food preparation pattern recognition: An innovative technique in food supplement quality control. *J. Food Sci. Technol. Mysore* **2016**, *53*, 1071–1083. [CrossRef]
28. Zhang, X.X.; Shi, Q.Q.; Ji, D.; Niu, L.X.; Zhang, Y.L. Determination of the phenolic content, profile, and antioxidant activity of seeds from nine tree peony (Paeonia section Moutan DC.) species native to China. *Food Res. Int.* **2017**, *97*, 141–148. [CrossRef]

29. Mailer, R.; Ayton, J. Effect of irrigation and water stress on olive oil quality and yield based on a four year study. *Acta Hortic.* **2011**, *888*, 63–72. [CrossRef]
30. Souza, R.T.D.A.; Silva, D.K.D.A.; Santos, M.V.F.D.; Naumann, H.D.; Magalhães, A.L.R.; Andrade, A.P.D. Association of edaphoclimatic characteristics and variability of condensed tannin content in species from Caatinga. *Rev. Cienc. Agron.* **2020**, *51*, e20196611. [CrossRef]
31. Fraser, K.; Harrison, S.J.; Lane, G.A.; Otter, D.E.; Hemar, Y.; Quek, S.Y.; Rasmussen, S. Analysis of low molecular weight metabolites in tea using mass spectrometry-based analytical methods. *Crit. Rev. Food Sci. Nutr.* **2014**, *54*, 924–937. [CrossRef] [PubMed]
32. Kang, K.B.; Woo, S.; Ernst, M.; van der Hooft, J.J.; Nothias, L.F.; da Silva, R.R.; Dorrestein, P.C.; Sung, S.H.; Lee, M. Assessing specialized metabolite diversity of Alnus species by a digitized LC-MS/MS data analysis workflow. *Phytochemistry* **2020**, *173*, 11229. [CrossRef]
33. Rocchetti, G.; Blasi, F.; Montesano, D.; Ghisoni, S.; Marcotullio, M.C.; Sabatini, S.; Cossignani, L.; Lucini, L. Impact of conventional/non-conventional extraction methods on the untargeted phenolic profile of Moringa oleifera leaves. *Food Res. Int.* **2019**, *115*, 319–327. [CrossRef]
34. Damiani, E.; Carloni, P.; Rocchetti, G.; Senizza, B.; Tiano, L.; Joubert, E.; de Beer, D.; Lucini, L. Impact of cold versus hot brewing on the phenolic profile and antioxidant capacity of rooibos (Aspalathus linearis) herbal tea. *Antioxidants* **2019**, *8*, 499. [CrossRef]
35. Zhang, C.; Zuo, T.; Wang, X.; Wang, H.; Hu, Y.; Li, Z.; Li, W.; Jia, L.; Qian, Y.; Yang, W.; et al. Integration of data-dependent acquisition (DDA) and data-independent high-definition MSE (HDMSE) for the comprehensive profiling and characterization of multicomponents from panax japonicus by UHPLC/IM-QTOF-MS. *Molecules* **2019**, *24*, 2708. [CrossRef]
36. Johnson, S.R.; Rikli, H.G. Aspartic acid isomerization characterized by high definition mass spectrometry significantly alters the bioactivity of a novel toxin from poeciloptheria. *Toxins* **2020**, *12*, 207. [CrossRef]
37. Rohdewald, P. A review of the French maritime pine bark extract (Pycnogenol (R)), a herbal medication with a diverse clinical pharmacology. *Int. J. Clin. Pharmacol. Ther.* **2002**, *40*, 158–168. [CrossRef]
38. Mármol, I.; Quero, J.; Jiménez-Moreno, N.; Rodríguez-Yoldi, M.J.; Ancín-Azpilicueta, C. A systematic review of the potential uses of pine bark in food industry and health care. *Trends Food Sci. Technol.* **2019**, *88*, 558–566. [CrossRef]
39. Fogacci, F.; Tocci, G.; Sahebkar, A.; Presta, V.; Banach, M.; Cicero, A.F.G. Effect of pycnogenol on blood pressure: Findings from a PRISMA compliant systematic review and meta-analysis of randomized, double-blind, placebo-controlled, clinical studies. *Angiology* **2020**, *71*, 217–225. [CrossRef]
40. Mello, B.C.B.S.; Petrus, J.C.C.; Hubinger, M.D. Concentration of flavonoids and phenolic compounds in aqueous and ethanolic propolis extracts through nanofiltration. *J. Food Eng.* **2010**, *96*, 533–539. [CrossRef]
41. EU. Directive 2009/32/EC of the European Parliament and of the Council of 23 April 2009 on the Approximation of the Laws of the Member States on Extraction Solvents Used in the Production of Foodstuffs and Food Ingredients. 2009. Available online: https://eur-lex.europa.eu/legal-content/EN/ALL/?uri=CELEX%3A32009L0032 (accessed on 3 November 2020).
42. Vos, F.; Crespy, V.; Chaffaut, L.; Mennen, L.; Knox, C.; Neveu, V. Original article phenol-explorer: An online comprehensive database on polyphenol contents in foods. *Database* **2010**, *2010*, bap024. [CrossRef]
43. Salehi, B.; Fokou, P.V.T.; Sharifi-Rad, M.; Zucca, P.; Pezzani, R.; Martins, N.; Sharifi-Rad, J. The therapeutic potential of naringenin: A review of clinical trials. *Pharmaceuticals* **2019**, *12*, 11. [CrossRef]
44. Mastino, P.M.; Mauro, M.; Jean, C.; Juliano, C.; Marianna, U. Analysis and potential antimicrobial activity of phenolic compounds in the extracts of cistus creticus subspecies from sardinia. *Nat. Prod. J.* **2018**, *8*, 166–174. [CrossRef]
45. Forney, L.; Lenard, N.; Stewart, L.; Henagan, T. Dietary quercetin attenuates adipose tissue expansion and inflammation and alters adipocyte morphology in a tissue-specific manner. *Int. J. Mol. Sci.* **2018**, *19*, 895. [CrossRef]
46. Rotelli, A.E.; Guardia, T.; Juárez, A.O.; De La Rocha, N.E.; Pelzer, L.E. Comparative study of flavonoids in experimental models of inflammation. *Pharmacol. Res.* **2003**, *48*, 601–606. [CrossRef]
47. Hameed, A.; Hafizur, R.M.; Hussain, N.; Raza, S.A.; Rehman, M.; Ashraf, S.; Ul-Haq, Z.; Khan, F.; Abbas, G.; Choudhary, M.I. Eriodictyol stimulates insulin secretion through cAMP/PKA signaling pathway in mice islets. *Eur. J. Pharmacol.* **2018**, *820*, 245–255. [CrossRef] [PubMed]

48. de Oliveira Ferreira, E.; Fernandes, M.Y.S.D.; de Lima, N.M.R.; Neves, K.R.T.; do Carmo, M.R.S.; Lima, F.A.V.; Fonteles, A.A.; Menezes, A.P.F.; de Andrade, G.M. Neuroinflammatory response to experimental stroke is inhibited by eriodictyol. *Behav. Brain Res.* **2016**, *312*, 321–332. [CrossRef]
49. Wang, Y.; Chen, Y.; Chen, Y.; Zhou, B.; Shan, X.; Yang, G. Biomedicine & pharmacotherapy eriodictyol inhibits IL-1β-induced in fl ammatory response in human osteoarthritis chondrocytes. *Biomed. Pharmacother.* **2018**, *107*, 1128–1134. [CrossRef] [PubMed]
50. Prakash, M.; Basavaraj, B.V.; Chidambara Murthy, K.N. Biological functions of epicatechin: Plant cell to human cell health. *J. Funct. Foods* **2019**, *52*, 14–24. [CrossRef]
51. Bernatova, I. Biological activities of (−)-epicatechin and (−)-epicatechin-containing foods: Focus on cardiovascular and neuropsychological health. *Biotechnol. Adv.* **2018**, *36*, 666–681. [CrossRef] [PubMed]
52. Wu, Q.; Needs, P.W.; Lu, Y.; Kroon, P.A.; Ren, D.; Yang, X. Different antitumor effects of quercetin, quercetin-3′-sulfate and quercetin-3-glucuronide in human breast cancer MCF-7 cells. *Food Funct.* **2018**, *9*, 1736–1746. [CrossRef]
53. Li, J.; Malakhova, M.; Mottamal, M.; Reddy, K.; Kurinov, I.; Carper, A.; Langfald, A.; Oi, N.; Kim, M.O.; Zhu, F.; et al. Norathyriol suppresses skin cancers induced by solar ultraviolet radiation by targeting ERK kinases. *Cancer Res.* **2012**, *72*, 260–271. [CrossRef]
54. Lin, H.; Tu, C.; Niu, Y.; Li, F.; Yuan, L.; Li, N.; Xu, A.; Gao, L.; Li, L. Dual actions of norathyriol as a new candidate hypouricaemic agent: Uricosuric effects and xanthine oxidase inhibition. *Eur. J. Pharmacol.* **2019**, *853*, 371–380. [CrossRef] [PubMed]
55. Li, J.; Liu, M.; Yu, H.; Wang, W.; Han, L.; Chen, Q.; Ruan, J.; Wen, S.; Zhang, Y.; Wang, T. Mangiferin improves hepatic lipid metabolism mainly through its metabolite-norathyriol by modulating SIRT-1/AMPK/SREBP-1c signaling. *Front. Pharmacol.* **2018**, *9*, 1–13. [CrossRef]
56. Lee, Y. Cancer chemopreventive potential of procyanidin. *Toxicol. Res.* **2017**, *33*, 273–282. [CrossRef] [PubMed]
57. Lopes, N.P. Natural product reports. *Nat. Prod. Rep.* **2016**, *33*. [CrossRef]
58. Pandey, R.; Chandra, P.; Arya, K.R.; Kumar, B. Development and validation of an ultra high performance liquid chromatography electrospray ionization tandem mass spectrometry method for the simultaneous determination of selected flavonoids in Ginkgo biloba. *J. Sep. Sci.* **2014**, *37*, 3610–3618. [CrossRef]
59. Hsieh, C.L.; Cheng, C.Y.; Tsai, T.H.; Lin, I.H.; Liu, C.H.; Chiang, S.Y.; Lin, J.G.; Lao, C.J.; Tang, N.Y. Paeonol reduced cerebral infarction involving the superoxide anion and microglia activation in ischemia-reperfusion injured rats. *J. Ethnopharmacol.* **2006**, *106*, 208–215. [CrossRef]
60. Kim, S.H.; Kim, S.A.; Park, M.K.; Kim, S.H.; Park, Y.D.; Na, H.J.; Kim, H.M.; Shin, M.K.; Ahn, K.S. Paeonol inhibits anaphylactic reaction by regulating histamine and TNF-α. *Int. Immunopharmacol.* **2004**, *4*, 279–287. [CrossRef]
61. Wu, J.B.; Song, N.N.; Wei, X.B.; Guan, H.S.; Zhang, X.M. Protective effects of paeonol on cultured rat hippocampal neurons against oxygen-glucose deprivation-induced injury. *J. Neurol. Sci.* **2008**, *264*, 50–55. [CrossRef]
62. Ye, S.; Liu, X.; Mao, B.; Yang, L.; Liu, N. Paeonol enhances thrombus recanalization by inducing vascular endothelial growth factor 165 via ERK1/2 MAPK signaling pathway. *Mol. Med. Rep.* **2016**, *13*, 4853–4858. [CrossRef]
63. Zhang, B.; Cai, J.; Duan, C.-Q.; Reeves, M.J.; He, F. A review of polyphenolics in oak woods. *Int. J. Mol. Sci.* **2015**, *16*, 6978–7014. [CrossRef]
64. Mill, O.L.; Antunes-ricardo, M.; García-cayuela, T.; Ibañez, E. Enzyme-assisted in situ supercritical fluid extraction of isorhamnetin conjugates from Opuntia ficus-indica (L.) Mill Marilena Antunes-Ricardo. *Inst. Food Sci. Res.* **2019**, *141*, 71–72. [CrossRef]
65. Arshadi, M.; Gref, R.; Geladi, P.; Dahlqvist, S.A.; Lestander, T. The influence of raw material characteristics on the industrial pelletizing process and pellet quality. *Fuel Process. Technol.* **2008**, *89*, 1442–1447. [CrossRef]

Publisher's Note: MDPI stays neutral with regard to jurisdictional claims in published maps and institutional affiliations.

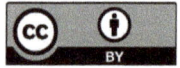

© 2020 by the authors. Licensee MDPI, Basel, Switzerland. This article is an open access article distributed under the terms and conditions of the Creative Commons Attribution (CC BY) license (http://creativecommons.org/licenses/by/4.0/).

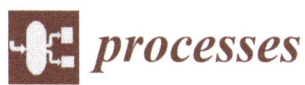

Article

Determination of the Total Polyphenols Content and Antioxidant Activity of *Echinacea Purpurea* Extracts Using Newly Manufactured Glassy Carbon Electrodes Modified with Carbon Nanotubes

Florin Banica [1], Simona Bungau [1,*], Delia Mirela Tit [1], Tapan Behl [2,*], Pavel Otrisal [3], Aurelia Cristina Nechifor [4], Daniela Gitea [1], Flavia-Maria Pavel [5] and Sebastian Nemeth [1]

1. Department of Pharmacy, Faculty of Medicine and Pharmacy, University of Oradea, 29 N. Jiga St., 410028 Oradea, Romania; florinbanica1@gmail.com (F.B.); mirela_tit@yahoo.com (D.M.T.); gitea_daniela@yahoo.co.uk (D.G.); sebinemeth@yahoo.com (S.N.)
2. Chitkara College of Pharmacy, Chitkara University, Punjab 140401, India
3. Faculty of the Physical Culture, Palacký University Olomouc, 77111 Olomouc, Czech Republic; pavel.otrisal@upol.cz
4. Department of Analytical Chemistry, Faculty of Applied Chemistry and Materials Science University Politehnica of Bucharest,1-7 Polizu St., 011061 Bucharest, Romania; aureliacristinanechifor@gmail.com
5. Department of Preclinical Disciplines, Faculty of Medicine and Pharmacy, University of Oradea, 410073 Oradea, Romania; flavia.bontze@gmail.com
* Correspondence: sbungau@uoradea.ro (S.B.); tapanbehl31@gmail.com (T.B.); Tel.: +40-726-776588 (S.B.); +91-852517931 (T.B.)

Received: 17 June 2020; Accepted: 8 July 2020; Published: 13 July 2020

Abstract: A sensitive electrochemical method was used for the determination of the total phenolic content and antioxidant activity of *Echinacea purpurea* extracts. In this study, 3 glassy carbon electrodes (GCE) were used: one unmodified and the other two newly manufactured glassy carbon electrodes modified with carbon nanotubes (CNTs) and chitosan (CS) in different concentrations, having the following composition: 1 mg/mL CNTs/CS 5%/GCE and 20 mg/mL CNTs/CS 0.5%/GCE. The determinations were performed on 3 different pharmaceutical forms (capsules, tablets and tincture), which contain *E. pururea* extract from the root or aerial part of the plant. Standard chicoric and caftaric polyphenolic acids, as well as food supplements extracts, were characterized using voltammetry, in a Britton-Robinson (B-R) electrolyte buffer. The modified 1 mg/mL CNTs/CS 5%/GCE electrode has superior properties compared to the other two (the unmodified and 20 mg/mL CNTs/CS 0.5%/GCE-modified) electrodes used in the study. *Echinacea* tincture had the highest antioxidant capacity and the biggest total amount of polyphenols (28.72 mg/equivalent of 500 mg powder). *Echinacea* capsules had the lowest antioxidant capacity, but also the lowest total amount of polyphenols (19.50 mg/500 mg powder); similarly, tablets had approximately the same values of polyphenols content (19.80 mg/500 mg powder), and also antioxidant capacity. The total polyphenol content was consistent with the one indicated by the manufacturers. Pulse-differential cyclic voltammetry represents a rapid, simple and sensitive technique to establish the entire polyphenolic amount and the antioxidant activity of the *E. purpurea* extracts.

Keywords: polyphenols; antioxidant activity; *Echinacea purpurea* extracts; glassy carbon electrode (GCE); carbon nanotubes (CNTs)

1. Introduction

Echinacea purpurea (L.) Moench, which is included in the Asteraceae (Compositae) family, is acknowledged to be one of the most significant medicinal plants worldwide. The extracts obtained from different parts of *Echinacea purpurea* were traditionally used in North America as remedies for wounds and different types of infections, and came to be extremely well-known herbal remedies [1]. Dietary supplements and extracts of this plant present antiviral, antibacterial, antifungal and antioxidant action, different parts of many plants being used from antiquity [2] to treat viral and inflammatory illnesses [1,3]. Many studies have revealed that *Echinacea* extracts promote the secretion of cytokines like interleukins (Il-1, Il-6, Il-8, Il-12), tumour necrosis factor alfa (TNF-α) and nitric oxide (NO), and an increased activation of macrophages [4–6]. The most significant potential active substances found in *E. purpurea* are represented by polyphenols—derivatives of caffeic acid, as follows: chicoric acid, chlorogenic acid, caftaric acid, echinacoside and cynarin [7,8].

All species of *Echinacea* that were studied presented radical scavenging action, the most efficient being *E. purpurea* [8]. The principal component of *Echinacea* root—chicoric acid (Figure 1A)—is considered a significant antioxidant in the plant, being a suitable marker for the quality of products containing this plant, due to its powerful immunostimulatory, antioxidant and antiviral characteristics and due to its degradation susceptibility [9,10]. Another important phenolic component in *E. purpurea* is caftaric acid (Figure 1B), which inhibits the oxidation of low-density lipoprotein (LDL) cholesterol isolated from human plasma and removes 2,2-diphenyl-1-picrylhydrazyl (DPPH) free radicals in a cell-free assay [11].

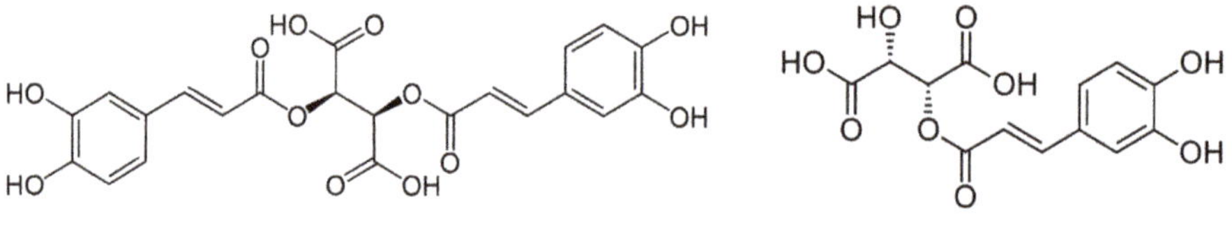

Figure 1. Structural formula: (**A**) Chicoric acid, (**B**) Caftaric acid.

Various researchers have focused on studying the antioxidant activity and polyphenolic composition of *Echinacea* extracts using different methods, such as High-Performance Liquid Chromatography (HPLC) and Ultra-High Performance Liquid Chromatography (UPLC) techniques [12–14], colorimetric methods—chemical 2,2-diphenyl-1-picrylhydrazyl (DPPH) and 2,2′-Azino-bis(3-ethyl-benzothiazoline-6-sulfonic acid) (ABTS)—radical scavenging techniques [3,8,10]. In general, chemical methods need various preparation stages and extended duration to finish the measurement. Nevertheless, prolonged steps and complexness in some of the methods above makes them inappropriate for precise determination. Therefore, rapid and simple techniques have become a significant requirement. Lately, it has been noted that electrochemical methods may be established to determine the polyphenolic composition [15–18]. Electrochemical methods that are used for the determination are simple and sensitive. Furthermore, voltammetric methods show very good functioning in terms of enhanced sensitivity, reduced overpotential and decreased detection limit [19,20]. Square Wave Voltammetry was used to determination of the antioxidant activity in *Echinacea purpurea* roots [21].

At present, carbon nanotubes (CNTs) are extensively used as modifiers due to their physicochemical attributes, distinctive structure and compatibility with biological molecules. CNTs are considered an essential category of nanomaterials. Because of their specific properties—mechanical, chemical and electrical—they have been seen as analytical tools, being considered as rolled up graphite sheets connected by Van der Waal's bonds [22]. The reactivity of graphene sheet as compared to the nanotubes' chemical reactivity improved as a direct outcome of the CNT surface curvature [23].

Recent studies showed that transforming electrodes by adding carbon CNTs makes the electrochemical processes that involve biomolecules easier and enhances the measured signal. The development of electrochemical sensors has attracted considerable attention as a low-cost method for the sensitive detection of a variety of pharmaceutical analytes. Since the discovery of CNTs in 1991 [24], research on them has grown rapidly. In recent years, CNTs have also been used as electrode-modified materials because they offer unique advantages, including enhanced electronic properties, a large edge plane/basal plane ratio, and electron transfer reactions [25]. Thus, CNTs-based sensors generally have higher sensitivities in a low concentration or in the complex matrix, lower limits of detection and faster electron transfer kinetics than traditional carbon electrodes.

Many factors need to be investigated in order to create an optimal CNTs-based sensor. Electrode performance can be influenced by the pretreatment of the nanotube, CNTs surface modification, the method of electrode attachment and the addition of electron mediators. With the further development of CNTs and nanotechnology, studies on preparation, properties and application of CNTs-based modified electrodes have still been a hot topic attracting lots of researchers around the world. This research focused on the application of CNTs-modified electrodes in different pharmaceutical analytes, which mainly includes the electrochemical studies on weak basic/acidic pharmaceuticals and other related small biological molecules. The physical and catalytic properties make CNTs ideal for use in sensors with extremely varied applications [26]. Most notably, CNTs display high electrical conductivity, chemical stability and mechanical strength [27]. A disadvantage of using CNTs can be considered the low wettability of their surface, which induces a weak surface bond [28]. This involves improving the mechanical properties of CNTs with chitosan (CS), a natural polysaccharide used in pharmaceutical [29] and medical applications [30,31], having the role of fixing CNTs to the glassy carbon electrode (GCE) surface and to functionalize the CNTs in order to increase their electroactive surface.

The aim of this study was to determine the total polyphenolic content and, secondary, the antioxidant capacity of commercial food supplements containing extracts of *Echinacea purpurea*, through differential pulse voltammetry, using both an unmodified glassy carbon electrode (GCE) and two modified with CNTs. The novelty of the paper consists precisely in the use of these glassy carbon electrodes modified with CNTs, newly manufactured by the authors, which, after being characterized by cyclic voltammetry, were observed to generate oxidation/reduction peaks, higher than other types of electrodes. The method of analysis with the modified electrode is original due to the fact that, to our knowledge, no voltammetric dosing of polyphenols has been performed using electrodes modified with CNTs and CS.

2. Materials and Methods

2.1. Reagents

In this research, standard chicoric and caftaric polyphenolic acids, as well as food supplement extracts, were characterized using voltammetry, in a Britton-Robinson (B-R) electrolyte buffer. The characteristics of the standard substances and reagents that were used are described in Table 1. Double-distilled water was used to prepare the solutions. The studied products are commercial and were purchased from pharmaceutical units, and they are presented in Table 2.

Table 1. Reagents used.

Reagent	Purity	CAS	Supplier	Purpose of Usage
1,1-diphenyl-2-picrylylhydrazyl	≥98% (HPLC)	1898-66-4	Sigma-Aldrich, USA	DPPH method
Acetone	p.a. ≥ 99%	67-64-1	Chempur, Poland	Solvent
Boric acid	p.a. ≥ 99%	10043-35-3	Micromchim, Romania	Buffer B-R preparation
Caftaric acid (2-Caffeoyl-L-tartaric acid)	≥97.0%	67879-58-7	Sigma-Aldrich, USA	Dosage

Table 1. Cont.

Reagent	Purity	CAS	Supplier	Purpose of Usage
Cichoric/Chicoric acid (2,3-Dicaffeoyl-L-tartaric acid)	≥95%, (HPLC)	6537-80-0	Sigma-Aldrich, USA	Dosage
Copper (II) sulphate pentahydrate	≥98%	7758-99-8	Sigma-Aldrich, USA	Interferent
D-(+)-glucose monohydrate	7.0–9.5% water	14431-43-7	Sigma-Aldrich, USA	Interferent
Ethanol	95%	64-17-5	Chempur, Poland	Solvent
Folin-Ciocalteu reagent	-	12111-13-6	Sigma-Aldrich, USA	Total content of polyphenolic compounds determination
Gallic acid	≥98% (HPLC)	5995-86-8	Sigma-Aldrich, USA	DPPH antioxidant activity determination
Glacial acetic acid	p.a. ≥ 99%	64-19-7	Chempur, Poland	Buffer B-R preparation
Chitosan	Low molecular weight	9012-76-4	Merck, Germany	Modified electrode preparation
L-ascorbic acid	≥99%	50-81-7	Sigma-Aldrich, USA	DPPH antioxidant activity determination
Magnesium chloride	Anhydrous, ≥98%	7786-30-3	Sigma-Aldrich, USA	Interferent
Methanol	≥99%	67-56-1	Chempur, Poland	Solvent
MWCNT	≤100%	308068-56-6	Sigma-Aldrich, USA	Modified electrode preparation
Nickel (II) sulphate hexahydrate	≥98%	10101-97-0	Chempur, Poland	Interferent
Phenol	99–100.5%	108-95-2	Sigma-Aldrich, USA	Interferent
Phosphoric acid	ACS reagent, ≥85 wt.% in H_2O	7664-38-2	Merck, Germany	Buffer B-R preparation
Potassium ferricyanide, Red prussiate	≥99%	13746-66-2	Merck, Germany	Redox couple
Potassium ferrocyanide, Yellow prussiate	≥98.5%	14459-95-1	Merck, Germany	Redox couple
Potassium nitrate	≥99%	7757-79-1	Merck, Germany	Interferent
Resorcinol	≥99%	108-46-3	Chempur, Poland	Interferent
Sodium carbonate	BioXtra, ≥99.0%	497-1908	Chempur, Poland	Total content of polyphenolic compounds determination
Sodium hydroxide	BioXtra, ≥98.0% (acidimetric), pellets (anhydrous)	1310-73-2	Chempur, Poland	Interferent
Sodium chloride	≥99%	7647-14-5	Sigma-Aldrich, USA	Interferent
Tartaric acid	≥99.5%	87-69-4	Sigma-Aldrich, USA	Interferent
Uric acid	≥99%	69-93-2	Chempur, Poland	Interferent

HPLC–High-Performance Liquid Chromatography; DPPH–2,2-diphenyl-1-picrylhydrazyl; MWCNT–Multiwall carbon nanotube; B-R–Britton-Robinson; ACS–American Chemical Society; H_2O–water.

Table 2. Pharmaceutical forms with Echinacea.

	Manufacturer	Content	Category
Capsules 500 mg	Cosmopharm, Bucharest, Romania	Concentrated *Echinacea* extract, 20 mg polyphenols	Natural immunostimulant
Tablets 500 mg	Alevia, Fălticeni, Romania	*Echinacea Purpurea* standardized extract, 4% polyphenols	Food supplement
Tincture 50 mL	Dacia Plant, Bod, Romania	Extract 1: 3.75 in hydroalcoholic solution (ethyl alcohol/water—35/65 by mass) from aerial parts of *Echinacea purpurea*	Food supplement

2.2. Solutions and Sample Preparation

The stock solutions of chicoric acid and caftaric acid, both 25 mmol/L, were prepared in a volumetric mixture of ethanol/water (1:1), and B-R buffer was used for the range of pH 2 to 10, with the buffer consisting of a mixture of 3 acids, as follows: H_3PO_4, H_3BO_3 and CH_3COOH, all of them at a concentration of 0.04 mol/L. pH adjustment was done with 0.01 mol/L NaOH.

Extraction of caffeic acid derivatives from the pharmaceutical forms was performed by dissolving/diluting a quantity/volume of powder/solution in a mixture of 20 mL acetone: water = 60:40, under continuous stirring, for 30 min, after which the mixture was centrifuged for 15 min at 5000 rpm. The acetone:water extract was dried in a rotary evaporator at 30 °C, then dissolved in a mixture of methanol:water = 1:1 [21]. The solution obtained is diluted with B-R buffer, obtaining solutions of different concentrations for which the voltammograms are recorded.

Stock solutions were stored at −5 °C, protected from light. When using the solutions, they are protected by wrapping the voltammetric cell with aluminum foil. Stock solutions can be stored for up to 5 weeks.

All measurements were performed in triplicate.

2.3. Apparatus

Voltammetric measurements were performed with an Autolab PGSTAT 128N electrochemical device (Utrecht, Kingdom of the Netherlands), using Nova 2.1.2 software, in a 20 mL electrochemical cell, equipped with 3 electrodes: reference electrode Ag/AgCl, auxiliary platinum (Pt) electrode wire and working glass carbon electrode (GCE, 3 mm diameter, Metrohm-Autolab, Switzerland). All of the measurements were performed at room temperature (25 ± 2 °C). The voltammetric peak intensities were measured using the baseline corresponding to each peak. The pH of the B-R buffer solution was adjusted with 0.01 M NaOH solution, using the Brinkmann Metrohm 632 pH-meter (Metrohm AG, Herisau, Switzerland) equipped with a combined pH electrode. Spectrophotometric determinations were performed using T70 ultraviolet-visible (UV-VIS) spectrometer with sequential automatic scanning (PG Instruments Ltd., Leicestershire, United Kingdom), controlled by UVWIN software.

2.4. Preparation of CNTs in CS

For the modification of the GCE, a solution of CS 5% in 2% acetic acid solution was prepared. CNTs were dispersed in this solution so as to obtain a solution of concentration 1 mg CNTs/mL, in an ultrasonication bath SONOREX SUPER (Bandelin-Electronic GmbH & Co. KG, Berlin, Germany), at a temperature of 25 ± 2 °C, for 30 min (1 mg/mL CNTs/CS 5%/GCE). Another suspension prepared for electrode modification contained 20 mg CNTs/mL 0.5% CS solution in 2% acetic acid solution (20 mg/mL CNTs/CS 0.5%/GCE) [32,33]. CS has the role of fixing the strong electroactive material of CNTs to the surface of the glassy carbon electrode.

2.5. Preparation of Modified GCE

Two types of methods (physical and chemical) were used to clean the electrode for every work phase. The physical treatment consisted of polishing the electrode manually, using alumina power (Ø = 0.3 micron), for one minute, then rinsing it using deionized water. The chemical treatment consisted of sonicating the electrode in 6 M HCl solution for three minutes and rinsing it using deionized water, followed by sonication in ethanol for three minutes, then rinsing with deionized water. The modification of the glass carbon electrode was performed by depositing 5 µL suspension of CNTs in CS, followed by air drying.

2.6. Determination of the Total Polyphenol Content

2.6.1. Differential Pulse Voltammetry

To calculate the amount of caffeic acid and catechins in pharmaceutical forms, the following steps were taken: knowing the current intensity for the mixture of standard solution of caffeic and chicoric acids, the current intensities for caffeic acid (approximately 0.203 ± 0.007 V), mixture of caffeic acid + chicoric (approximately 0.520 ± 0.024 V) and catechins (approximately 0.690 ± 0.005 V) were combined, and a proportionality calculation determined the respective compounds. These calculations were performed due to the fact that in *Echinacea* extracts, there are polyphenols that could be attributed to caffeic acid and catechins.

2.6.2. Spectrophotometry

The total content of polyphenolic compounds in *Echinacea purpurea* extracts was colorimetrically determined, using Folin-Ciocalteu reagent and gallic acid (GA) [34]. The selection of GA as a standard was based on its availability to be stable in the pure substance state. Folin-Ciocalteu reagent is used for colorimetric analysis of phenolic and polyphenolic antioxidants. Basically, a sample of 0.2 mL of *Echinacea purpurea* extract was added to a test tube and mixed with 2 mL of Folin-Ciocalteu reagent; after 5 min of reaction, 1.8 mL of sodium carbonate (7.5%) was added. The absorbance was measured at 750 nm, using the UV-VIS spectrophotometer. The curve was established for analysis using GA. The polyphenolic content was determined using the standard GA calibration curve and expressed in mg of GA equivalents (GAE).

2.7. Antioxidant Activity Determination

2.7.1. Cyclic Voltammetry

To draw a calibration line, a 10^{-2} M ascorbic acid (AA) solution was prepared and was used to record the differential pulse voltammograms for 7 AA solutions (with concentrations between 0.25 and 4.59 mM) in B-R buffer. Similarly, a 10^{-2} M GA solution was prepared for tracing a calibration line that was used to record differential pulse voltammograms for 10 GA solutions (with concentrations between 0.25 and 6.55 mM) in B-R buffer.

2.7.2. DPPH Method

The antioxidant activity of the standardized *Echinacea purpurea* extract was measured with a stable free radical 1,1-diphenyl-2-picrilhydrazyl (DPPH) according to the Briefly method [35]. The method involves reducing the DPPH staining (from purple to yellow) in the presence of a phenolic antioxidant (FeOH), in methanolic solution, according to the reactions:

$$DPPH\cdot + FeOH \rightarrow DPPH\text{-}H + FeO\cdot$$

$$DPPH\text{-}H + FeO\cdot \rightarrow Degradation/oxidation\ products$$

The DPPH method is based on the reaction with electron donors or hydrogen radicals (H·) producing antioxidant compounds. It was found that the ability to capture free radicals from extracts increases with increasing concentrations of antioxidants. The reduction in DPPH is directly proportional to the amount of antioxidant present in the reaction mixture.

Each analyzed extract (0.20 mL of the previously prepared solutions) was mixed with 2.80 mL 0.1 mM of freshly prepared solution of DPPH radical in methanol. The mixture was kept in the dark for 15 min at 37 °C, after which its absorbance was read at 517 nm in 1 cm quartz cuvettes, compared to a solution of DPPH radical in methanol. Antioxidant activity was expressed as mM equivalents of AA per g dry weight (DW), using the calibration curve constructed with 0.05, 0.1, 0.2, 0.3, 0.4 and

0.5 mM AA dissolved in methanol and with the same concentrations of GA (0.05, 0.1, 0.2, 0.3, 0.4 and 0.5 mM) also dissolved in methanol.

3. Results

3.1. Electrochemical Characterization of Electrodes by Cyclic Voltammetry

In order to characterize the modified electrode, cyclic voltammetry was used for a redox probe, consisting of 2 electroactive species $K_3[Fe(CN)_6]/K_4[Fe(CN)_6]$, in the form of a 10 mM solution in B-R buffer. Scanning voltammetry was performed in the range −0.500 to 0.800 V in anodic direction, returning to the initial point in the cathodic direction with a scanning speed of 0.1 V/s (Figure 2).

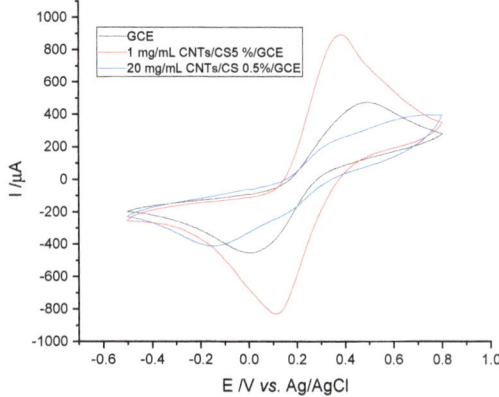

Figure 2. Cyclic voltammograms of electrodes in $K_3[Fe(CN)_6]/K_4[Fe(CN)_6]$ 10 mM solution in Britton-Robinson (B-R) buffer (pH 3), 0.100 V/s scan rate.

An intensity of the oxidation peak for 1 mg/mL CNTs/CS 5%/GCE-modified electrode can be observed at 803 µA, for GCE, at 349 µA, and for 20 mg/mL CNTs/CS 0.5%/GCE electrode, at 114 µA. This indicates a clearly superior electroactive surface of 1 mg/mL CNTs/CS 5%/GCE-modified electrode compared to the other two electrodes. It is a fact also confirmed by the calculation of the electroactive surface with the Randels–Sevcik Equation (Equation (1)) [36], for all three electrodes investigated in the cyclic voltammograms recorded in the redox probe $K_3[Fe(CN)_6]/K_4[Fe(CN)_6]$ 10 mM, in B-R buffer, as follows:

$$I_p = 2.69 \times 10^5 \times n^{3/2} AD^{1/2}v^{1/2}C \tag{1}$$

where I_p is current intensity (A), n is number of electrons transferred (usually 1), A is the electroactive surface of the electrode (cm^2), D is the diffusion coefficient (cm^2/s), C is concentration (mol/mL) and v is scan speed (V/s).

For the anodic peak, the largest electroactive surface is at the electrode 1 mg/mL CNTs/CS 5%/GCE (0.342 cm^2) and the smallest at the electrode 20 mg/mL CNTs/GCE (0.048 cm^2), increasing by 7.125 times. In these calculations, the unmodified GCE is intermediate (0.149 cm^2) in terms of signal. Regarding the cathodic peak, the signal difference is no longer very different due to the higher cathodic peak of the electrode 20 mg/mL CNTs/CS 0.5%/GCE. In the following, the best performing electrode 1 mg/mL CNTs/CS 5%/GCE will be denoted as CNTs/CS/GCE.

3.1.1. Influence of Scanning Speed on the Intensity of the Anodic/Cathodic Peak

Cyclic voltammograms were recorded in the range −0.500 to 0.800 V for a 10 mM chicoric acid solution, at different scanning speeds (0.010, 0.025, 0.050, 0.075, 0.100, 0.150, 0.200 and 0.300 V/s), in solution of B-R buffer (Figure 3A). As the scanning speed intensifies, voltammograms describe a sharp increase in oxidation peaks, and the potential of these peaks shifts to higher values. Also, the maximum potentials moved to increased (0.610 ± 0.060 V) and decreased (0.435 ± 0.055 V) values for the oxidation and reduction processes. The intensities of oxidation and reduction currents also vary in direct proportion with the square root of the scanning speed (Figure 3B). This is demonstrated by linear regression equations:

$$I_{pa}(\mu A) = -28.52645 + 0.0076 \times v^{1/2} \text{ (V/s)} \quad (2)$$

$$I_{pc}(\mu A) = 32.45163 - 0.0081 \times v^{1/2} \text{ (V/s)} \quad (3)$$

with a correlation coefficient of 0.98191 and 0.98067, which indicates that the electrochemical reaction is a controlled diffusion process that occurs in all solutions and is due to unequal local concentrations of reagents.

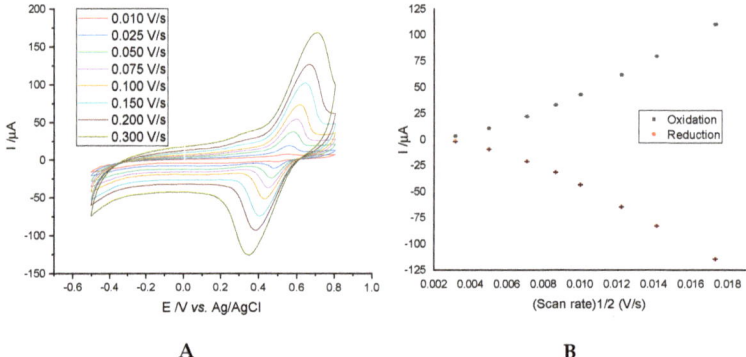

Figure 3. (**A**) Cyclic voltammograms for a 10 mM chicoric acid solution with scan speeds of 0.010, 0.025, 0.050, 0.075, 0.100, 0.150, 0.200 and 0.300 V/s, in B-R buffer (pH = 3) with modified electrode containing 20 mg CNTs/mL 0.5% CS solution in 2% acetic acid solution (20 mg/mL CNTs/CS 0.5%/GCE) denoted CNTs/CS/GCE. (**B**) The linearity between the peak current (Ip) and the square root of the scan rate $v^{1/2}$.

At a slow scanning speed, the diffusion layer will develop at a greater distance from the electroactive surface of the sensor compared to a rapid scanning of the potential. Electron flux at the electrode is lower at slow scanning speeds versus faster scanning speeds.

3.1.2. Optimization of the pH Value

The solution with 10 mM concentration of chicoric acid in B-R buffer, at different pH values, was tested. Differential pulse voltammograms recorded in the range 0 to 1.0 V are shown in Figure 4A. A high current intensity is observed for a solution with pH = 3 intensity that decreases with increasing pH of the B-R buffer. Moreover, the shift of the oxidation peak to lower potential values can be observed simultaneously with the increase of the pH values of the B-R solution (except the pH = 2 B-R solution) (Figure 4B).

3.1.3. Calibration lines

The calibration lines were determined by differential pulse voltammetry in the range 0.0 to 1.0 V. Stock solutions of caftaric and chicoric acids were prepared, both with a concentration of 25 mM, in a mixture of ethanol:water (1:1). Aliquots of acids were successively added over 10 mL of B-R electrolyte solution. The measurements were recorded with the same system of three electrodes: Ag/AgCl electrode (reference electrode), platinum wire electrode (counter electrode) and CNTs/CS/GCE (working electrode). Differential pulse voltammograms are shown in Figure 5A,B. The calibration diagrams resulted in arranging the peak amplitude against the standard solutions concentration.

The peak current amplitude against concentration dependence was registered in the concentration interval of the analyte (Figure 5C,D).

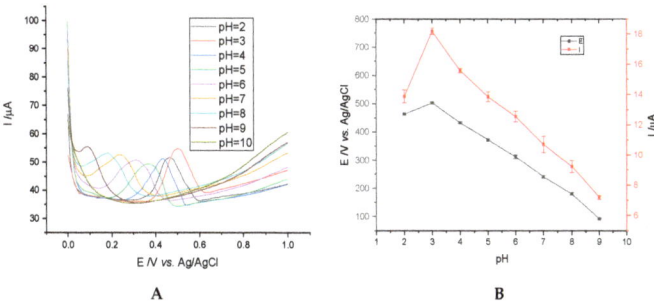

Figure 4. (**A**) Differential pulse voltammograms for a 10 mM chicoric acid solution in Britton-Robinson buffer at different pH values. (**B**) Plot of anodic peak potential and peak current vs. pH.

The two calibration lines are expressed through the following equations:

$$I(\mu A) = -0.96521 + 6.8482\ °C\ (mM) \tag{4}$$

$$I(\mu A) = 24.85987 + 1.0636\ °C\ (mM) \tag{5}$$

having values of R = 0.99500 and R = 0.98484, respectively. The amplitude of the peak current was considered as the interval between the baseline and the maximum value of the current.

In Figure 5A,B, the oxidation peak of caftaric acid occurs at 0.505 ± 0.002 V, and that of chicoric acid at 0.515 ± 0.001 V.

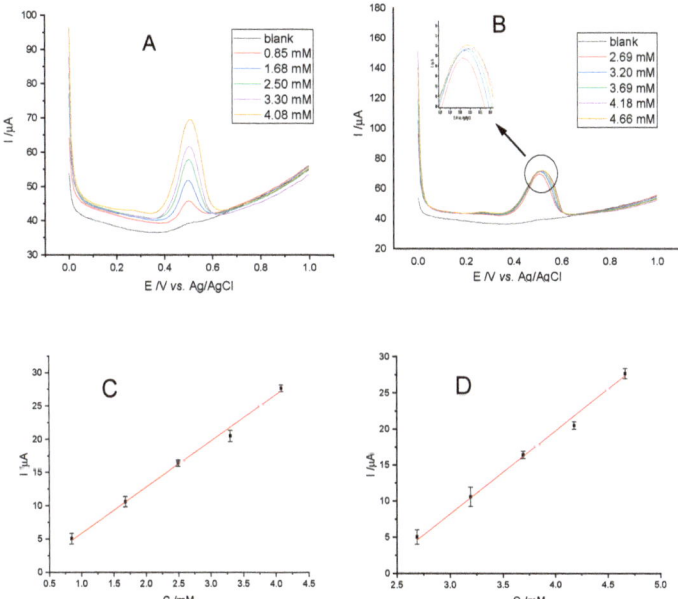

Figure 5. Differential pulse voltammograms for (**A**) caftaric acid: 0.85, 1.68, 2.50, 3.30 and 4.08 mM, (**B**) chicoric acid: 2.69, 3.20, 3.69, 4.18 and 4.66 mM in Britton-Robinson buffer (pH = 3), (**C**) calibration curve for A, (**D**) calibration curve for B.

The amplitude of the peak current was considered as the interval between the baseline and the maximum value of the current. Limits of detection (LOD) were calculated using the 3σ/S ratio, (σ—standard deviation of the response, S—slope of the calibration curve) and limits of quantification (LOQ) were specified using the 10σ/S ratio, and their values are summarized in Table 3.

Table 3. Detection and quantification limits for caftaric and chicoric acids.

Acid	Linearity Range	Limit of Detection (mM)	Limit of Quantification
Caftaric	0.850–4.084	0.283	0.850
Chicoric	2.691–4.661	0.897	2.691

3.1.4. Electrode Stability

The reproducibility of the modified electrode with CNTs was investigated. Thus, differential pulse voltammograms were recorded for a 10 mM chicoric acid solution for two consecutive weeks (Figure 6). The standard deviation of the oxidation peaks measured 3 times for each day was 2.69%, which means that the CNTs/CS/GCE electrode has a good reproducibility.

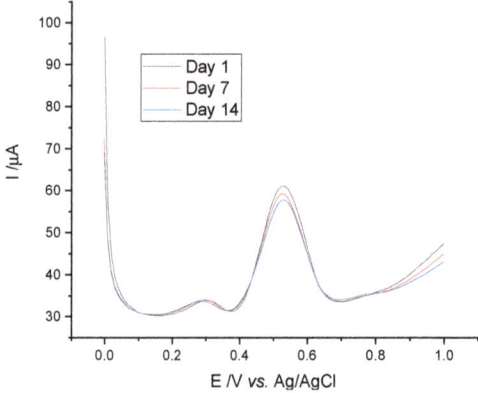

Figure 6. Differential pulse voltammograms for a 10 mM chicoric acid solution measured on days 1, 7 and 14 using the CNTs/CS/GCE electrode in Britton-Robinson buffer (pH = 3).

3.1.5. Interference Studies

For a solution containing both caftaric and chicoric acids, in concentrations of 6.40 and 5.55 mM, the influence of interferences was studied. Organic substances (such as resorcinol, glucose, uric acid, phenol and tartaric acid) with a concentration of 10 mM in solution, brought an increase in the intensity of the oxidation peaks corresponding to caftaric acid and caffeic acid, with a maximum of 3.2%. Inorganic ions (i.e., Na^+, K^+, Mg^{2+}, Ni^{2+}, Cu^{2+}, Cl^-, NO_3^- and SO_4^{2-}, Table 1), having concentrations of 100 mM in the solution of caftaric acid and chicoric acid, also did not significantly alter the signal of the oxidation peak. So, the CNTs/CS/GCE electrode had a good selectivity in determining the two acids (caftaric and chicoric).

3.2. Voltammetric Study of Echinacea Purpurea in Pharmaceutical Forms

Differential pulse voltammograms were recorded in the same range of 0.0 to 1.0 V in B-R buffer.

Figure 7 shows the differential pulse voltammograms for a solution of caftaric acid and chicoric acid (concentration of 6.40 and 5.55 mM) along with 3 other solutions of *Echinacea purpurea* extract 3.00 mg/mL from capsules/tablets/tincture in B-R buffer. The presence of strong oxidation peaks at 0.515 ± 0.025 V, due to the oxidation of 3,4-dihydroxyl substituents (caftaric acid and chicoric acid), is noted.

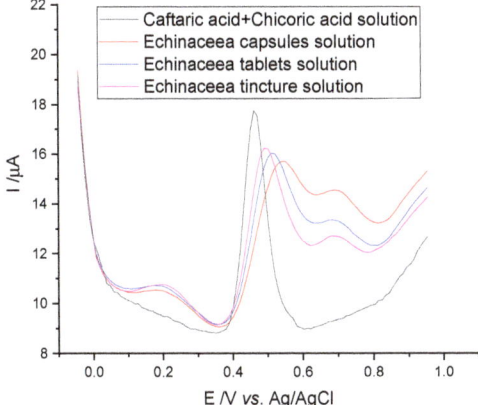

Figure 7. Differential pulse voltammograms for caftaric acid solution (6.40 mM) and chicoric acid (5.55 mM), for *Echinacea purpurea* extracts (capsules, tablets, tincture) 3 mg/mL in Britton-Robinson buffer (pH 3).

The presence of the other two oxidation peaks from 0.209 ± 0.002 V and 0.697 ± 0.005 V of the studied pharmaceutical forms can be attributed to caffeic acid or quercetin [21] respectively, to malvidin-3-glucoside, catechin or chlorogenic acid [37,38]. Amounts of polyphenols have similar values to those found by Oniszczuk et al. [39].

By correlating the oxidation peaks for both caftaric and chicoric acids with the current intensities for the oxidation peaks of the analyzed pharmaceutical forms, the quantities of polyphenols existing in the *Echinacea* extracts were obtained. The polyphenolic content was determined by the spectrophotometric method, and the standard GA calibration curve (expressed in GAE) was used. The values obtained are specified in Table 4.

Table 4. The amounts of acids present in the analyzed pharmaceutical forms with Echinacea.

Pharm. Form	Total Phenolic Derivatives Theoretically	Voltammetry				Spectrophotometry
		Caffeic Acid	Caftaric + Cichoric Acids	Catechins	Total Content of Polyphenols Found	Total Content of Polyphenols Found mg GAE/500 mg Powder
			mg/500 mg Powder			
Capsules	20	2.006 ± 0.214 *	16.129 ± 0.159	1.366 ± 0.583	19.501 ± 0.483	2.638 ± 0.258
Tablets	20	1.958 ± 0.348	16.222 ± 0.291	1.622 ± 0.794	19.802 ± 0.678	2.682 ± 0.592
Tincture	30	2.161 ± 0.287	22.701 ± 0127	3.866 ± 0.927	28.728 ± 0.826	3.890 ± 0.156

* SD: standard deviation for 3 determinations; GAE: gallic acid equivalents.

3.3. Antioxidant Activity

The differential pulse voltammograms for the gallic and ascorbic polyphenolic acids standards are shown in Figure 8A,B. Characteristic irreversible oxidation processes were registered for both compounds, similar to those observed for other antioxidant compounds (with one anodic peak E_{pa} = 0.515 ± 0.035 V for ascorbic acid [40–43], and two anodic peaks $E(I)_{pa}$ = 0.370 ± 0.040 V, $E(II)_{pa}$ = 0.550 ± 0.030 V for gallic acid [44,45]).

The equations of the calibration lines (Figure 8C,D) of AA (Equation (6)) and GA (Equation (7)) are:

$$I(\mu A) = 21.42588 + 1376.17861 \,°C(mol/L); R = 0.99806 \quad (6)$$

$$I(\mu A) = 1.12068 + 2708.14749 \,°C(mol/L); R = 0.99827 \quad (7)$$

Using the equations of the calibration lines for the two acids, the equivalent concentration was calculated for the three pharmaceutical forms analyzed in relation to the respective acids. Thus, the antioxidant capacity of *Echinacea* extract powder, relative to AA and GA, is shown in Table 5.

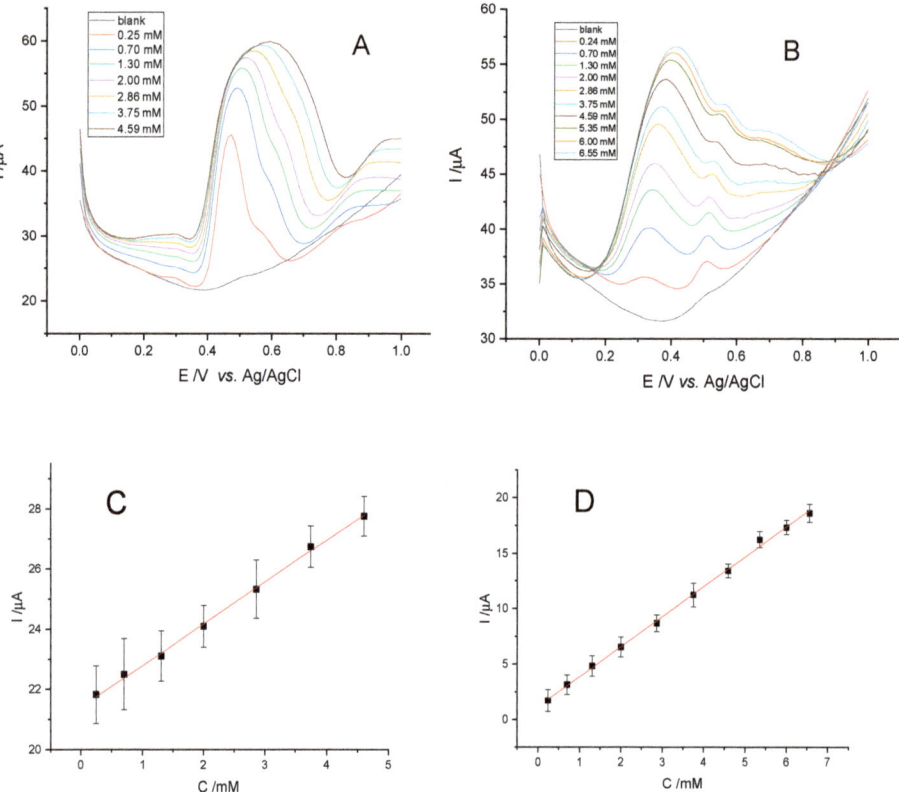

Figure 8. Differential pulse voltammograms for (**A**) ascorbic acid solutions 0.25, 0.70, 1.30, 2.00, 2.86, 3.75 and 4.59 mM, and (**B**) gallic acid 0.24, 0.70, 1.30, 2.00, 2.86, 3.75, 4.59, 5.35, 6.00 and 6.55 mM, in Britton-Robinson buffer (pH = 3). (**C**) Calibration curve for A, (**D**) calibration curve for B.

Table 5. Antioxidant capacity equivalent to ascorbic/gallic acid (AA/GA).

Pharmaceutical Form	Antioxidant Activity, mg acid/g Extract			
	Voltammetry		Spectrophotometry	
	AA	GA	AA	GA
Capsules	6.125 ± 0.428 [a]	0.952 ± 0.819	8.917 ± 0.482	3.009 ± 0.294
Tablets	6.354 ± 0.181	1.133 ± 0.103	9.477 ± 0.024	3.191 ± 0.326
Tincture	6.722 ± 0.537	1.245 ± 0.724	9.826 ± 0.624	3.457 ± 0.753

[a] SD: standard deviation for 3 determinations.

In the case of determination by the DPPH method, the calibration curves for AA and GA are linear (with a correlation coefficient >0.99), which indicates a good correspondence between the concentration of the analyzed solutions and the respective absorbance: $A_{AA} = 0.02079 + 1.0937\ C\ (mM)$, $R = 0.99663$ and $R^2 = 0.99579$, and $A_{GA} = 0.10301 + 1.26575\ C\ (mM)$, $R = 0.99290$ and $R^2 = 0.99112$, as it is also shown in Figure 9.

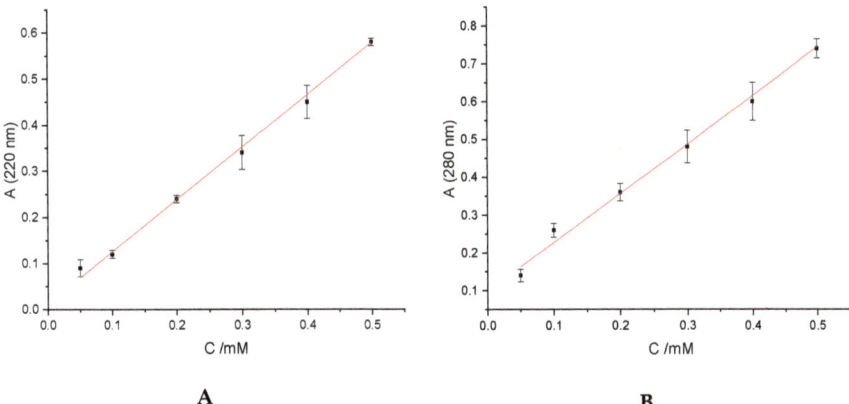

Figure 9. Calibration lines for (**A**) ascorbic acid and (**B**) gallic acid.

The possible association between the total polyphenol content and the antioxidant activity was tested, and it resulted in a direct, positive and strong association in intensity, regardless of the report (r = 0.93542, R^2 = 0.87502, p = 0.23—equivalent to AA; r = 0.880797, R^2 = 0.65282, p = 0.4—equivalent to GA).

4. Discussion

The determination of total content of polyphenols and antioxidant activity of natural pharmaceutical products is a difficult goal, being both selective and sensitive at the same time. For this purpose, simple and fast techniques are needed. Our research presented a sensitive electrochemical method of determination (both for the total polyphenols content and for the antioxidant activity of *Echinacea purpurea* extracts), benefiting from a newly manufactured glassy carbon electrode, modified with CNTs. CNTs are the most relevant representatives of the nanomaterials that are used in the manufacturing process of the electrochemical sensors, having high performance. Multiwalled CNTs are usually selected, taking into account their many advantages (high electrocatalytic activity and rapid electron transfer rate).

The structure of the caffeic acid derivatives that have ortho-dihydroxyl groups is highly connected to their reaction of oxidation [46]. The oxidation process of the catechol moiety implies a two-electron transfer that takes place stepwise through one-electron processes, succeeded by a permanent/unchangeable chemical reaction for every stage to yield an o-quinone end-product [47]. Accordingly, at the glassy carbon electrode (GCE) surface, the *Echinacea* extracts, chicoric or caftaric acid, that have comparable moiety of caffeic acid, will be oxidized. The modification of glassy carbon electrodes increases the redox peak current; also, it could be used with higher sensitivity.

For the electrode characterization, a redox system was used, with 2 electroactive species, which offers the advantage of showing a peak of oxidation, and respectively, a peak of reduction, regardless of the scanning direction of the cyclic voltammetry. Thus, if scanned to positive potentials, the oxidation peak of $K_4[Fe(CN)_6]$ will be observed, and if the scanning direction is changed to negative potentials, the reduction peak of $K_3[Fe(CN)_6]$ will be observed. If only $K_3[Fe(CN)_6]$ is used, under conditions of scanning to positive potentials, no signal will be observed in the anodic half-cycle, but a $K_3[Fe(CN)_6]$ reduction signal will appear in the cathodic half-cycle as well as the oxidation of $K_4[Fe(CN)_6]$ generated in the next anodic half-cycle. The results indicated that the tested electrode has a higher sensitivity than the other two electrodes used and can be used to determine the number of polyphenols and antioxidant activity.

In cyclic voltammetry, Ip depends on several factors: scanning speed, concentration of electroactive species, diffusion properties of electroactive species at the electrode surface, etc. Based on these considerations, and the first two factors listed above being identical for the three electrodes used, it is obvious that a net higher value of Ip for the electrode CNTs/CS/GCE is due to a very good electroactive surface compared to the other two electrodes used. If referring to the two modified electrodes, it can be stated that a smaller amount of added CS cannot fix a large quantity of CNTs to the electrode surface (based on the Ip values corresponding to the two modified electrodes).

Voltammetry studies have shown the presence of oxidation peaks at 0.505 V for caftaric acid and 0.515 V for chicoric acid, and they increase in direct proportion with the increase of the acid concentration in the range of 0.85–4.08 mM, and respectively in the range of 2.69–4.66 mM (Figure 5). These peaks are due to the oxidation of the -OH groups to the quinoline form, oxidation that consumes 2 electrons and 2 protons to form o-quinone for the studied acids [48].

Oxidation peaks in voltammograms demonstrate the existence of electroactive phenolic species in the extract and can be used to determine the total polyphenol content. This finding confirms that, based on the current intensities, the two acids mentioned above are the main polyphenols existing in the extract, because similar results were obtained for the standard phenolic compounds of caftaric and chicoric acid. Oxidation potentials that occur at 0.505 V (Figure 7) and 0.515 V (Figure 7) for both acids have close values that cannot be split by the electrode used. It should be noted that the shift of the oxidation peak towards more negative and positive potential values for the analyzed forms is due to the presence of other polyphenolic compounds in the studied extracts.

The antioxidant activity was examined by comparing and reporting two substances with strong antioxidant effects: ascorbic acid and gallic acid. Of the three pharmaceutical forms studied, Echinacea tincture had the highest antioxidant capacity (relative to ascorbic acid and gallic acid) and the total amount of polyphenols (28.72 mg/equivalent of 500 mg powder). Echinacea capsules had the lowest antioxidant capacity, but also the lowest total amount of polyphenols (19.50 mg/500 mg powder). Similarly, the tablets had approximately the same values of polyphenols content (19.80 mg/500 mg powder), and also antioxidant capacity. The positive association between total polyphenol content and antioxidant activity demonstrates the importance of polyphenolic compounds that contribute to the antioxidant activity of echinacea extracts, but also to the total antioxidant effect. These results are consistent with other studies that evaluated the antioxidant activity of *Echinacea purpurea* by spectrophotometric or electrochemical methods [21,49].

5. Conclusions

The results of this study indicate that the pulse-differential cyclic voltammetry represents a rapid, simple and sensitive technique to establish the entire polyphenolic amount and the antioxidant activity of the *E. purpurea* extracts. The modified 1 mg/mL CNTs/CS 5%/GCE electrode has superior properties compared to the other two (the unmodified and 20 mg/mL CNTs/CS 0.5%/GCE-modified) electrodes used and can be operated with to determine the polyphenol content and antioxidant capacity of natural extracts, supplements and foods. Due to the very good correlation between the antioxidant action obtained and the total polyphenolic content, it is considered that the antioxidant activity of the studied products containing *Echinacea* comes largely from the derivatives of caffeic acid that are present in the extracts of this plant. The use of dietary supplements containing *Echinacea* extracts, due to their action in preventing oxidative reactions induced by free radicals, may bring health benefits.

Author Contributions: All authors contributed equally to this paper. Conceptualization, F.B., D.M.T. and S.N.; Data curation, P.O., A.C.N. and D.G.; Formal analysis, F.B.; Investigation, F.B., T.B., D.G., F.-M.P. and S.N.; Methodology, S.B. and T.B.; Software, F.B. and T.B.; Supervision, S.B. and T.B.; Validation, P.O. and F.-M.P.; Writing—original draft, F.B., S.B., D.M.T., P.O., A.C.N. and S.N.; Writing—review and editing, S.B., D.M.T. and A.C.N. All authors have read and agreed to the published version of the manuscript.

Funding: This research received no external funding.

Acknowledgments: The authors are thankful to the University of Oradea for all the laboratory facilities.

Conflicts of Interest: The authors declare no conflict of interest.

References

1. Hudson, J.B. Applications of the Phytomedicine Echinacea Purpurea (Purple Coneflower) in Infectious Diseases. *J. Biomed. Biotechnol.* **2012**, *2012*, 1–16. [CrossRef] [PubMed]
2. Bungau, S.G.; Popa, V.C. Between Religion and Science Some Aspects Concerning Illness and Healing in Antiquity. *Transylv. Rev.* **2015**, *24*, 3–18.
3. Hu, C.; Kitts, D.D. Studies on the Antioxidant Activity of Echinacea Root Extract. *J. Agric. Food Chem.* **2000**, *48*, 1466–1472. [CrossRef]
4. Vimalanathan, S.; Arnason, J.T.; Hudson, J.B. Anti-inflammatory Activities of Echinacea Extracts Do Not Correlate with Traditional Marker Components. *Pharm. Biol.* **2009**, *47*, 430–435. [CrossRef]
5. Burns, J.J.; Zhao, L.; Taylor, E.W.; Spelman, K. The Influence of Traditional Herbal Formulas on Cytokine Activity. *Toxicology* **2010**, *278*, 140–159. [CrossRef] [PubMed]
6. Mishima, S.; Saito, K.; Maruyama, H.; Inoue, M.; Yamashita, T.; Ishida, T.; Gu, Y. Antioxidant and Immuno-Enhancing Effects of Echinacea Purpurea. *Biol. Pharm. Bull.* **2004**, *27*, 1004–1009. [CrossRef] [PubMed]
7. Zhang, Y.; Tang, T.; He, H.; Wu, H.; Hu, Z. Influence of several postharvest processing methods on polyphenol oxidase activity and cichoric acid content of Echinacea purpurea roots. *Ind. Crops Prod.* **2011**, *34*, 873–881. [CrossRef]
8. Pellati, F.; Benvenuti, S.; Magro, L.; Melegari, M.; Soragni, F. Analysis of Phenolic Compounds and Radical Scavenging Activity of Echinacea Spp. *J. Pharm. Biomed. Anal.* **2004**, *35*, 289–301. [CrossRef]
9. Zolgharnein, J.; Niazi, A.; Afiuni-Zadeh, S.; Zamani, K. Determination of Cichoric Acid as a Biomarker in Echinacea Purpurea Cultivated in Iran Using High Performance Liquid Chromatography. *Chin. Med.* **2010**, *1*, 23–27. [CrossRef]
10. Thygesen, L.; Thulin, J.; Mortensen, A.; Skibsted, L.H.; Molgaard, P. Antioxidant Activity of Cichoric Acid and Alkamides from Echinacea purpurea, Alone and in Combination. *Food Chem.* **2007**, *101*, 74–81. [CrossRef]
11. Villaño, D.; Fernández-Pachón, M.S.; Moyá, M.L.; Troncoso, A.M.; García-Parrilla, M.C. Radical Scavenging Ability of Polyphenolic Compounds Towards DPPH Free Radical. *Talanta* **2007**, *71*, 230–235. [CrossRef] [PubMed]
12. Bauer, R.; Remiger, P.; Wagner, H. Comparative TLC and HPLC analysis of herbal drugs from Echinacea purpurea, E. pallida and E. angustifolia. *Dtsch. Apoth. Ztg.* **1988**, *128*, 174–180.
13. Perry, N.B.; Burgess, E.J.; Glennie, V.L. Echinacea Standardization: Analytical Methods for Phenolic Compounds and Typical Levels in Medicinal Species. *J. Agric. Food Chem.* **2001**, *49*, 1702–1706. [CrossRef] [PubMed]
14. Brown, P.N.; Chan, M.; Paley, L.; Betz, J.M. Determination of Major Phenolic Compounds in Echinacea Spp. Raw Materials and Finished Products by High-Performance Liquid Chromatography With Ultraviolet Detection: Single-Laboratory Validation Matrix Extension. *J. AOAC Int.* **2011**, *94*, 1400–1410. [CrossRef] [PubMed]
15. Kilmartin, P.A. Electrochemistry applied to the analysis of wine: A mini-review. *Electrochem. Commun.* **2016**, *67*, 39–42. [CrossRef]
16. Karaosmanoglu, H.; Suthanthangjai, W.; Travas-Sejdic, J.; Kilmartin, P.A. Electrochemical analysis of beverage phenolics using an electrode modified with poly(3,4-ethylenedioxythiophene). *Electrochim. Acta* **2016**, *201*, 366–373. [CrossRef]
17. Abdel-Hamid, R.; Newair, E.F. Adsorptive stripping voltammetric determination of gallic acid using an electrochemical sensor based on polyepinephrine/glassy carbon electrode and its determination in black tea sample. *J. Electroanal. Chem.* **2013**, *704*, 32–37. [CrossRef]
18. Makhotkina, O.; Kilmartin, P.A. The use of cyclic voltammetry for wine analysis: Determination of polyphenols and free sulfur dioxide. *Anal. Chim. Acta* **2010**, *668*, 155–165. [CrossRef]
19. Zhao, Y.; Tang, Y.; He, J.; Xu, Y.; Gao, R.; Zhang, J.; Chong, T.; Wang, L.; Tang, X. Surface Imprinted Polymers Based on Amino-Hyperbranched Magnetic Nanoparticles for Selective Extraction and Detection of Chlorogenic Acid in Honeysuckle Tea. *Talanta* **2018**, *181*, 271–277. [CrossRef]
20. Ribeiro, C.M.; Miguel, E.M.; Silva, J.D.S.; Silva, C.B.D.; Goulart, M.O.F.; Kubota, L.T.; Gonzaga, F.B.; Santos, W.J.R.; Lima, P.R. Application of a Nanostructured Platform and Imprinted Sol-Gel Film for Determination of Chlorogenic Acid in Food Samples. *Talanta* **2016**, *156–157*, 119–125. [CrossRef]

21. Newair, E.F.; Kilmartin, P.A.; Garcia, F. Square wave voltammetric analysis of polyphenol content and antioxidant capacity of red wines using glassy carbon and disposable carbon nanotubes modified screen-printed electrodes. *Eur. Food Res. Technol.* **2018**, *244*, 1225–1237. [CrossRef]
22. Daniel, S.; Rao, T.P.; Rao, K.S.; Rani, S.U.; Lee, H.Y.; Kawai, T.; Naidu, G.R.K. A review of DNA functionalized/grafted carbon nanotubes and their characterization. *Sens. Actuators B Chem.* **2007**, *122*, 672–682. [CrossRef]
23. Ovádeková, R.; Labuda, J. Electrochemical DNA biosensors for the investigation of dsDNA host-guest interactions and damage. *Curr. Opin. Electrochem.* **2006**, *11*, 21–56.
24. Iijima, S. Helical Microtubules of Graphitic Carbon. *Nature* **1991**, *354*, 56–58. [CrossRef]
25. Wang, Y.R.; Hu, P.; Liang, Q.L.; Luo, G.A.; Wang, Y.M. Application of Carbon Nanotube Modified Electrode in Bioelectroanalysis. *Chin. J. Anal. Chem.* **2008**, *36*, 1011–1016. [CrossRef]
26. Otrisal, P.; Obsel, V.; Forus, S.; Bungau, C.; Aleya, L.; Bungau, S. Protecting emergency workers and armed forces from volatile toxic compounds: Applicability of reversible conductive polymer-based sensors in barrier materials. *Sci. Total Environ.* **2019**, *694*. [CrossRef]
27. Qu, L.; Yang, S. Application of Carbon Nanotubes Modified Electrode in Pharmaceutical Analysis. In *Carbon Nanotubes—Growth and Applications*; Naraghi, M., Ed.; IntechOpen: Rijieka, Croatia, 2011.
28. Zhao, L.; Gao, L. Novel In Situ Synthesis of MWNTs–Hydroxyapatite Composites. *Carbon* **2004**, *42*, 423–426. [CrossRef]
29. Ruel-Gariépy, E.; Chenite, A.; Chaput, C.; Guirguis, S.; Leroux, J. Characterization of Thermosensitive Chitosan Gels for the Sustained Delivery of Drugs. *Int. J. Pharm.* **2000**, *203*, 89–98. [CrossRef]
30. Cirillo, G.; Vittorio, O.; Kunhardt, D.; Valli, E.; Voli, F.; Farfalla, A.; Curcio, M.; Spizzirri, U.G.; Hampel, S. Combining Carbon Nanotubes and Chitosan for the Vectorization of Methotrexate to Lung Cancer Cells. *Materials* **2019**, *12*, 2889. [CrossRef]
31. Sengiz, C.; Congur, G.; Eksin, E.; Erdem, A. Multiwalled Carbon Nanotubes-Chitosan Modified Single-Use Biosensors for Electrochemical Monitoring of Drug-DNA Interactions. *Electroanalysis* **2015**, *27*, 1855–1863. [CrossRef]
32. Fritea, L.; Bănică, F.; Costea, T.O.; Moldovan, L.; Iovan, C.; Cavalu, S. A gold nanoparticles-Graphene based electrochemical sensor for sensitive determination of nitrazepam. *J. Electroanal. Chem.* **2018**, *830–831*, 63–71. [CrossRef]
33. Cavalu, S.; Simon, V.; Banica, F. In vitro study of collagen coating by electrodeposition on acrylic bone cement with antimicrobial potential. *Dig. J. Nanomater. Biostruct.* **2010**, *6*, 89–97.
34. Singleton, V.L.; Rossi, J.A. Colorimetry of Total Phenolics with Phosphomolybdic-Phosphotungstic Acid Reagents. *Am. J. Enol. Vitic.* **1965**, *16*, 144–158.
35. Bondet, V.; Brand-Williams, W.; Berset, C. Kinetics and Mechanisms of Antioxidant Activity using the DPPH.Free Radical Method. *LWT Food Sci. Technol.* **1997**, *30*, 609–615. [CrossRef]
36. Zanello, P. *Inorganic Electrochemistry: Theory, Practice and Application*; The Royal Society of Chemistry, Thomas Graham House: Cambridge, UK, 2003.
37. Hernanz-Vila, D.; Jara-Palacios, M.J.; Escudero-Gilete, M.L.; Heredia, F.J. Applications of Voltammetric Analysis to Wine Products. In *Applications of the Voltammetry*; Stoitcheva, M., Zlatev, R., Eds.; IntechOpen: Rijieka, Croatia, 2017.
38. Sloley, B.D.; Urichuk, L.J.; Tywin, C.; Coutts, R.T.; Pang, P.K.; Shan, J.J. Comparison of Chemical Components and Antioxidants Capacity of Different Echinacea Species. *J. Pharm. Pharmacol.* **2001**, *53*, 849–857. [CrossRef]
39. Oniszczuk, T.; Oniszczuk, A.; Gondek, E.; Guz, L.; Puk, K.; Kocira, A.; Kusz, A.; Kasprzak, K.; Wójtowicz, A. Active Polyphenolic Compounds, Nutrient Contents and Antioxidant Capacity of Extruded Fish Feed Containing Purple Coneflower (*Echinacea purpurea* (L.) Moench.). *Saudi J. Biol. Sci.* **2019**, *26*, 24–30. [CrossRef]
40. Cosio, M.S.; Buratti, S.; Mannino, S.; Benedetti, S. Use of an electrochemical method to evaluate the antioxidant activity of herb extracts from the Labiatae family. *Food Chem.* **2006**, *97*, 725–731. [CrossRef]
41. Dar, R.A.; Brahman, P.K.; Khurana, N.; Wagay, J.A.; Lone, Z.A.; Ganaie, M.A.; Pitre, K.S. Evaluation of antioxidant activity of crocin, podophyllotoxin and kaempferol by chemical, biochemical and electrochemical assays. *Arab. J. Chem.* **2017**, *10*, S1119–S1128. [CrossRef]
42. Badea, M.; Chiperea, S.; Balan, M.; Floroian, L.; Restani, P.; Marty, J.L.; Iovan, C.; Tit, D.M.; Bungau, S.; Taus, N. New approaches for electrochemical detection of ascorbic acid. *Farmacia* **2018**, *66*, 83–87.

43. Fritea, L.; Tertiş, M.; Cristea, C.; Cosnier, S.; Săndulescu, R. Simultaneous Determination of Ascorbic and Uric Acids in Urine Using an Innovative Electrochemical Sensor Based on β-Cyclodextrin. *Anal. Lett.* **2015**, *48*, 89–99. [CrossRef]
44. Badea, M.; di Modugno, F.; Floroian, L.; Tit, D.M.; Restani, P.; Bungau, S.; Iovan, C.; Badea, G.E.; Aleya, L. Electrochemical Strategies for Gallic Acid Detection: Potential for Application in Clinical, Food or Environmental Analyses. *Sci. Total Environ.* **2019**, *672*, 129–140. [CrossRef]
45. Abdel-Hamid, R.; Bakr, A.; Newair, E.F.; Garcia, F. Simultaneous Voltammetric Determination of Gallic and Protocatechuic Acids in Mango Juice Using a Reduced Graphene Oxide-Based Electrochemical Sensor. *Beverages* **2019**, *5*, 17. [CrossRef]
46. Glevitzky, I.; Dumitrel, G.A.; Glevitzky, M.; Pasca, B.; Otrisal, P.; Bungau, S.; Cioca, G.; Pantis, C.; Popa, M. Statistical Analysis of the Relationship Between Antioxidant Activity and the Structure of Flavonoid Compounds. *Rev. de Chim.* **2019**, *70*, 3103–3107. [CrossRef]
47. Hottaa, H.; Uedaa, M.; Naganoa, S.; Tsujinob, Y.; Koyamac, J.; Osakaia, T. Mechanistic Study of the Oxidation of Caffeic Acid by Digital Simulation of Cyclic Voltammograms. *Anal. Biochem.* **2002**, *303*, 66–72. [CrossRef] [PubMed]
48. Newair, E.F.; Abdel-Hamid, R.; Kilmartin, P.A. Mechanism of Chicoric Acid Electrochemical Oxidation and Identification of Oxidation Products by Liquid Chromatography and Mass Spectrometry. *Electroanalysis* **2016**, *28*, 1–12. [CrossRef]
49. Zayova, E.; Stancheva, I.; Geneva, M.; Petrova, M.; Vasilevska-Ivanova, R. Morphological evaluation and antioxidant activity of in vitro- and in vivo-derived *Echinacea purpurea* plants. *Open Life Sci.* **2012**, *7*, 698–707. [CrossRef]

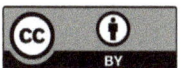

© 2020 by the authors. Licensee MDPI, Basel, Switzerland. This article is an open access article distributed under the terms and conditions of the Creative Commons Attribution (CC BY) license (http://creativecommons.org/licenses/by/4.0/).

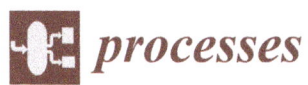

Article

Moringa oleifera—Storage Stability, *In Vitro*-Simulated Digestion and Cytotoxicity Assessment of Microencapsulated Extract

Cecilia Castro-López [1,2], Catarina Gonçalves [3], Janeth M. Ventura-Sobrevilla [4], Lorenzo M. Pastrana [3], Cristóbal N. Aguilar-González [2] and Guillermo C. G. Martínez-Ávila [1,*]

- [1] School of Agronomy, Autonomous University of Nuevo Leon, Nuevo León 66050, Mexico; caslopcec28@hotmail.com
- [2] School of Chemistry, Autonomous University of Coahuila, Coahuila 25280, Mexico; cristobal.aguilar@uadec.edu.mx
- [3] Food Processing Group, International Iberian Nanotechnology Laboratory, Av. Mestre José Veiga S/N, 4715-330 Braga, Portugal; catarina.goncalves@inl.int (C.G.); lorenzo.pastrana@inl.int (L.M.P.)
- [4] School of Health Sciences, Autonomous University of Coahuila, Coahuila 26090, Mexico; janethventura@uadec.edu.mx
- [*] Correspondence: guillermo.martinezavl@uanl.edu.mx; Tel.: +52-81-83294000 (ext. 3512)

Received: 1 June 2020; Accepted: 28 June 2020; Published: 1 July 2020

Abstract: Moringa extract was microencapsulated for the first time by spray-drying technique using tragacanth gum (MorTG) to improve its stability under gastrointestinal and storage conditions, assessing total polyphenolic content (TPC) and antioxidant activity. Additionally, cytotoxicity of the microencapsulated components was evaluated after contact with Caco-2 cells. Results showed that TPC was released as follows—oral (9.7%) < gastric (35.2%) < intestinal (57.6%). In addition, the antioxidant activity in *in vitro* digestion reached up to 16.76 ±0.15 mg GAE g^{-1}, which was 300% higher than the initial value. Furthermore, microencapsulated moringa extract presented a half-life up to 45 days of storage, where the noticeably change was observed at 35 °C and 52.9% relative humidity. Finally, direct treatment with 0.125 mg mL^{-1} MorTG on Caco-2 cells showed a slight antiproliferative effect, with a cell viability of approx. 87%. Caco-2 cells' viability demonstrated non-cytotoxicity, supporting the safety of the proposed formulation and potential use within the food field.

Keywords: *Moringa oleifera*; microencapsulation; cell viability; storage; *in vitro* digestion; polyphenols

---

1. Introduction

The increasing demand for healthy foods has led current research to the development of new and natural additives or ingredients that can provide a benefit beyond nutrition [1]. In this sense, *Moringa oleifera* Lam (Moringaceae) has been documented as a rich plant of bioactive compounds (e.g., polyphenols, carbohydrates, fatty acids and biofunctional peptides) with several advantages for human health and food applications [2]. Earlier studies focused mainly in the polyphenol content since it has been reported that these compounds have antioxidant abilities that may be used for human consumption [3–5]. However, they are sensitive to several factors used in food processing operations (pH, water activity, light conditions, oxygen and temperature). Thus, it is necessary to prevent their degradation and improve their stability in those conditions. Within these, encapsulation technology is a method that can provide a good physical barrier against the above-mentioned factors [6,7]. And even, some authors report that encapsulation may also decrease their unpleasant taste and improve sensory properties [8,9]. Additionally, from a technological point of view, it would be most applicable to benefit from Moringa phenolics in powder form due to the easiest handling in food and pharmaceutical industries [10].

In this respect, in a previous study we reported a comprehensive characterization of the polyphenols present in *M. oleifera* extract, as well as its antioxidant properties [11]. Hence, in a later study, three different, suitable, novel, natural and generally recognized as safe (GRAS) wall materials (tragacanth gum, locust bean gum and carboxymethyl-cellulose) were explored for Moringa spray-drying microencapsulation followed by several physicochemical analyses (data under submission). Among the three materials, microencapsulates produced with Tragacanth gum (TG) showed better performance in antioxidant properties retention, aside from good particle size distribution and morphological, thermal and crystallinity characteristics. Nevertheless, there is no available information of either bioaccessibility and storage stability, controlling release and/or enhancing solubility. Thus, the aim of this paper was to determine the stability of microencapsulated Moringa's activity in *in vitro*-simulated digestion and at different storage conditions. Additionally, Caco-2 cells' viability after incubation with the microencapsulated Moringa or with the individual components was also evaluated, as a first safety assessment of the proposed formulation envisaging its potential use in the food industry.

2. Materials and Methods

2.1. Chemicals and Reagents

All the chemicals used were analytical grade and purchased from Sigma-Aldrich (Toluca, México). Tragacanth gum was obtained from a domestic supplier (Deiman S.A. de C.V., Puebla, México); while minimum essential medium (MEM) was obtained from Thermo-Scientific (Portugal) and penicillin/streptomycin, fetal bovine serum (FBS) and non-essential amino-acids were acquired from Millipore (Oeiras, Portugal).

2.2. Plant Material and Extraction of Polyphenolic Compounds

Moringa leaves (*Moringa oleifera* Lam.) were provided from a producer from General Escobedo, Nuevo León, México. They were leafed off manually, washed in water, dried in an air-forced oven (60 °C for 24 h), grounded using an electric grinder until having a particle size between 3–5 mm and finally stored in a dry place. Then, the polyphenolic compounds were extracted by microwave-assisted extraction with a solid—liquid ratio of 1:50 w/v, using water as solvent. The conditions used for the extraction method were reported in a previous study [11]. Briefly, the extraction conditions were microwave power, 550 W; extraction time, 90 s; and controlled temperature, 70 °C.

2.3. Microencapsulation Process

Moringa polyphenol-rich extract was microencapsulated with tragacanth gum (TG), as encapsulating agent. The dispersion was prepared using the raw extract (200 mL) and adding 1% w/v of TG. The resulting mixture was stirred by a constant speed stirrer at 300 rpm for 90 min at 30 °C until a homogenized system was obtained. The liquid feed was spray dried in a Büchi B-290 Mini Spray Dryer (Büchi Laboratoriums-Technik AG, Flawil, Switzerland) under the following experimental conditions—drying air inlet temperature, 120 °C; outlet temperature, 68–71 °C; atomization air volumetric flow rate, 601 L h^{-1}; feed volumetric flow rate, 2 mL min^{-1}; nozzle diameter, 0.7 mm; and aspirator, 100% [12].

2.4. Stability During Storage

For stability tests, the microencapsulates (200 mg) were put in plastic cups, uniformly spreaded and stored in airtight plastic containers filled with saturated $MgCl_2$ and $Mg(NO_3)_2$ solutions to produce a relative humidity (RH) with values of 32.8% and 52.9%, respectively. These containers were stored at three different temperatures—(a) 5 °C (refrigeration), (b) 25 °C (room temperature) and (c) 35 °C (temperature recommended for accelerated shelf life studies) [13]. The samples were analyzed after the following storage times—0, 5, 10, 15, 20, 25, 30 and 35 days, where the total polyphenol content and the antioxidant capacity were the parameters evaluated to determine stability. The first-order reaction rate constants (k) and half-lives ($t_{1/2}$) were calculated as follows:

$$-\ln(C_t/C_0) = kt \tag{1}$$

$$t_{1/2} = (\ln(2))/k \tag{2}$$

where C_0 is the initial content of the microencapsulated compound and C_t is the content of the microencapsulated compound in the time-point (t).

Also, the values of Q_{10} (meaning that this coefficient reflects the number of times the deterioration of the particles accelerates or decreases depending on whether the temperature increases or decreases 10 degrees Celsius) were determined at a specific temperature (T_x) by Equations (2) and (3), where kT is the constant reaction rate at a temperature T_x and kT-10 is the constant reaction rate at a temperature 10 °C lower than the temperatures tested. For purpose of this analysis values of 25 and 35 °C were used in order to determine Q_{10} [14].

$$Q_{10} = kT/kT - 10. \tag{3}$$

2.5. Release of Compounds during In Vitro Digestion

The simulated *in vitro* digestion was prepared according to the method of Ahmad et al. [15]. First, the simulated gastric fluid (SGF) was prepared from a NaCl solution (0.2%) to pH ≈ 3 (adjusted by the addition of HCl 1 M). Later, the simulated intestinal fluid (SIF) was prepared by dissolving KH_2PO_4 (0.68 g) in deionized water (75 mL) and then by adjusting the pH to 7.1 (with KOH 0.2 M) and topping up the final volume to 100 mL. Finally, the saliva fluid was prepared by dissolving NaCl (4.68 mg), KCl (5.96 mg), $NaHCO_3$ (0.084 g) and α-amylase (7.0 mg) in deionized water (40 mL). The pH of this solution was adjusted to 6.8. Afterwards, samples (200 mg) were placed in a flask, incubated at 37 °C under constant agitation and digested sequentially as follows—(a) mouth: 10 mL of salivary juice was added and mixed for 5 minutes and an aliquot (2 mL) was collected; (b) stomach: 10 mL of SGF were added and mixed for 1 h, aliquots (2 mL) were collected after 30 minutes and 1 h of incubation; and (c) intestine: 10 mL of SIF were added and mixed for 3 h. Aliquots (2 mL) were collected after 2 h, 3 h and 4 h.

2.6. Activities Assessment

2.6.1. Preparation of Samples

Powder from storage stability was dissolved in 2 mL ethanol: water solution (50:50 v/v). This mixture was agitated for 3 min and centrifuged at 10,000 rpm for 10 min at 4 °C. Finally, the supernatant containing the Moringa extract was collected and stored at −20 °C until measured. Aliquots from simulated *in vitro* digestion received the same treatment of centrifugation and supernatant recollection.

2.6.2. Determination of Total Polyphenol Content (TPC)

The total polyphenol content (TPC) was measured to evaluate the release during *in vitro* digestion or degradation under storage conditions and was determined according to the method proposed by Georgé et al. [16]. Briefly, 250 µL of supernatant was mixed with 250 µL of Folin-Ciocalteu's reagent for 1 min, after 250 µL of sodium carbonate (75 g L^{-1}) were added. The final solution was mixed and incubated at 40 °C for 30 minutes. Subsequently, 2 mL of distilled water were added and the absorbance at 750 nm was recorded. TPC was calculated using a calibration curve performed with gallic acid in the concentration range 20 to 150 ppm.

2.6.3. DPPH radical Scavenging Activity

The antioxidant capacity of the supernatant after *in vitro* digestion or after being subjected to different storage conditions, was evaluated by the methodology proposed by Brand-Williams et al. [17]. Briefly, 50 µL of each supernatant was added to 2950 µL DPPH• radical methanol (60 µM) solution. After 30 minutes of incubation in the dark, the absorbance of the samples was recorded at a wavelength of 517 nm. The capability of inhibition was calculated with the following equation and expressed as percentage of inhibition of DPPH• radical comparing to the control (distilled water):

$$\text{Inhibition (\%)} = [(A_{control} - A_{sample})/A_{control}] \times 100. \tag{4}$$

The antioxidant capacity was calculated using a calibration curve performed with gallic acid in the concentration range 20 to 150 ppm.

2.7. Cell Toxicity

2.7.1. Cell Culture

Caco-2 human colon epithelial cancer cells (ATCC, HTB-37, LGC Standards S.L.U., Barcelona, Spain) were routinely cultured in minimum essential medium (MEM), supplemented with 20% fetal bovine serum (FBS), 1% non-essential amino acids, 1 mM sodium pyruvate and 1% penicillin/streptomycin. These cells were maintained in T75 cell culture flasks, at 37 °C, in a humidified 5% CO_2 atmosphere and harvested at 80% of confluency using Trypsin/EDTA solution 0.25%/0.02% (w/v). Cells were used in passage 20–40.

2.7.2. Cell Viability Assay

The resazurin salt was used to assess the cellular compatibility of encapsulating agent, raw extract and microencapsulates diluted in the culture medium, at different concentrations: 0.125, 0.075, 0.050 and 0.025 mg mL^{-1}. Caco-2 cells were seeded onto 96-well plates at a density of 10,000 cells per well and left adhering overnight. After that, the culture medium was eliminated and replaced by the samples. Then, the cells were incubated for 24 and 48 h with resazurin (0.01 mg mL^{-1}). The fluorescence intensity, was measured at an excitation wavelength of 530 nm and an emission wavelength of 590 nm. The percentage of cell viability was expressed as the percentage of fluorescence in treated cells compared with the fluorescence of cells growing in the culture medium (considered as 100% cell viability). A positive control with 30% of DMSO was performed [18]. For each condition, the fluorescence intensity of samples without cells (background) was measured to assess any interference of samples with resazurin and subtracted to the fluorescence obtained with cells, in each time-point.

2.8. Statistical Analysis

The Minitab 17 Statistical Software (Minitab, Inc., State College, PA, USA) was used to analyze all results. Data are representative of two independent experiments, each containing three biological replicates and expressed as mean ± standard deviation (SD).

3. Results and Discussion

3.1. Influence of Storage Conditions on the Polyphenolic Content

The stability of the total polyphenolic content (TPC) in the microencapsulated Moringa was estimated under different storage conditions and the half-life values of the reactions were calculated. In addition, the degradation kinetics of the polyphenols were monitored during the storage period and the rate constants and the degradation of the polyphenols were calculated. A first-order reaction model was adjusted under all the conditions evaluated (Table 1). Microencapsulated moringa microparticles stored at 5 and 25 °C at 32.8% RH showed the lowest total polyphenol loss, about 42.47%–45.28%

of the initial total content (23.24 mg GAE g^{-1}), suggesting that microencapsulation, combined with storage at refrigeration or room temperature, help to maintain part of the polyphenols contained in the particle (Figure 1a). As expected, increasing the storage temperature (35 °C) led to an increased degradation of the compounds with a loss of 53.58%, since they are sensitive to temperature. It was also observed that the effect of temperature on degradation rates was greater for samples stored at higher RH (52.9%). This indicates that the activity of water also has a significant role in the degradation of tested compounds, given that the higher the water content, the greater the molecular mobility within the microparticles, which facilitates the physicochemical degradation reactions [13]. In the same way, according to Desobry et al. [19], the interval that presents a higher degradation rate corresponds to the degradation of compounds present on the surface of the microcapsules or compounds within the microcapsules that are in contact with oxygen, which is present in the pores of the particle or trapped inside it in the form of bubbles, which allows their easy oxidation.

Table 1. Degradation kinetic parameters of Moringa microencapsulates (MorTG) stored at different conditions.

Storage Conditions		k (days^{-1})	$t_{1/2}$ (days)	R^2	Q_{10}
Temperature (°C)	Water Activity (a_w)				
5	0.328	0.0170	40.75	0.989	
	0.529	0.0175	39.42	0.971	
25	0.328	0.0155	44.47	0.978	1.26
	0.529	0.0175	39.42	0.986	
35	0.328	0.0197	35.04	0.961	1.24
	0.529	0.0218	31.65	0.983	

On the other hand, the parameters of the reaction rate constant (k), half-life time ($t_{1/2}$) and factor Q_{10} are shown in Table 1. The Moringa microparticles have first-order kinetics, showing a linear degradation with respect to time. Storage at 35 °C showed a higher value of k (0.0218) in the degradation of the polyphenol content than the samples stored at 5 and 25 °C. The half-life data ($t_{1/2}$) showed an inverse relation with the storage temperature. The longest half-life for microencapsulated MorTG was verified for storage at 25 °C (32.8% RH) presenting up to 44.47 days of stability. The values of Q_{10} calculated for 25 and 35 °C, were higher than 1, which means that the degradation rate of polyphenols increases with temperature due to the high sensitivity of these compounds. This negative effect of high temperature and humidity on the stability of such compounds has already been reported in many studies available in the literature [10,20–22].

3.2. Influence of Storage Conditions on Antioxidant Activity

As already mentioned, one of the most important criteria for evaluating polyphenol microencapsulation quality is the length of time during which the powder retains its bioactivity [23]. In this context, the antioxidant activity was monitored during the storage conditions as shown in Figure 1b. The data obtained showed that microparticles presented a moderate decrease of original antioxidant activity along storage time, which was enhanced by higher temperature and water activity.

At all temperatures tested, with 32.8% RH, the microparticles were stable up to 30 days of storage, while at 52.9% RH a notable tendency to decrement was found after 25 days; thus, it was observed that the retained activity was in a range between 39.7% and 75.32% regarding the initial activity (18.60 mg GAE g^{-1}). These results suggested that the stability of microencapsulated extract is seriously compromised when exposed to higher temperature and humidity environments, which is in agreement with the results obtained by Wang et al. [24], Zheng et al. [25] and Bakowska-Barczak & Kolodziejczyk [7] who reported changes in the antioxidant activity of encapsulated tea polyphenols, bayberry polyphenols and polyphenols extracted from black currant pomace, when the storage temperature was increased.

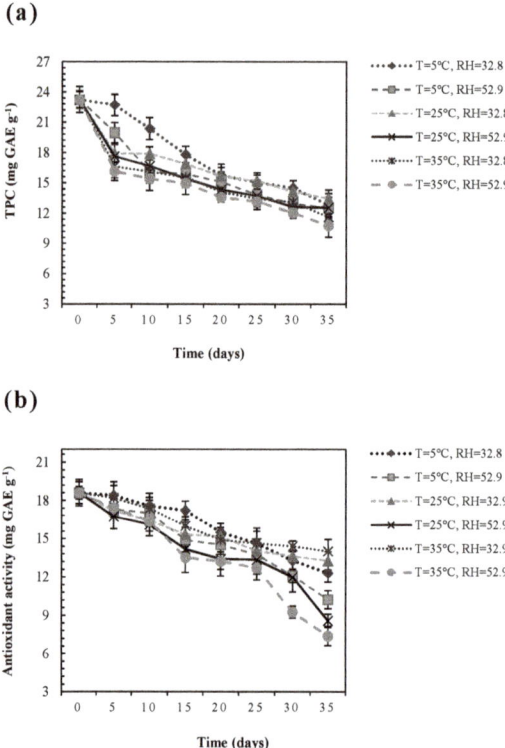

Figure 1. Total polyphenol content (**a**) and antioxidant activity (**b**) of Moringa microencapsulates (MorTG) subject to different storage temperatures and relative humidities for 35 days.

Nevertheless, the antioxidant activity presents less variation during storage compared with the reduction of TPC. Regarding this, several studies have tried to correlate the antioxidant potential and the polyphenolic content of microparticles submitted to different storage conditions. Fracassetti et al. [26] and Moser et al. [22] studied the influence of storage on antioxidant activity of freeze-dried wild blueberry powder and violeta grape juice microencapsulates. They reported a decreased of the antioxidant activity with increasing temperature but the reduction does not seem directly correlated with the observed decrease in the total polyphenol content, which showed linear degradation. In accordance with these authors, such behavior may be attributed to many factors which can influence hydrolysis, oxidation and condensation reactions that take place during storage of phenolic compounds which bring out formation of new antioxidant polymers.

2.3. Release of Polyphenolic Compounds during In Vitro Digestion

As previously reported by our group, extracts of *Moringa oleifera* are a potential source of antioxidant compounds that must be protected by microencapsulation to preserve their bioactivity after biological processes such as digestion [11]. Nevertheless, it has been reported that the stability and bioaccessibility (fraction of the compound that is released from its matrix after digestion and become available for absorption) of these compounds greatly affect their possible benefits (bioactivity) [15]. So, it is important to study and understand how these compounds are released from the encapsulated structures during the digestion process, in the gastrointestinal conditions [15].

The impact of gastrointestinal digestion on the release of polyphenolic compounds from the microencapsulated structures (MorTG) to the supernatant (micellar phase, potentially absorbable) obtained, after low-speed centrifugation, is shown in Figure 2. The results revealed that the TPC in the supernatant increased during the digestion phases (oral < gastric < intestinal) and the highest value was recorded in the intestinal phase. As can be seen, the release of polyphenols under salivary conditions was found to be 9.7%; while, after 30 and 60 minutes under gastric conditions 27.2 and 35.2% were released, respectively. Finally, afterwards 2, 3 and 4 h in intestinal conditions, 44.1, 51.8 and 57.6% were released into the micellar phase. Hence, this behavior indicate that the encapsulated compounds were protected against the condition changes of *in vitro* digestion such as the pH variations and the presence of enzymes (e.g., α-amylase in saliva fluid).

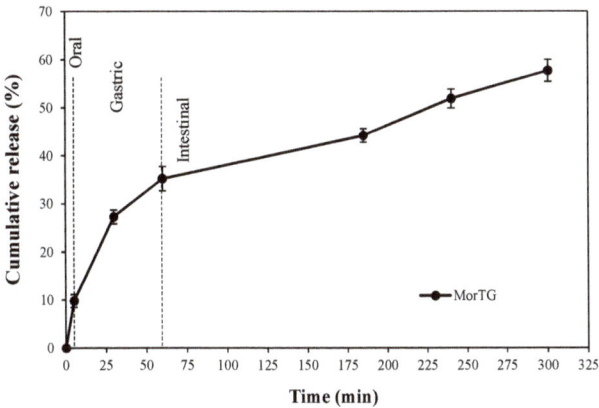

Figure 2. Polyphenol cumulative release during *in vitro* digestion of Moringa microencapsulates (MorTG) determined by Folin-Ciocalteu's method.

Regarding the low values of TPC observed in the oral and gastric phases, it has been reported that this behavior may be associated to the low solubility of these compounds in the aforementioned fluids, their molecular binding mechanisms with polymer or also because they were released only from the microcapsules surface pores [27]. Notably, the more complete release of TPC in intestinal phase may be attributed to the enhanced swelling of the microcapsules in the simulated intestinal fluid, that might have increased the diffusion path length of polyphenols within the particles [28]. Furthermore, it has been described that the release properties depend on the type of polymer used for encapsulation. Since the higher solubility of wall materials in solvent, the higher the release of encapsulated compounds [29]. In this sense, a characteristic of tragacanth gum is that it is composed of water-soluble and insoluble fractions which provide it swelling properties that have an impact on the disintegration rate of the powder. So, the water-soluble fraction might cause the fast release of surface polyphenols (during the first minutes with solvent contact); while the water-insoluble fraction might form, gel leading to slow and gradual release (remaining polyphenols with a more possible strong molecular binding) [29–31]. Finally, it has also been described that tragacanth structural relaxation can influences compound diffusivity within microcapsules and thus modulate polyphenol release [32]. One of the main factors affecting this relaxation is the environmental pH since both under or above the isoelectric point of tragacanth, this gum may either take or give protons (protonation or ionization of carboxyl groups) and lead to a decreased (lower pH) or increased (higher pH) polyphenol diffusion from the matrix [33,34].

3.4. Antioxidant Activity During in Vitro Digestion

The antioxidant potential of plant extracts is mainly attributed to the phenolic contents. However, the antioxidant properties of phenolic compounds might change due to the chemical transformations resulting from different mechanisms during the gastrointestinal digestion [27]. Therefore, to evaluate the effect of *in vitro* digestion on the antioxidant potential of microencapsulated Moringa, DPPH• assay was performed.

The obtained results, which are shown in Table 2, agree with the measurements of TPC, being the highest antioxidant activity associated to the intestinal phase. It can be seen that in the first two phases there was an antioxidant cumulative activity of 5.23 ± 0.36 mg GAE g^{-1} (oral) and 11.07 ± 0.46 mg GAE g^{-1} (gastric). Whereas in the intestinal phase 16.76 ± 0.15 mg GAE g^{-1} was obtained. Clearly, the results found in this study indicated that antioxidant activity increased gradually (up to >300% more activity) during and at the end of *in vitro* digestion (initial activity of 5.12 mg GAE g^{-1}). In this regard, Flores et al. [35] and Ahmad et al. [36], mentioned that DPPH• scavenging values increased significantly after the gastric phase of digestion for encapsulated blueberry (*Vaccinium ashei*) extracts and saffron anthocyanins, respectively. Furthermore, according to You et al. [37] this increment in antioxidant activity could be attributed to the formation of some components with stronger antioxidant activities during the simulated gastrointestinal digestion. Besides, pH of fluid may affect the racemization of molecules, which probably creates enantiomers with different reactivities [38]. Additionally, during the *in vitro* digestion process, antioxidant compounds could be more reactive depending on the acidic pH (gastric medium) or neutral pH (intestinal medium) since it was confirmed that the susceptibility of these compounds to pH strongly depends on the phenol's structure [39]. Interestingly, this hypothesis can be associated with previous work [11] in which we characterized the polyphenolic compounds present in Moringa extracts, determining a main presence of flavonoids, which may be more resistant to pH degradation than the monocyclic polyphenolic compounds (e.g., phenolic acids).

Table 2. Antioxidant activity of Moringa microencapsulates (MorTG) during *in vitro* digestion by DPPH• assay.

Digestion Phase	Duration of Digestion	DPPH [1]
		MorTG
Oral	5 min	5.23 (±0.36)
Gastric	30 min	8.54 (±0.51)
	60 min	11.07 (±0.46)
Intestinal	2 h	13.19 (±0.73)
	3 h	15.20 (±0.51)
	4 h	16.76 (±0.15)

[1] Cumulative antioxidant activity expressed as mg GAE g^{-1}.

Finally, it is necessary to add that the increase antioxidant activity can also be associated with the phenolics released from the microcapsules after the digestive process. The weak activity recorded in oral and gastric phases may be related to the low phenolic compounds content, while the higher activity in the intestinal phase confirms the maximum release of compounds in intestinal conditions.

3.5. Effect in Caco-2 Cells Viability

Usually, the biocompatibility of materials is normally evaluated using *in vitro* methods. Cell lines are frequently cultivated in contact with test materials and after a variable period, the proliferation and death rates are measured. Thus, viability of Caco-2 cells under exposure to different concentrations of non-encapsulated and microencapsulated Moringa extract was determined, as an *in vitro* model to assess safety of the proposed formulation. Furthermore, in order to exclude the possible cytotoxicity of the wall material, tragacanth gum was also evaluated.

As shown in Figure 3, cell viability did not decrease after incubation with the wall material, at all concentrations tested, showing approximately 99.5% (48 h) of cell viability compared to the control (cells growing in the culture medium). Regarding to the non-encapsulated Moringa extract and microcapsules (MorTG), after 48 h of incubation, they presented above 82 and 87% of cell viability, at the highest concentration (0.125 mg mL^{-1}), respectively. Based on these data, it can be established that, the effect on Caco-2 viability was dose-and time-dependent. Comparing wall material, raw extract and Moringa microencapsulated results it seems that the effect on cell viability should be exert by raw extract. According to the ISO 10993-5:2009 standard [40], if the relative cell viability for the highest concentration of the test sample is >70% of the control group, then the material shall be considered non-cytotoxic. Consequently, further studies may be performed if Moringa microencapsulated in higher concentrations are needed for nutraceutical and/or therapeutic applications.

Our findings are consistent with reports showing antiproliferative and/or toxic effects of polyphenols or polyphenol rich extracts in Caco-2 cells and other cell lines, such as Courtney et al. [41], Sánchez-Vioque et al. [42] and Szewczyk et al. [43] with *Terminalia carpentariae* and *Terminalia grandiflora* extracts, *Oenothera paradoxa* seed extract and *Crocus sativus* L. leaf extract, respectively. However, it is important to note that the authors reported concentrations between 0.5 to 1 mg mL^{-1} to exert a more potent inhibition of Caco-2 cell proliferation, which are 4–8 times higher compared to the highest concentration (0.125 mg mL^{-1}) proved in this study. This could be explained by the potential presence of mixtures of polyphenol compounds in *Moringa oleifera*, as previously reported by our group [11]. Since it has been associated that high doses of polyphenolic compounds (>100 mg) such as hydroxycinnamic acids, hydroxybenzoic acids and flavonoids mostly (maybe due to the synergistic action), can act as pro-oxidants in cell culture systems and induce selective cytotoxicity [44,45]. Finally, to the best of our knowledge, this is the first report on Caco-2 viability after incubation with Moringa polyphenol extract (free or microencapsulated form).

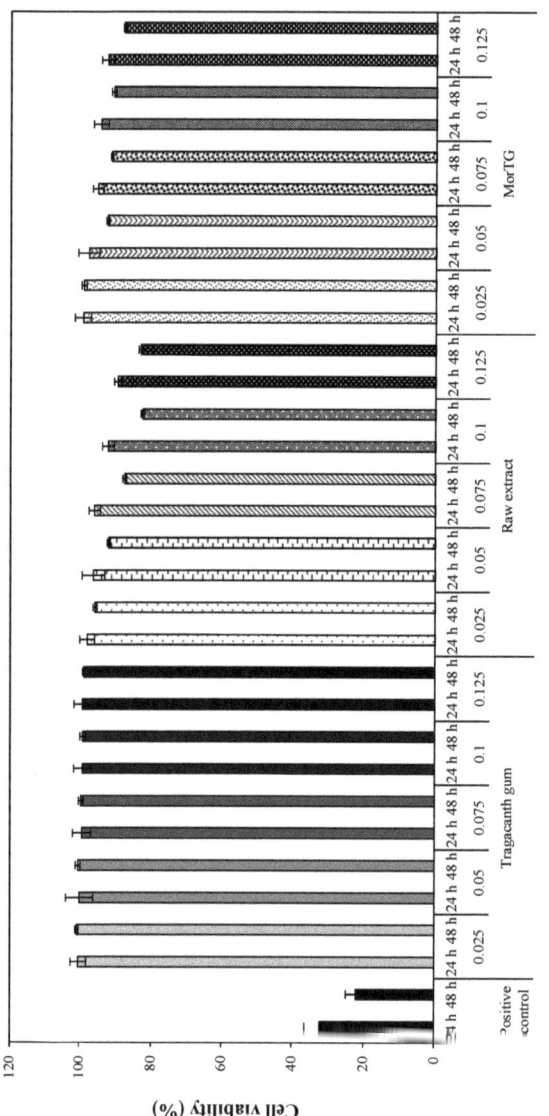

Figure 3. Cell viability (□) of Caco-2 cells incubated with bioactive (raw extract), wall material (tragacanth) and Moringa microencapsulates (MorTG) for 24 and 48 h. Positive control (cell death) was performed with cells incubated with 30% of DMSO.

4. Conclusions

This study proposed the microencapsulation of Moringa polyphenols with the utilization of tragacanth gum as wall material. The Moringa microencapsulates were found to be stable in salivary and gastric digestion phases (up to 35.2%); while most of the compounds resulted in higher percent release in intestinal phase, reaching a maximum value of 57.6%. Besides, under a relative humidity of 32.8% and storage temperatures of 5 and 25 °C, the TPC and DPPH• radical scavenging activity showed the lowest total polyphenol losses (between 42.47%–45.28%, respectively). Additionally, Caco-2 cells treated with MorTG presented a cell viability of 87% at the highest concentration (0.125 mg mL^{-1}), thereby confirming the lack of toxicity of microencapsulates. These promising results suggest that MorTG may be an interesting polyphenol source for incorporation into other products. Nevertheless, further studies must be performed since the possible inclusion of other adjuvant materials could improve their stabilization and antioxidant properties when subjected to adverse conditions.

Author Contributions: Conceptualization, investigation and writing—original draft preparation, C.C.-L.; conceptualization, methodology and resources, C.G. and L.M.P.; resources, writing—review and editing, J.M.V.-S.; visualization and supervision, C.N.A.-G.; resources, supervision and writing—review and editing, G.C.G.M.-Á. All authors have read and agreed to the published version of the manuscript.

Funding: This work was funded by MICRODIGEST project (grant agreement 037716) co-funded by FCT and ERDF through COMPETE2020.

Acknowledgments: Cecilia Castro-López thanks to Mexican Council for Science and Technology (CONACYT) for the postgraduate scholarship.

Conflicts of Interest: The authors declare no conflict of interest.

References

1. Onwulata, C.I. Encapsulation of new active ingredients. *Annu. Rev. Food Sci. Technol.* **2011**, *3*, 183–202. [CrossRef]
2. Saucedo-Pompa, S.; Torres-Castillo, J.A.; Castro-López, C.; Rojas, R.; Sánchez-Alejo, E.J.; Ngangyo-Heya, M.; Martínez-Ávila, G.C.G. Moringa plants: Bioactive compounds and promising applications in food products. *Food Res. Int.* **2018**, *111*, 438–450. [CrossRef] [PubMed]
3. Bholah, K.; Ramful-Baboolall, D.; Neergheen-Bhujun, V.S. Antioxidant activity of polyphenolic rich Moringa oleifera Lam. Extracts in food Systems. *J. Food Biochem.* **2015**, *39*, 733–741. [CrossRef]
4. Nadeem, M.; Abdullah, M.; Hussain, I.; Inayat, S.; Javid, A.; Zahoor, Y. Antioxidant potential of *Moringa oleifera* leaf extract for the stabilisation of butter at refrigeration temperature. *Czech J. Food Sci.* **2013**, *31*, 332–339. [CrossRef]
5. Sreelatha, S.; Padma, P.R. Antioxidant activity and total phenolic content of Moringa oleifera leaves in two stages of maturity. *Plant Foods Hum. Nutr.* **2009**, *64*, 303–311. [CrossRef]
6. Sun-Waterhouse, D.; Wadhwa, S.S.; Waterhouse, G.I.N. Spray-drying microencapsulation of polyphenol bioactives: A comparative study using different natural fibre polymers as encapsulants. *Food Bioprocess Technol.* **2013**, *6*, 2376–2388. [CrossRef]
7. Bakowska-Barczak, A.M.; Kolodziejczyk, P.P. Black currant polyphenols: Their storage stability and microencapsulation. *Ind. Crop. Prod.* **2011**, *34*, 1301–1309. [CrossRef]
8. Fang, Z.; Bhandari, B. Encapsulation of polyphenols-A review. *Trends Food Sci. Technol.* **2010**, *21*, 510–523. [CrossRef]
9. Munin, A.; Edwards-Lévy, F. Encapsulation of natural polyphenolic compounds: A review. *J. Pharm.* **2011**, *4*, 793–829. [CrossRef]
10. Laine, P.; Kylli, P.; Heinonen, M.; Jouppila, K. Storage stability of microencapsulated cloudberry (*Rubus chamaemorus*) phenolics. *J. Agric. Food Chem.* **2008**, *56*, 11251–11261. [CrossRef]
11. Castro-López, C.; Ventura-Sobrevilla, J.M.; González-Hernández, M.D.; Rojas, R.; Ascacio-Valdés, J.A.; Aguilar, C.N.; Martínez-Ávila, G.C.G. Impact of extraction techniques on antioxidant capacities and phytochemical composition of polyphenol-rich extracts. *Food Chem.* **2017**, *237*, 1139–1148. [CrossRef] [PubMed]

12. Medina-Torres, L.; Santiago-Adame, R.; Calderas, F.; Gallegos-Infante, J.A.; González-Laredo, R.F.; Rocha-Guzmán, N.E.; Núñez-Ramírez, D.M.; Bernad-Bernad, M.J.; Manero, O. Microencapsulation by spray-drying of laurel infusions (*Litsea glaucescens*) with maltodextrin. *Ind. Crop. Prod.* **2016**, *90*, 1–8. [CrossRef]
13. Tonon, R.V.; Brabet, C.; Hubinger, M.D. Anthocyanin stability and antioxidant activity of spray-dried acai (Euterpe oleracea Mart.) juice produced with different carrier agents. *Food Res. Int.* **2010**, *43*, 907–914. [CrossRef]
14. Ferrari, C.C.; Germer, S.P.M.; Alvim, I.D.; de Aguirre, J.M. Storage stability of spray-dried blackberry powder produced with maltodextrin or gum arabic. *Dry. Technol.* **2013**, *31*, 470–478. [CrossRef]
15. Ahmad, M.; Qureshi, S.; Maqsood, S.; Gani, A.; Masoodi, F.A. Micro-encapsulation of folic acid using horse chestnut starch and β-cyclodextrin: Microcapsule characterization, release behavior & antioxidant potential during GI tract conditions. *Food Hydrocoll.* **2017**, *66*, 154–160.
16. George, S.; Brat, P.; Alter, P.; Amiot, M.J. Rapid determination of polyphenols and vitamin C in plant-derived products. *J. Agric. Food Chem.* **2005**, *53*, 1370–1373. [CrossRef]
17. Brand-Williams, W.; Cuvelier, M.E.; Berset, C. Use of a free radical method to evaluate antioxidant activity. *LWT Food Sci. Technol.* **1995**, *28*, 25–30. [CrossRef]
18. Emter, R.; Natsch, A. A fast Resazurin-based live viability assay is equivalent to the MTT-test in the keratino sens assay. *Toxicol. In Vitro* **2015**, *29*, 688–693. [CrossRef] [PubMed]
19. Desobry, S.A.; Netto, F.M.; Labuza, T.P. Comparison of spray-drying, drum-drying and freeze-drying for β-carotene encapsulation and preservation. *J. Food Sci.* **1997**, *62*, 1158–1162. [CrossRef]
20. Díaz, D.I.; Beristain, C.I.; Azuara, E.; Luna, G.; Jimenez, M. Effect of wall material on the antioxidant activity and physicochemical properties of *Rubus fruticosus* juice microcapsules. *J. Microencapsul.* **2015**, *32*, 247–254. [CrossRef] [PubMed]
21. Mahdavi, S.A.; Jafari, S.M.; Assadpour, E.; Ghorbani, M. Storage stability of encapsulated barberry's anthocyanin and its application in jelly formulation. *J. Food Eng.* **2016**, *181*, 59–66. [CrossRef]
22. Moser, P.; Telis, V.R.N.; de Andrade Neves, N.; García-Romero, E.; Gómez-Alonso, S.; Hermosín-Gutiérrez, I. Storage stability of phenolic compounds in powdered BRS Violeta grape juice microencapsulated with protein and maltodextrin blends. *Food Chem.* **2017**, *214*, 308–318. [CrossRef] [PubMed]
23. Wilkowska, A.; Ambroziak, W.; Adamiec, J.; Czyżowska, A. Preservation of antioxidant activity and polyphenols in chokeberry juice and wine with the use of microencapsulation. *J. Food Process. Preserv.* **2016**, *41*, 1–9. [CrossRef]
24. Wang, J.; Li, H.; Chen, Z.; Liu, W.; Chen, H. Characterization and storage properties of a new microencapsulation of tea polyphenols. *Ind. Crop. Prod.* **2016**, *89*, 152–156. [CrossRef]
25. Zheng, L.; Ding, Z.; Zhang, M.; Sun, J. Microcapsulation of bayberry polyphenols by ethyl cellulose: Preparation and characterization. *J. Food Eng.* **2011**, *104*, 89–95. [CrossRef]
26. Fracassetti, D.; Del Bo, C.; Simonetti, P.; Gardana, C.; Klimis-Zacas, D.; Ciappellano, S. Effect of time and storage temperature on anthocyanin decay and antioxidant activity in wild blueberry (*Vaccinium angustifolium*) powder. *J. Agric. Food Chem.* **2013**, *61*, 2999–3005. [CrossRef]
27. Ydjedd, S.; Bouriche, S.; López-Nicolás, R.; Sánchez-Moya, T.; Frontela-Saseta, C.; Ros-Berruezo, G.; Rezgui, F.; Louaileche, H.; Kati, D.E. Effect of *in vitro* gastrointestinal digestion on encapsulated and no encapsulated phenolic compounds of Carob (*Ceratonia siliqua* L.) pulp extracts and their antioxidant capacity. *J. Agric. Food Chem.* **2017**, *65*, 827–835. [CrossRef]
28. Wongsasulak, S.; Pathumban, S.; Yoovidhya, T. Effect of entrapped α-tocopherol on mucoadhesivity and evaluation of the release, degradation, and swelling characteristics of zein-chitosan composite electrospun fibers. *J. Food Eng.* **2014**, *120*, 110–117. [CrossRef]
29. Asghari-Varzaneh, E.; Shahedi, M.; Shekarchizadeh, H. Iron microencapsulation in gum tragacanth using solvent evaporation method. *Int. J. Biol. Macromol.* **2017**, *103*, 640–647. [CrossRef]
30. Hostler, A.C. Hydrocolloids: Practical guides for the food industry. In *Proceedings of the International Conference on Harmonisation of Technical Requirements for Registration of Pharmaceuticals for Human Use. Stability Testing of New Drug Substances and Products Q 1A (R2), Geneva, Switzerland*; Eagan Press Handbook Series; Eagan Press: St. Paul, MI, USA, 2004.

31. Sansone, F.; Picerno, P.; Mencherini, T.; Russo, P.; Gasparri, F.; Giannini, V.; Lauro, M.R.; Puglisi, G.; Aquino, R.P. Enhanced technological and permeation properties of a microencapsulated soy isoflavones extract. *J. Food Eng.* **2013**, *115*, 298–305. [CrossRef]
32. Allison, S.D. Effect of structural relaxation on the preparation and drug release behavior of poly (lactic-co-glycolic) acid microparticle drug delivery systems. *J. Pharm. Sci.* **2008**, *97*, 2022–2035. [CrossRef]
33. Nur, M.; Vasiljevic, T. Insulin inclusion into a tragacanth hydrogel: An oral delivery system for insulin. *Materials* **2018**, *11*, 79. [CrossRef] [PubMed]
34. Verma, C.; Pathania, D.; Anjum, S.; Gupta, B. Smart designing of tragacanth gum by graft functionalization for advanced materials. *Macromol. Mater. Eng.* **2020**, 1900762. [CrossRef]
35. Flores, F.P.; Singh, R.K.; Kerr, W.L.; Phillips, D.R.; Kong, F. In vitro release properties of encapsulated blueberry (*Vaccinium ashei*) extracts. *Food Chem.* **2015**, *168*, 225–232. [CrossRef] [PubMed]
36. Ahmad, M.; Ashraf, B.; Gani, A.; Gani, A. Microencapsulation of saffron anthocyanins using β-glucan and β-cyclodextrin: Microcapsule characterization, release behaviour & antioxidant potential during in vitro digestion. *Int. J. Biol. Macromol.* **2018**, *109*, 435–442. [PubMed]
37. You, L.J.; Zhao, M.M.; Regenstein, J.M.; Ren, J.Y. Changes in the antioxidant activity of loach (*Misgurnus anguillicaudatus*) protein hydrolysates during a simulated gastrointestinal digestion. *Food Chem.* **2010**, *120*, 810–816. [CrossRef]
38. Wootton-Beard, P.C.; Moran, A.; Ryan, L. Stability of the total antioxidant capacity and total polyphenol content of 23 commercially available vegetable juices before and after *in vitro* digestion measured by FRAP, DPPH, ABTS and Folin-Ciocalteu methods. *Food Res. Int.* **2011**, *44*, 217–224. [CrossRef]
39. Friedman, M.; Jürgens, H.S. Effect of pH on the stability of plant phenolic compounds. *J. Agric. Food Chem.* **2000**, *48*, 2101–2110. [CrossRef] [PubMed]
40. ISO (International Organization for Standardization). ISO 10993–5:2009 Standard "Biological Evaluation of Medical Devices—Part 5: Tests for In Vitro Cytotoxicity". Available online: https://www.iso.org/standard/36406.html (accessed on 15 June 2020).
41. Courtney, R.; Sirdaarta, J.; White, A.; Cock, I.E. Inhibition of Caco-2 and HeLa proliferation by *Terminalia carpentariae* C. T. white and *Terminalia grandiflora* benth. extracts: Identification of triterpenoid components. *Pharmacogn. J.* **2017**, *9*, 441–451. [CrossRef]
42. Sánchez-Vioque, R.; Santana-Méridas, O.; Polissiou, M.; Vioque, J.; Astraka, K.; Alaiz, M.; Herraiz-Peñalver, D.; Tarantilis, P.A.; Girón-Calle, J. Polyphenol composition and in vitro antiproliferative effect of corm, tepal and leaf from *Crocus sativus* L. on human colon adenocarcinoma cells (Caco-2). *J. Funct. Foods* **2016**, *24*, 18–25. [CrossRef]
43. Szewczyk, K.; Lewandowska, U.; Owczarek, K.; Sosnowska, D.; Gorlach, S.; Koziołkiewicz, M.; Hrabec, Z.; Hrabec, E. Influence of polyphenol extract from evening primrose (*Oenothera paradoxa*) seeds on proliferation of Caco-2 cells and on expression, synthesis and activity of matrix metalloproteinases and their inhibitors. *Pol. J. Food Nutr. Sci.* **2014**, *64*, 181–191. [CrossRef]
44. Baeza, G.; Amigo-Benavent, M.; Sarriá, B.; Goya, L.; Mateos, R.; Bravo, L. Green coffee hydroxycinnamic acids but not caffeine protects human HepG2 cells against oxidative stress. *Food Res. Int.* **2014**, *62*, 1038–1046. [CrossRef]
45. Wang, S.; Mateos, R.; Goya, L.; Amigo-Benavent, M.; Sarriá, B.; Bravo, L. A phenolic extract from grape by-products and its main hydroxybenzoic acids protect Caco-2 cells against pro-oxidant induced toxicity. *Food Chem. Toxicol.* **2016**, *88*, 65–74. [CrossRef] [PubMed]

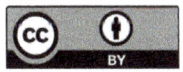

© 2020 by the authors. Licensee MDPI, Basel, Switzerland. This article is an open access article distributed under the terms and conditions of the Creative Commons Attribution (CC BY) license (http://creativecommons.org/licenses/by/4.0/).

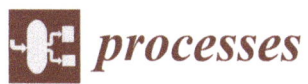

Article

Preliminary Testing of Ultrasound/Microwave-Assisted Extraction (U/M-AE) for the Isolation of Geraniin from *Nephelium lappaceum* L. (Mexican Variety) Peel

Cristian Hernández-Hernández [1], Cristóbal Noé Aguilar [1], Adriana Carolina Flores-Gallegos [1], Leonardo Sepúlveda [1], Raúl Rodríguez-Herrera [1], Jesús Morlett-Chávez [2], Mayela Govea-Salas [3] and Juan Ascacio-Valdés [1,*]

[1] Bioprocesses and Bioproducts Research Group, Food Research Department, School of Chemistry, Autonomous University of Coahuila, Saltillo 25280, Mexico; hernandezcristian@uadec.edu.mx (C.H.-H.); cristobal.aguilar@uadec.edu.mx (C.N.A.); carolinaflores@uadec.edu.mx (A.C.F.-G.); leonardo_sepulveda@uadec.edu.mx (L.S.); raul.rodriguez@uadec.edu.mx (R.R.-H.)
[2] Laboratory of Molecular Biology, School of Chemistry, Autonomous University of Coahuila, Saltillo 25280, Mexico; antoniomorlett@uadec.edu.mx
[3] Laboratory of Nanobiosciences, School of Chemistry, Autonomous University of Coahuila, Saltillo 25280, Mexico; m.govea.salas@uadec.edu.mx
* Correspondence: alberto_ascaciovaldes@uadec.edu.mx; Tel.: +52-84-4416-1238; Fax: +52-84-4416-9213

Received: 20 March 2020; Accepted: 3 May 2020; Published: 12 May 2020

Abstract: The rambutan peel (RP) is a relevant source of bioactive molecules, which could be used for application in cosmetics, food, and pharmaceutical areas. Total soluble polyphenol content was extracted from Mexican variety rambutan peels using an emergent ultrasound/microwave-assisted extraction (U/M-AE) technology. Five extractions were performed using different mass/volume and ethanol/water ratios; 1:16-0; 1:16-70; 1:8-0; 1:8-70; 1:12-30. Condition 1:16-0 was defined as the best extraction condition with 0% ethanol percentage (only water). The content of total soluble polyphenols was 307.57 mg/g. The total bound polyphenol content was 26.53 mg/g. Besides, two separation processes were made with the soluble fraction; the first one was performed using Amberlite XAD-16 (Sigma-Aldrich, Saint Louis, MO, USA), and seven polyphenolic compounds were obtained. The second one was performed using a preparative HPLC (Varian, Palo Alto, CA, USA) equipment obtained fraction where three compounds were obtained: geraniin (main compound), ellagic acid, and ellagic acid pentoside. The major compound isolated in the two separations was geraniin, according to HPLC/ESI/MS (High Performance Liquid Chromatography/ElectroSpray Ionization/Mass) analysis.

Keywords: U/A-AE; *Nephelium lappaceum* L.; separation; ellagitannins; geraniin

1. Introduction

The rambutan (*Nephelium lappaceum* L.) is an exotic fruit that is grown in Southeast Asia (Malaysia, Thailand, Indonesia). Currently, its cultivation is spread in several countries in the humid tropics of America, such as Colombia, Ecuador, Honduras, Costa Rica, Trinidad and Tobago, Cuba, and, mainly, Mexico. (In Mexico, the rambutan was introduced in the 1950s.) The rambutan is consumed fresh, and the peel is discarded, generating waste [1]. In recent research, it has been reported that rambutan peel (RP) contains bioactive molecules such as polyphenols (mainly ellagitannins) that have great potential as an ingredient in functional foods due to their biological properties, such as immune-modulatory, cytoprotective, anticancer, antimicrobial and antioxidant (Figure 1). As well as their therapeutic effects, besides our understanding of their biosynthesis and their interest in the body system, polyphenols also have analgesic properties and prevent cardiovascular diseases [2].

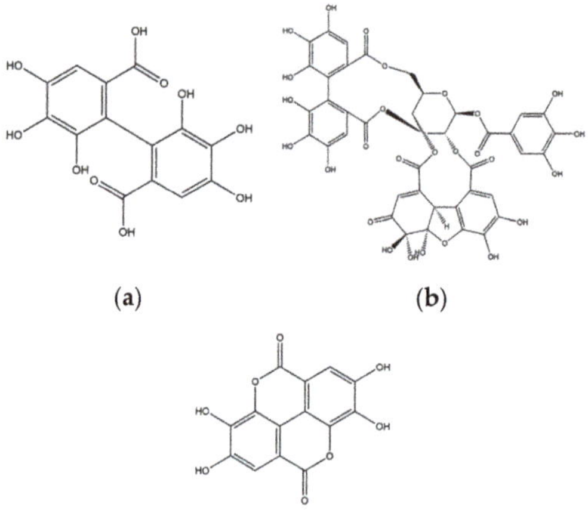

Figure 1. (a) HHDP (Hexahydroxydiphenic acid) group, the particular group of ellagitannins; (b) geraniin, an ellagitannin; (c) ellagic acid, a compound derived from ellagitannins.

Currently, there are several techniques for bioactive compound extraction implementing new extraction technologies, such as microwave-assisted extraction (MAE) and ultrasound-assisted extraction (UAE), among others. These are considered "green" techniques as they reduce the use of organic solvents and obtain higher yields from the extracts, as well as taking care of the environment [3]. The ultrasound can be associated with microwaves, a combination that can act as an emergent hybrid technology: ultrasound/microwave-assisted extraction (U/M-AE) [4]. U/M-AE, compared to conventional methods, has more advantages by reducing extraction time, giving higher yields, and consuming fewer solvents. This technology, supported by HPLC/MS (High Performance Liquid Chromatography/Mass) analysis, has advantages for the identification of bioactive molecules because the use of this extraction technology allows a better interaction between the solvent and the compounds of interest due to the cavitation phenomenon produced by ultrasound. This interaction is also favored by the temperature of the microwave treatment and temperature is an essential factor in promoting the extraction and solubility of the compounds. It is important to mention that this occurs at the same time using U/M-AE, and that all this represents an important advantage for the use of HPLC/MS in the identification of the obtained compounds, since fractions of specific compounds of interest are obtained. [5]. Actually, HPLC is a chromatographic technique used in phytochemistry to identify, quantify, and purify components. The resolution power of HPLC is ideal for the characterization and quantification of secondary metabolites in plant extracts: mainly phenolic compounds, steroids, flavonoids, alkaloids. The combination of HPLC and MS facilitates the identification of chemical compounds in medicinal plants. The HPLC/MS technique has advantages when it provides the molecular structure of the MS and has become a powerful technique for the identification of bioactive compounds due to its operational simplicity [4,5]. Therefore, in this study, the extraction of polyphenols from Mexican variety rambutan peel was performed using U/M-AE technology and testing some selected parameters to obtain the best extraction conditions. Soluble and bound polyphenols were determined, as well as the separation and identification of the main bioactive molecules (geraniin), by liquid chromatography and mass spectrometry (HPLC/ESI/MS).

2. Materials and Methods

2.1. Raw Material

The rambutan peels (RP) were obtained in the Soconusco region of Chiapas state in Mexico. The peel was washed with distilled water and dehydrated in a conventional oven at 50 °C for 48 h (5% moisture after dehydration). Subsequently, the RP was milled using a Thomas-Wiley mill of knives, model 4 Arthur H (particle size 2 mm), Thomas Company (Philadelphia, PA, USA). It was then stored at room temperature in a glass container in the dark for subsequent analysis.

2.2. Experimental Design

The experimental design for the extraction of bioactive molecules from the rambutan peel was carried out by applying a factorial fractioned design with two evaluated factors, the mass/volume ratio (m/v) and the ratio of ethanol/water (e/w), to determine the best extraction condition. All rambutan peel extractions were carried out on the same extraction equipment. The conditions used in the extraction equipment were 20 min at room temperature for ultrasound, 5 min at 70 °C for microwave. The five evaluated extraction conditions are shown in Table 1. Subsequently, the extracts were analyzed to determine the total content of soluble and bound polyphenols.

Table 1. Extraction condition of polyphenolic compounds in RP.

ID	Mass/Volume Ratio (g/mL)	Water/Ethanol Ratio (%)
1	1:16	0
2	1:16	70
3	1:8	0
4	1:8	70
5	1:12	30

2.3. Ultrasound/Microwave-Assisted Extraction (U/M-AE) of Soluble Polyphenols

For the extraction of soluble polyphenol compounds from RP, a hybrid technology system was used: An Ultrasound/Microwave Cooperative Workstation (Nanjing ATPIO Instruments Manufacture Co., Ltd. company, Nanjing, China) operating at a microwave frequency of 2450 MHz and 25 kHz ultrasound (Figure 2). The ground rambutan peel with a particle size of 2 mm was placed in a reactor of the extraction equipment. Subsequently, a volume of 700 mL was added with the five extraction conditions, as shown in Table 1. The extracts obtained were stored for subsequent analysis of the total polyphenol content.

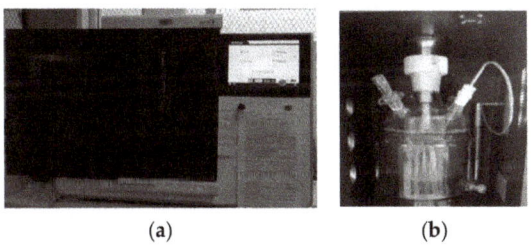

(a) (b)

Figure 2. (a) Ultrasound/Microwave Cooperative Workstation; (b) Reactor for extractions.

2.4. Separation of Bound Polyphenol Fractions

The bound polyphenol fractions were obtained from the solid residue after the extraction of soluble polyphenols using the five conditions shown in Table 1, usingthe methods reported by Zhang et al. [6] with slight modifications. For the extraction of the bound phenols, 1 g of the RP residue was used and digested with 50 mL of 2 M sodium hydroxide at room temperature for 4 h. The mixture was acidified with concentrated hydrochloric acid at pH 2.0. The mixture was filtered with Whatman No. 41 (Sigma-Aldrich, Saint Louis, MO, USA) filter paper, and the lipids were removed with 30 mL of hexaneusing a separation funnel. The remaining mixture was extracted three times with 75 mL ethyl acetate by liquid–liquid separation. The ethyl acetate fractions were collected and evaporated to dryness by a rotatory evaporator. The bound phenolic compounds were dissolved in 5 mL using the m/v and e/w ratios performed for soluble polyphenols. The fractions obtained were used as bound phenols in RP.

2.5. Determination of Total Polyphenol Content

The content of hydrolyzable and condensed polyphenols in RP extracts were determined by the Folin–Ciocalteu method [7] and HCl-Butanol described by Nitao et al. [8] for soluble and bound polyphenol samples. The experiment was carried out in triplicate. Gallic acid and catechin were used as reference standards. Total soluble and bound polyphenol content was obtained by summing hydrolyzable and condensed polyphenols. The analysis of soluble and bound polyphenols was carried out in a dark place in the absence of light. For the total soluble polyphenol content, a Tukey test was performed to determine significant differences ($p \leq 0.05$). The response variable was the content of total soluble polyphenolic compounds. Additionally, a contour diagram and analysis of the Pareto chart was performed under an exploratory (Box Hunter, and Hunter) design with Statistica program (StartSoft, version 7.0, Dell, Austin, TX, USA).

2.6. Separation and Partial Purification of Soluble Polyphenol Fractions Using Amberlite XAD-16

The separation of phenolic fractions from RP with Amberlite XAD-16 was prepared using the methodology described by Ascacio-Valdés et al. [9]. The phenolic extracts obtained by U/M-AE were filtered through Whatman No.41 filter paper. Afterward, Amberlite XAD-16 resin was used for subsequent packaging in a chromatography column. The phenolic extracts were passed through the chromatography column with Amberlite XAD-16. Distilled water was used as an eluent for discarding undesirable compounds such as carbohydrates, lipids, and other impurities. Later, ethanol was used as eluent to recover the molecules of interest retained in the Amberlite XAD-16 resin and to recover the phenolic fraction. The phenolic fraction was evaporated in an oven at 50 °C and recovered as a fine powder; an 8% yield was obtained, a high yield compared to materials reported as the best sources of ellagitannins, such as pomegranate peels (6%) [9].

2.7. Separation and Isolation of Ellagitannins by Preparative HPLC

The soluble polyphenol fractions of RP were separated by high-resolution preparative scale chromatography for the purification of the extracts using the method described by Aguilar-Zárate et al. [10]. Posteriorly, 300 mg of polyphenols were weighed and prepared in a 2 mL solution with 50% ethanol, then gauged to 10 mL of distilled water and filtered with 0.45 µm membranes. The extracts were separated using liquid chromatography equipment, (Varian ProStar 3300, Varian, Palo Alto, CA, USA) and a Dynamax column, Microsorb300 C18 (250 mm × 21.4 mm, 10 µm). A flow rate of 8 mL/min was used and the conditions were as follows: as mobile phase, (A) CH3COOH (3% v/v in water) and (B) methanol. The method used for the separation of the molecules was isocratic: 5% initial B; 0–45 min, 5–90% B; 45–50 min, 90% B; 50–70 min, 90–5% B; 70–95 min. The elution of the compounds (ellagitannins) was monitored at 280 nm. The column was washed with 90% methanol (45–60 min) and reconditioned to the initial conditions (60–80 min). The fractions were recovered and characterized by HPLC/ESI/MS analysis.

2.8. Identification of Polyphenolic Compounds by HPLC/ESI/MS Analysis

The identification and characterization of the polyphenolic compounds of the RP extract were carried out by the method described by Sepulveda et al. [11] with some slight modifications.

The ethanolic fraction of RP was filtered using 0.45 μm nylon membranes and placed in a 2 mL vial. The analyses by reversed-phase high-performance liquid chromatography were performed on a Varian HPLC system, including an auto-sampler (ProStar 410, Varian, Palo Alto, CA, USA), a ternary pump (ProStar 230I, Varian, Palo Alto, California, USA) and a PDA detector (ProStar 330, Varian, Atlanta, GA, USA). A chromatography ion trap mass spectrometer (Varian 500-MS IT Mass Spectrometer, Palo Alto, CA, USA) equipped with an electrospray ion source was also used. Samples (5 μL) were injected onto a Denali C18 column (150 mm × 2.1 mm, 3μm, Grace, Albany, OR, USA) and the oven temperature was maintained at 30 °C. The eluents were formic acid (0.2%, v/v; solvent A) and acetonitrile (solvent B). The following gradient was applied: initial, 3% B; 0–5 min, 9% B linear; 5–15 min, 16% B linear; 15–45 min, 50% B linear. Then, the column was washed and reconditioned; the flow rate was maintained at 0.2 mL/min and elution was monitored at 245, 280, 320 and 550 nm. The whole effluent (0.2 mL/min) was injected into the source of the mass spectrometer without splitting. All MS experiments were carried out in the negative mode [M-H]-nitrogen was used as nebulizing gas and helium as damping gas. The ion source parameters were spray voltage 5.0 kV and capillary voltage and temperature were 90.0 V and 350 °C respectively. Data were collected and processed using MS Workstation software (V 6.9). Samples were firstly analyzed in full scan mode acquired in the m/z range 50–2000. MS/MS analyses were performed on a series of selected precursor ions. Finally, the compounds were compared using a database of bioactive compounds (WorkStation version 2.0 database, VARIAN, Palo Alto, CA, USA).

3. Results and Discussion

3.1. Soluble Polyphenol Content in RP Extract

The extractions performed with samples 1:16-0, 1:16-70, and 1:12-30 showed a higher content of soluble polyphenols (Figure 3). Generally, the solvent extraction system is selected by the polarity of interest compounds, the amount of solvent used, the safety of the extraction, and the cost [12]. The samples 1:16-0, 1:16-70, and 1:12-30 are not significantly different ($p \leq 0.05$) insoluble polyphenol content. Therefore, the sample 1:16-0 was taken as the best extraction condition using water as the solvent, and was neither toxic nor harmful to the environment. Water is an excellent solvent for the extraction of polyphenols such as ellagitannins [13]. For this reason, ratio 1:16-0 was established as the best extraction condition with a content of 307.57 mg/g ± 20.27 mg/g dry matter of total soluble polyphenols. Moreover, the content of bound polyphenols was lower than the soluble polyphenols.

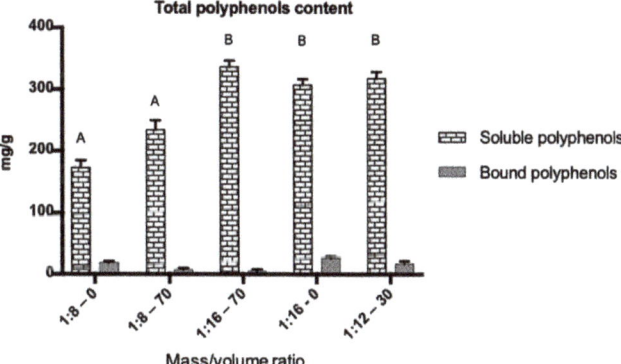

Figure 3. The total content of soluble and boundpolyphenolsin RP. The best extraction conditions were 1:16-0 with 307.57 mg/g ± 20.27 mg/g, then 1:16-70 with 318.55 mg/g ± 18.96 mg/g and 1:12-30 with 311.09 mg/g ± 29.36mg/g. According to Tukey's test means with the same letter are not significantly different ($p \leq 0.05$).

Figure 4 shows the effect of the evaluated factors in this study. The response variable was total soluble polyphenols, the representation of extraction mass/volume (m/v), and water/ethanol percentage (e/w) effects. The m/v factor has a more substantial effect on w/e factor. Therefore, at higher m/v ratios, higher soluble polyphenol content is found, indicating that changes in m/v ratio may increase or decrease the content of polyphenolic compounds. Besides, the (e/w) factor has a low effect on the total soluble polyphenol content. The contour diagram shown in Figure 2 indicates that the best extraction condition of total phenolic compounds is achieved with a 1:16-0 ratio. Using 43.75 g of RP sample and 0% ethanol (water), a total of 307.57 mg/g dry matter of total soluble polyphenols is obtained. Sun et al. [12] obtained optimal conditions to find the maximum extraction efficiency of phenolic content in RP (213.76 mg/g dry matter).

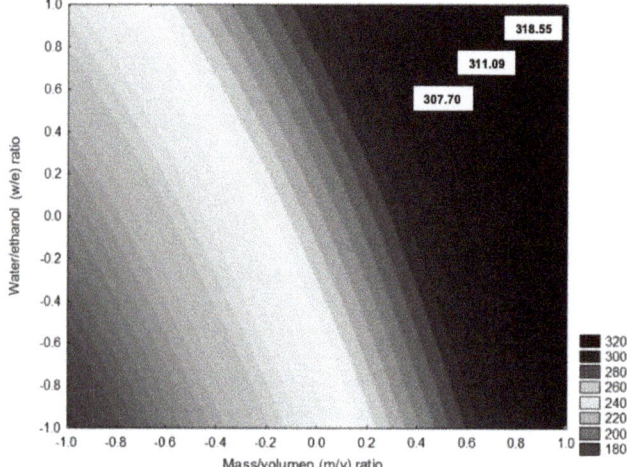

Figure 4. Contour diagram of the total polyphenol content in function of m/v ratio and w/e percentage. Polyphenol extraction ranges are between 180 and 320 mg/g of rambutan peel extract. The highest extraction conditions were 1:16-0 with 307.57 mg/g, 1:12-30 with 311.09 mg/g and 1:16-70 with 318.55 mg/g.

The standardized Pareto chart (Figure 5) is a representation of the effect of both variables, water/ethanol (e/w) and mass/volume (m/v), and their interactions. Each variable that crosses the vertical line is considered significant. However, a positive effect was observed in the m/v ratio, i.e., the increase in this ratio may contribute to a higher content of extracted polyphenols. In contrast the increase in the e/w ratio decreases the total number of extracted polyphenols. The positive effect observed in the m/v ratio could be explained by the types of polyphenols extracted since most are soluble and the solubility of the polyphenols in the solvent exerts high diffusivities of mass transfer at different temperatures. On the other hand, the e/w ratio may only have led more solvents to enter the cells to penetrate with a higher solid/liquid ratio, which seems to be the most plausible for this behavior for the e/w ratio [14].

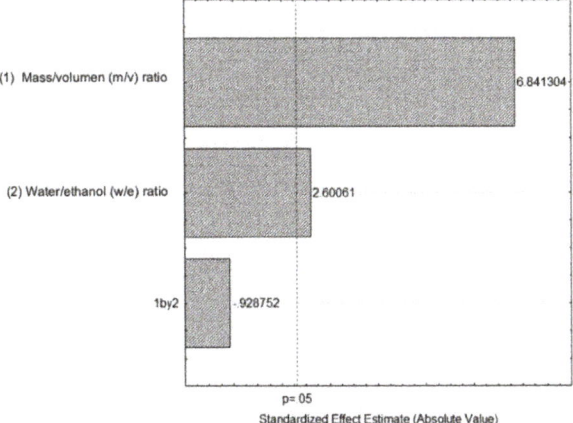

Figure 5. Standardized Pareto chart of the total polyphenol content in function of m/v ratio and e/w percentage.

3.2. Bound Polyphenol Content in RP Extract

The extraction of bound phenolic compounds at room temperature was carried out by alkaline hydrolysis. The content of total bound polyphenols was 26.53 ± 0.13 mg/g, with the best extraction condition 1:16-0. Comparing the results, soluble total polyphenol content was higher than the total polyphenols bound ($p \leq 0.05$) (Figure 3). Sun et al. [12] reported soluble and bound polyphenol content of rambutan peel using microwave-assisted extraction at 213.76 and 9.37 mg/g respectively.

3.3. Isolation of Ellagitannin

After partial purification with Amberlite XAD-16, a second purification with preparative HPLC was performed for ellagitannins isolation. The recovered fraction (41.2 mg) was identified as ellagitannins: Geraniin, ellagic acid, and ellagic acid pentoside according to HPLC/ESI/MS analysis. Finally, geraniin was the main compound present in the sample, with 13.8% of the total of the fraction recovered and 42.5% of abundance in preparative HPLC. Palanisamy et al. [15] recovered less than 3.79% geraniin because geraniin may have degraded to ellagic acid or corilagin.

3.4. Identification of Bioactive Compounds Present in RP Extract

HPLC/ESI/MS analysis was used to identify compounds present after the first partial purification with Amberlite XAD-16, and the second purification with preparative HPLC, as shown in Table 2. The identification profile of the main compounds was carried out using negative ionization modes as MS operating conditions, with molecular mass (MS) and their fragments (MS/MS) being obtained.

After the first partial purification with Amberlite XAD-16, a total of seven compounds were identified: six ellagitannins and one hydroxybenzoic acid. Mendez-Flores et al. [16] recovered 12 polyphenolic compounds in RP Mexican variety, also using Amberlite XAD-16. In the second purification with preparative HPLC, three compounds were identified: Geraniin, ellagic acid, and ellagic acid pentoside. Geraniin was the main identified compound (Figure 6). Palanisamy et al. [15] reported that geraniin was also the main compound identified using methanol and ethanol as the extraction solvent in rambutan peel. The relevance of obtaining these compounds is due to their important biological properties applicable in different industrial areas such as cosmetics, pharmaceuticals, and food.

Table 2. Compounds identified by HPLC/ESI/MS.

Purification	ID	Retention Time (min)	Compounds	Mass(m/z) [M-H]⁻	MS²	Group/Family
Amberlite XAD-16	1	25.66	Corilagin	634	481,301,275	Ellagitannin
	2	26.55	Geraniin	952	933,301,169	Ellagitannin
	3	28.5	Punigluconin	802	649,347,348	Ellagitannin
	4	29.85	Ellagicacidpentoside	433	299,300,287,125	Ellagitannin
	5	31.65	Ellagicacid	302	257, 229,185	Ellagitannin
	6	33.07	Tetragalloyglucose	789	617,465,635	Hydroxybenzoic acid
	7	33.5	Pedunculagin	785	301,481,765	Ellagitannin
Preparative HPLC	1	27.45	Geraniin	952	933,301,169	Ellagitannin
	2	30.55	Ellagicacid	302	257,229,185	Ellagitannin
	3	32.75	Ellagicacidpentoside	433	299,300,287,125	Ellagitannin

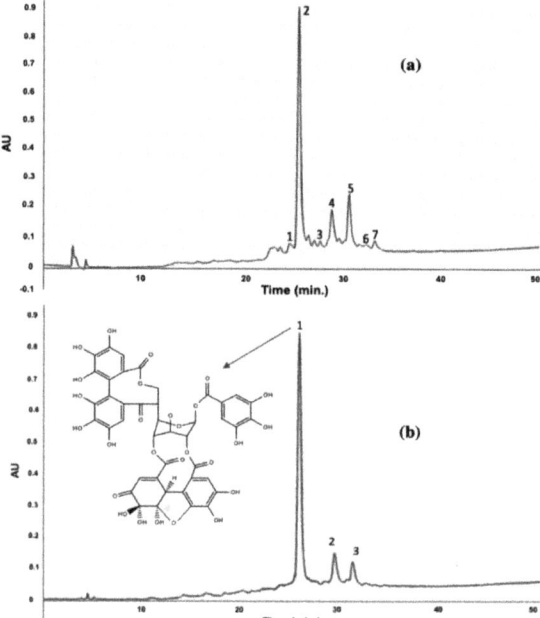

Figure 6. Chromatogram of the best extraction condition of RP 1:16-0 with the first and the second purification (a) 1 corilagin; 2 geraniin; 3 punigluconin; 4 ellagic acid pentoside; 5 ellagic acid; 6 tetragalloy glucose; 7 pedunculagin. (b) 1 geranin; 2 ellagic acid; 3 ellagic acid pentoside at 280 nm.

Author Contributions: Conceptualization, J.A.-V. and C.N.A.; methodology, C.H.-H., A.C.F.-G., and M.G.-S.; formal analysis, R.R.-H., L.S., J.M.-C.; investigation, J.A.-V. and C.N.A.; writing—Original draft preparation, C.H.-H.; writing—Review and editing, C.H.-H., J.A.-V., C.N.A.; supervision, J.A.-V., C.N.A. All authors have read and agreed to the published version of the manuscript.

Funding: This research was funded by the Autonomous University of Coahuila, Mexico. Cristian Hernández received a scholarship from CONACyT for his postgraduate studies.

Conflicts of Interest: The authors declare no conflict of interest.

References

1. Castillo-Vera, A.; López-Guillén, G.; Sandoval-Esquivez, A. La historia del cultivo de rambutan (*Nepheliumlapacceum* L.) en México. *Agroproductividad* **2017**, *10*, 53–57.
2. Hernández-Hernández, C.; Aguilar, C.; Rodríguez-Herrera, R.; Flores-Gallegos, A.; Morlett-Chávez, J.; Govea-Salas, M.; Ascacio-Valdés, J. Rambutan (*Nepheliumlappaceum* L.): Nutritional and functionalproperties. *Trends Food Sci. Technol.* **2019**, *85*, 201–210. [CrossRef]
3. Sagar, N.; Pareek, S.; Sharma, S.; Yahia, E.; Lobo, M. Fruit and Vegetable Waste: Bioactive Compounds, Their Extraction, and Possible Utilization. *Compr. Rev. Food Sci. Food Saf.* **2018**, *17*, 512–531. [CrossRef]
4. De Monte, C.; Carradori, S.; Granese, A.; Di Pierro, G.; Leonardo, C.; De Nunzio, C. Modern extraction techniques and their impact on the pharmacological profile of *Serenoarepens* extracts for the treatment of lower urinary tract symptoms. *BMC Urol.* **2014**, *14*, 1–11. [CrossRef] [PubMed]
5. Carniel, N.; Filippi, D.; DellossGullich, L.; Bilibio, D.; Bender, J.; Priamo, W. Recovery of Total Polyphenols from Pomegranate and Butia: A Study of Ultrasound-assisted Extraction and Antioxidant Activity. *Indian J. Adv. Chem. Sci.* **2017**, *5*, 112–117. [CrossRef]
6. Zhang, M.; Zhang, R.; Zhang, F.; Liu, R. Phenolic Profiles and Antioxidant Activity of Black Rice Bran of Different Commercially Available Varieties. *J. Agric. Food Chem.* **2010**, *58*, 7580–7587. [CrossRef] [PubMed]
7. Sinlgeton, V.; Rossi, J. Colorimetry of total phenolics with phosphomolybdic-phosphotungstic acid reagents. *Am. J. Enol. Vitic.* **1965**, *16*, 144–158.
8. Nitao, J.; Birr, B.; Nair, M.; Herms, D.; Mattson, W. Rapid Quantification of Proanthocyanidins (Condensed Tannins) with a Continuous Flow Analyzer. *J. Agric. Food Chem.* **2001**, *49*, 2207–2214. [CrossRef] [PubMed]
9. Ascacio-Valdés, J.; Aguilera-Carbó, A.; Buenrostro, J.; Prado-Barragán, A.; Rodríguez-Herrera, R.; Aguilar, C. The complete biodegradation pathway of ellagitanninsby *Aspergillusniger* in solid-state fermentation. *J. Basic Microbiol.* **2016**, *56*, 329–336. [CrossRef] [PubMed]
10. Aguilar-Zárate, P.; Wong-Paz, J.; Michel, M.; Buenrostro-Figueroa, J.; Díaz, H.; Ascacio, J.; Contreras-Esquivel, J.; Gutiérrez-Sánchez, G.; Aguilar, C. Characterization of Pomegranate-Husk Polyphenols and Semi-Preparative Fractionation of Punicalagin. *Phytochem. Anal.* **2017**, *28*, 433–438. [CrossRef] [PubMed]
11. Sepúlveda, L.; Wong-Paz, J.; Buenrostro-Figueroa, J.; Ascacio-Valdés, J.; Aguilera-Carbó, A.; Aguilar, C. Solid-state fermentation of pomegranate husk: Recovery of ellagic acid by SEC and identification of ellagitannins by HPLC/ESI/MS. *Food Biosci.* **2018**, *22*, 99–104. [CrossRef]
12. Sun, L.; Zhang, H.; Zhuang, Y. Preparation of Free, Soluble Conjugate, and Insoluble-Bound Phenolic Compounds from Peels of Rambutan (*Nepheliumlappaceum*) and Evaluation of Antioxidant Activitiesin vitro. *J. Food Sci.* **2012**, *77*, 198–204. [CrossRef] [PubMed]
13. Soquetta, M.; Terra, L.; Bastos, C. Green technologies for the extraction of bioactive compounds in fruits and vegetables. *CyTA-J. Food* **2018**, *16*, 400–412. [CrossRef]
14. Liao, X.; Hu, F.; Chen, Z. Identification and Quantitation of the Bioactive Components in *Osmanthusfragrans* Fruits by HPLC-ESI-MS/MS. *J. Agric. Food Chem.* **2018**, *66*, 359–367. [CrossRef] [PubMed]
15. Palanisamy, U.; Ling, L.; Manaharan, T.; Appleton, D. Rapid isolation of geraniin from *Nepheliumlappaceum* rind waste and its anti-hyperglycemic activity. *Food Chem.* **2011**, *127*, 21–27. [CrossRef]
16. Mendez-Flores, A.; Hernández-Almanza, A.; Sáenz-Galindo, A.; Morlett-Chávez, J.; Aguilar, C.; Ascacio-Valdés, J. Ultrasound-assisted extraction of antioxidant polyphenolic compounds from *Nepheliumlappaceum* L. (Mexican variety) husk. *Asian Pac. J. Trop. Med.* **2018**, *11*, 676–681. [CrossRef]

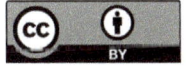

© 2020 by the authors. Licensee MDPI, Basel, Switzerland. This article is an open access article distributed under the terms and conditions of the Creative Commons Attribution (CC BY) license (http://creativecommons.org/licenses/by/4.0/).

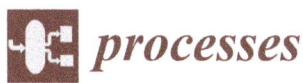

Article

Industrial-Scale Study of the Chemical Composition of Olive Oil Process-Derived Matrices

Haifa Jebabli [1,2], Houda Nsir [3], Amani Taamalli [2,4,*], Ibrahim Abu-Reidah [5,6], Francisco Javier Álvarez-Martínez [7], Maria Losada-Echeberria [7], Enrique Barrajón Catalán [7] and Ridha Mhamdi [2]

[1] Faculty of Mathematical, Physical and Natural Sciences of Tunis, University of Tunis El Manar, Tunis 2092, Tunisia; jebebli@hotmail.com
[2] Laboratory of Olive Biotechnology, Center of Biotechnology of Borj-Cedria, P.O. Box 901, Hammam-Lif 2050, Tunisia; ridha.mhamdi@cbbc.rnrt.tn
[3] Mediterranean Institute of Technology (Medtech), South Mediterranean University, Les Berges du Lac II 1053, Tunisia; houda.nsir@gmail.com
[4] Department of Chemistry, College of Sciences, University of Hafr Al Batin, P.O. Box 1803, Hafr Al Batin 39524, Saudi Arabia
[5] Industrial Chemistry Department, Faculty of Sciences, Arab American University, P.O. Box 240, Zababdeh-Jenin 13, Palestine; iabureidah@yahoo.com
[6] Department of Environmental Science/Boreal Ecosystem Research Initiative, Memorial University of Newfoundland, 20 University Drive, Corner Brook, NL A2H 5G4, Canada
[7] Instituto de Biología Molecular y Celular (IBMC) and Instituto de Investigación, Desarrollo e Innovación en Biotecnología Sanitaria de Elche (IDiBE), Universidad Miguel Hernández (UMH), 03202 Elche, Spain; f.alvarez@umh.es (F.J.Á.-M.); mlosada@umh.es (M.L.-E.); e.barrajon@umh.es (E.B.C.)
* Correspondence: ataamalli@uhb.edu.sa

Received: 2 May 2020; Accepted: 15 June 2020; Published: 17 June 2020

Abstract: The effect of the industrial process and collecting period on produced olive oil and by-products was evaluated. Obtained results showed significant variations for the majority of quality indices before and after vertical centrifugation between all samples from the three collecting periods. All samples were rich in monounsaturated fatty acid: Oleic acid (C18:1) with a maximum of 69.95%. The total polyphenols and individual phenolic compounds varied significantly through the extraction process, with a significant variation between olive oil and by-products. Notably, the percentage of secoiridoids and their derivatives was significant in paste and olive oil, highlighting the activity of many enzymes released during the different extraction steps. Regarding antioxidant capacity, the most remarkable result was detected in olive oil and olive mill wastewater samples.

Keywords: olive oil; olive paste; by-product; industrial process; phenolic compounds

1. Introduction

Olive oil represents the main ingredient of the traditional Mediterranean diet, thanks to its numerous beneficial effects on human health. The health benefits attributed to this product are mainly due to its richness in antioxidants [1]. Indeed, many scientific studies confirm that antioxidant compounds (tocopherols and polyphenols) are responsible for the reduction of the risk of coronary disease and degenerative diseases such as atherosclerosis, cancer, and strokes [2]. On the other hand, olive oil production represents an essential agro-industrial activity in the economic sector of many Mediterranean countries. Currently, the production of olive oils uses the continuous two-and three-phase processing systems because of their higher capacity, shorter processing, and reduced storage time and workforce costs [3]. This sector results in a high production of waste that can reach 30 million tons per year [4]. Olive oil extraction generates two main by-products: A solid residue (pomace) and an effluent known as olive mill wastewater (omww) [5]. Pomace represents a raw material for the extraction of pomace oil and is also used as fuel and for generation of biomass by microbiological processes. Olive mill wastewater has no economic value, representing a worthless by-product of the extra virgin olive oil industry and an additional cost for disposal pretreatment [6]. Such by-products are responsible for severe environmental problems because of their high concentration in organic acid that turns them into phototoxic materials [7]. Particularly, omww has a substantial level of polyphenols that have a toxic effect on individual plants and microorganisms [8]. However, these by-products may represent a promising source of bioactive molecules [9]. Several researchers have reviewed literature data concerning the composition of olive oil by-products in terms of phenolic compounds and have highlighted interesting results regarding the antioxidant and biological activity of phenolic extracts from wastewater and pomace [10]. As an approach to reduce the negative impact of olive oil industry by-products, the phenolic compounds derived from olive oils and by-products are now used in food, cosmetic, and pharmaceutical industries. Olive by-products show a high concentration in secoiridoid derivatives [11].

Interestingly, omww has high levels of phenolic compounds, which could be transformed into a natural source of valuable and powerful antioxidants [12]. Additionally, the phenolic compounds present in the omww have registered a potent biological activity. In particular, hydroxytyrosol is considered a protective agent of blood lipids against oxidation according to the European Food Safety Authority [12,13]. According to literature, the phenolic compounds present in the dry olive residues have antiproliferative activities against breast cancer [14]. Regarding olive pomace, it represents a high potential in the production of a functional food because of its low-cost and richness in phenolic compounds. In fact, the anti-inflammatory effect of olive pomace extract has been clearly demonstrated where the polyphenols have expressed a high therapeutic potential in intestinal bowel disease [15].

The principal aim of this work is to screen the quality of some olive oils produced in Tejerouine (Kef region, in the north-west of Tunisia) and to study the effect of production process on the chemical composition of olive products and by-products using a three-phase industrial scale system for three harvesting dates.

2. Materials and Methods

2.1. Sampling

All samples (paste, olive oil, omww, and pomace) were obtained from a three-phase continuous chain olive mill in Tejerouin in the Kef region (north-west of Tunisia). The collected samples come from the following cultivars: Sample one: Chetoui, samples two, three, five, and seven: Chetoui and Chemlali, sample four: Chetoui and Gerboui, and sample six: Chetoui and Koroneiki. In blended samples, the dominant cultivar was Chetoui which is the autochthonous cultivar of the Kef region. Sampling was carried out in the beginning (d1: 22/11/2017), middle (d2: 19/12/2017), and the end (d3: 19/01/2018) of the crop's season. From the non-centrifuged oil, omww and pomace were obtained after horizontal decantation step. From the centrifuged oil and omww were collected after the vertical centrifugation step.

For each sample, the same orchard and the same percentage of the different cultivars in the blend were considered for the three collecting dates.

2.2. Solvent-Extraction of the Polar Fraction

2.2.1. Extraction of Polar Fraction from omww

Two methods were used for the extraction of the polar fraction from omww.

Method (1) was as described in literature [16] with some modifications. The omww mixed with hexane was agitated and centrifuged. Then the delipidated omww (aqueous phase) was collected for the liquid–liquid extraction. At this point, ethyl acetate was added (v/v). After agitation and centrifugation, two phases were obtained representing a supernatant, rich in polyphenols, and a base, which was omww. The recovered organic phase was evaporated under vacuum in a rotary evaporator at 38 °C. The obtained residue was dissolved in methanol for further analysis.

Method (2) consisted of evaporating 8.33 mL of omww under vacuum in a rotary evaporator at 40 °C. The residue was mixed with methanol/water then dried by rotary evaporator at 40 °C, then methanol was added to the residue before analysis.

2.2.2. Extraction of Polar Fraction from Olive Pomace and Paste

Phenolic extracts from dry pomace and paste were obtained by the conventional method described in the literature [17]. Briefly, 1 g of dry matter was dissolved in 10 mL methanol. The samples were maintained for 24 h in the dark under agitation at room temperature. The extract was then filtered and evaporated under vacuum in a rotary evaporator at 38 °C.

2.2.3. Extraction of Polar Fraction from Virgin Olive Oil Samples

The phenolic extract of olive oil was obtained as follows: 2.5 g of olive oil was dissolved in 5 mL of hexane. Subsequently a mixture of methanol:water (60:40, v/v) was added. After that, the mixture was agitated and centrifuged at 3500 rpm for 10 min. The polar phase, was recovered for analysis.

2.3. Quality Indices

Determination of free fatty acids (FFAs) given as % of oleic acid, peroxide value (PV), absorbance in the UV (K_{232} and K_{270}) was carried out according to the standard methods described by the International Olive Council (IOC) [18]. The free acidity was determined by titration of a solution of oil dissolved in ethanol/ether (1:1) with 0.1 M potassium hydroxide in ethanol. Peroxide content was established by the reaction of a mixture of 1 g of oil and chloroform/acetic acid with a solution of potassium iodide in darkness. The free iodine was then titrated with a sodium thiosulfate solution. PV was expressed as milliequivalents of active oxygen per kilogram (meq O_2 kg^{-1}). K_{270} and K_{232} extinction coefficients were calculated from the absorbance at 270 and 232 nm, respectively, with a UV spectrophotometer using a 0.1 g of olive oil in cyclohexane and a path length of 1 cm.

2.4. Pigment Content

Chlorophylls and carotenoids were determined colorimetrically. The absorbance at 670 nm was specific to the chlorophyll fraction, and that at 470 nm was specific to carotenoids. The applied values of the specific extinction coefficients were E1 = 613 for pheophytin as a major component in the chlorophyll fraction, and E2 = 2000 for lutein as a major component in the carotenoid fraction. The pigment contents were calculated as follows:

$$\text{Chlorophyll (mg/kg)} = (A670 \times 10^6) / (E1 \times 100 \times d)$$

$$\beta\text{-carotene content} = (A470 \times 10^6) / (E2 \times 100 \times d)$$

E1: The specific extinction for pheophetin
E2: The specific extinction for lutein
where, A is the absorbance and d denotes the spectrophotometer cell thickness (1 cm).

2.5. Trolox Equivalent Antioxidant Capacity (TEAC)

TEAC was performed by preparing a solution of 2,2'-azinobis (3-ethylbenzothiazoline 6-sulfonate (ABTS) in distilled water and a solution of potassium persulfate. After that, in a 96-well plate, 200 µL of ABTS was added in all the well plate then 20 µL trolox with different dilutions already prepared, and 20 µL of extract were added to the first line well plate. Measures were finally performed using a plate reader. TEAC was expressed as mmol of trolox equivalent (TE) per 100 g of dry weight of extract (d.w.).

2.6. Determination of Total Polyphenols

The total polyphenol contents were determined in each extract using Folin–Ciocalteu's method adapted to a 96-well plate assay and expressed as percent of gallic acid equivalent (% GAE per extract) [19]. A calibration curve of gallic acid was prepared. Then, 10 μL of the extract was mixed with 50 μL of Folin–Ciocalteu. Then after addition of 100μL of sodium carbonate (Na_2CO_3), 840 μL of distilled water was added. After 20 min in the dark. The reading was accomplished at 700 nm.

2.7. HPLC-MS Analysis of the Polar Fraction

The polar fractions of the paste, olive oil, and by-products were analyzed using high-performance liquid chromatography coupled to mass spectrometry (HPLC-MS). An analytical technique that combines the physical separation capabilities of liquid chromatography and the mass analysis capabilities [20]. The phenolic compounds of the different extracts were separated using Agilent LC 1100 series (Agilent Technologies, Inc., Palo Alto, CA, USA) controlled by the Chemstation software and equipped with a pump, autosampler, column, and UV-Vis diode array detector. The HPLC instrument was coupled to an Esquire 3000+ (Bruker Daltonics, GmbH, Germany) mass spectrometer equipped with an electrospray ionization (ESI) source and ion-trap mass analyzer and operated by Esquire control and data analysis software. The column used was an Agilent Poroshell 120 RP-C_{18} (4.6 by 150 mm, 2.7 μm). The sample separation was carried out using a linear gradient using 1 % formic acid (A) and acetonitrile (B). The gradient started with 5% B, 25% at 30 min, 45% B at 45 min, then 5% at 51 min and 5 min more for rebalancing. The flow rate was 0.5 mL/min [21]. The diode-array detector was programmed at 280, 320, and 340 nm. The operating conditions of the mass spectrometer were optimized to achieve maximum sensitivity values. The ESI system operated in negative mode to generate ions [M-H]$^-$ under the following conditions: Desolvation temperature at 360°C, vaporizer temperature at 400 °C, drying gas (nitrogen), and nebulizer at 12 L per minute and 70 psi, respectively. The data was acquired as full exploration mass spectra from 50 to 1400 m/z using 200 ms for the collection of the ions in the trap.

2.8. Analysis of Fatty Acids

The analysis of the fatty acid composition was carried out according to the International Olive Council method [18] with some modifications. Methylated esters were obtained from the mixture of 0.1 g of oil with 3 mL of hexane and 0.5 KOH in methanol 0.2 N. Fatty acid determination was performed using a gas chromatography GC (Agilent 7890B technology) equipped with a capillary column CP –sil 88 model CP6173 (50 m of length and 250 μm of internal diameter). The film thickness was 250 μm, and the temperature was maintained at 225 °C throughout the analysis time. The temperature of the injector was 230 °C while the detector temperature was 300 °C and the oven temperature was set at 240°C. Hydrogen was used as a carrier gas.

2.9. Statistical Analysis

Statistical significance was tested through a one-way ANOVA and Duncan test at 5% confidence level using SPSS statistical package (Version 13.0 for Window, SPSS Inc. Chicago, IL., 2003).

3. Results

3.1. Quality Indices, Pigments, and Fatty Acid Composition of Olive Oil Samples

Table 1 shows the variation of quality indices of olive oil samples from the three collecting dates before and after vertical centrifugation. After vertical centrifugation, all final-produced olive oil samples conformed to the norms fixed by the IOC for extra virgin olive oil class except for samples 4d1 and 6d1 (after vertical centrifugation).

Table 1. Quality indices of olive oil samples.

			22-11-2017		
	Sample	FFAs	PV	K_{232}	K_{270}
before vertical centrifugation	1	0.4 ± 0.8 a,b	6 ± 0.8 a	1.90 ± 0.02 a	0.1 ± 0.1 a,b
	2	0.4 ± 0.1 a,b	9.70 ± 1.15 a,b,c,d	1.9 ± 0.4 a	0.07 ± 0.04 a
	3	0.5 ± 0.1 a,b	16.0 ± 1.5 e	2.10 ± 0.05 a	0.10 ± 0.01 a,b
	4	0.40 ± 0.02 a,b	13 ± 4.6 d	2.17 ± 0.10 a	0.14 ± 0.02 c,d
	5	0.4 ± 0.1 a,b	9 ± 0.6 a,b,c	2.3 ± 0.3 a,b	0.17 ± 0.04 b,c,d
	6	0.40 ± 0.01 a,b	13.0 ± 1.5 d	2.13 ± 0.22 a	0.15 ± 0.03 d
after vertical centrifugation	1	0.43 ± 0.06 a,b	10 ± 1 b,c,d	2.12 ± 0.1 a	0.12 ± 0.02 a,b,c
	2	0.30 ± 0.01 a	6.7 ± 2.3 a,b	1.87 ± 0.03 a	0.06 ± 0.01 a
	3	0.40 ± 0.01 a,b	10 ± 1 c,d	2.1 ± 0.2 a	0.07 ± 0.01 a
	4	0.3 ± 0.1 a	9.00 ± 0.01 a,b,c	2.6 ± 0.5 a	0.18 ± 0.10 b,c,d
	5	0.40 ± 0.15 a,b	10 ± 2 cd	2.3 ± 0.1 a,b	0.14 ± 0.02 c,d
	6	0.3 ± 0.1 a,b	13.0 ± 2.1 d	2.6 ± 0.2 b	0.20 ± 0.04 b,c,d

			19-12-2018		
	Sample	FFAs	PV	K_{232}	K_{270}
before vertical centrifugation	1	0.5 ± 0.0 a,b,c	7.0 ± 1.2 a,b	1.9 ± 0.1 a,b	0.18 ± 0.02 b
	2	1.2 ± 0.1 e	9 ± 2 b,c,d	2.47 ± 0.05 d	0.3 ± 0.1 c
	3	0.4 ± 0.0 a	5.7 ± 1.5 a	1.92 ± 0.02 a,b	0.18 ± 0.01 b
	4	0.4 ± 0.1 a,b	9.0 ± 1.2 b,c	1.85 ± 0.1 a,b	0.18 ± 0.01 b
	5	0.5 ± 0.1 a,b,c	18.0 ± 1.5 g	1.82 ± 0.04 a,b	0.180 ± 0.004 b
	6	0.4 ± 0.1 a,b	7.0 ± 1.2 a,b	1.71 ± 0.03 a	0.19 ± 0.01 b,c
	7	0.5 ± 0.2 a,b	8.0 ± 0.6 a,b	2.07 ± 0.05 c	0.25 ± 0.05 c
after vertical centrifugation	1	0.6 ± 0.2 b,c	12 ± 0.6 e,f	1.9 ± 0.1 a,b	0.15 ± 0.01 a,b
	2	0.9 ± 0.1 d	13.7 ± 1.5 f	2.3 ± 0.1 c,d	0.19 ± 0.01 b,c
	3	0.5 ± 0.1 ab	9 ± 1 b,c,d	1.99 ± 0.05 a,b	0.19 ± 0.01 b
	4	0.7 ± 0.1 c	12 ± 0.6 e,f	1.9 ± 0.1 a,b	0.11 ± 0.01 a
	5	0.6 ± 0.1 a,b,c	10 ± 0.6 c,d,e	1.98 ± 0.03 a,b	0.14 ± 0.03 a,b
	6	0.6 ± 0.1 a,b,c	11 ± 1 d,e	1.88 ± 0.01 a,b	0.14 ± 0.02 a,b
	7	0.5 ± 0.1 a,b,c	8 ± 1 b,c	1.9 ± 0.2 a,b	0.14 ± 0.03 a,b

			19-01-2018		
	Sample	FFAs	PV	K_{232}	K_{270}
before vertical centrifugation	1	0.4 ± 0.1 a,b	6.0 ± 1.5 a	1.8 ± 0.1 a,b	0.15 ± 0.02 a,b,c
	2	0.4 ± 0.1 a,b	4.0 ± 2.3 a	1.7 ± 0.1 a	0.11 ± 0.03 a
	3	0.4 ± 0.1 a,b	11 ± 2 b	1.9 ± 0.1 bc	0.16 ± 0.01 b,c
	4	0.5 ± 0.1 a	6.0 ± 1.5 a	1.7 ± 0.2 a	0.14 ± 0.03 a,b
after vertical centrifugation	1	0.4 ± 0.1 a,b	6.0 ± 1.5 a	1.7 ± 0.1 a,b	0.14 ± 0.01 a,b
	2	0.4 ± 0.1 a	4 ± 2.3 a	1.91 ± 0.13 b,c	0.16 ± 0.03 b,c
	3	0.4 ± 0 a	12.0 ± 2.1 b	1.9 ± 0.1 b,c	0.18 ± 0.01 c
	4	0.43 ± 0.06 a,b	6.0 ± 1.5 a	2.02 ± 0.04 a	0.17 ± 0.01 b,c

(a–g) The different letters indicate a significant difference (Duncan's test, $p = 0.05$). Values are expressed as mean values and standard deviations over three repetitions. Free fatty acids (FFAs): Expressed as % of C18:1 and peroxide value (PV): Expressed as meq O_2 kg^{-1}.

Regarding pigments, a significant difference ($p < 0.05$) was observed between centrifuged and non-centrifuged oils. Interestingly, higher contents in chlorophylls and carotenoids were registered for centrifuged olive oil in comparison to non-centrifuged ones (Figure 1).

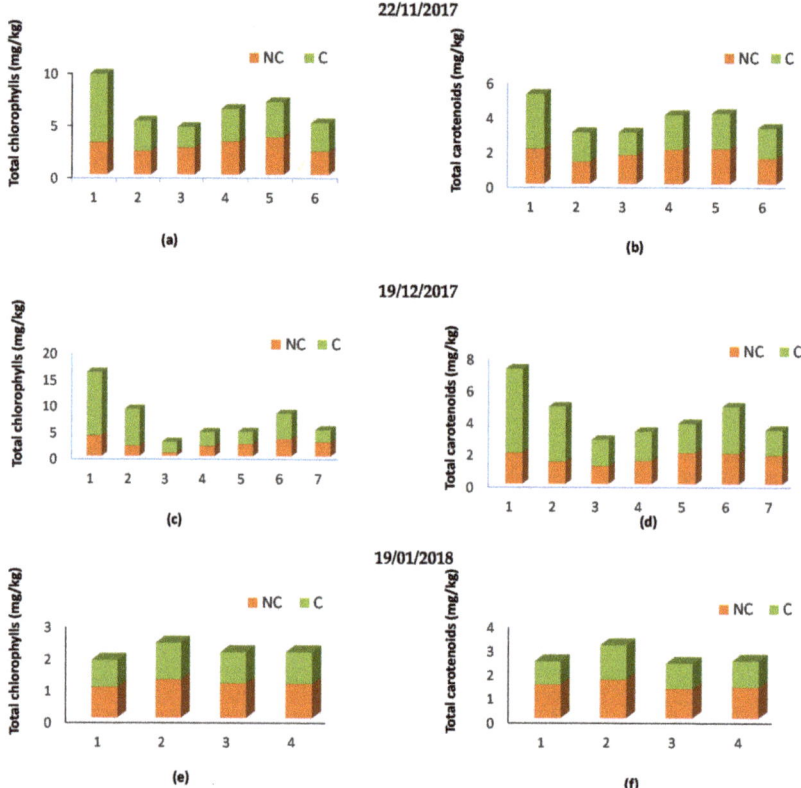

Figure 1. Pigment content variation according to vertical centrifugation and collecting period. (**a**) chlorophyll content variation in olive oils of 22/11/2017; (**b**) carotenoid content variation in olive oils collected at 22/11/2017; (**c**) chlorophyll content variation in olive oils at 19/12/2017; (**d**) carotenoid content variation in olive oils of 19/12/2017; (**e**) carotenoid content variation in olive oils collected at 19/01/2018; and (**f**) carotenoid content variation in olive oils of 19/01/2018. NC: Before vertical centrifugation, C: After vertical centrifugation.

The fatty acid composition of the studied samples is reported in Table 2. All obtained fatty acid percentages were conform to the International Olive Council standards for extra virgin olive oil class [18]. All samples were rich in monounsaturated acid (oleic acid) C18:1 with a maximum of 69.95% (sample six at the second collecting date Table 2).

Table 2. Fatty acid composition of olive oil samples (% m/m methyl esters).

	Sample	C16:0	C16:1	C17:0	C17:1	C18:0	C18:1	C18:2	C18:3	C20:0	C20:1
d1	1	12.87	0.59	0.13	0.21	3.00	64.6	16.31	-	0.43	0.40
	2	12.11	0.52	0.19	0.35	2.81	65.62	15.17	0.75	0.38	0.42
	3	13.70	0.56	0.29	0.40	2.98	64.54	14.62	0.51	0.45	0.36
	4	12.71	0.52	0.11	0.13	3.00	64.32	16.97	-	0.45	0.36
	5	12.92	-	0.16	-	2.96	64.80	17.44	0.61	0.45	0.47
	6	12.05	0.39	0.47	0.21	2.92	62.88	19.17	-	0.46	-
d2	1	13.07	0.51	-	-	3.12	64.94	16.48	0.49	0.41	0.45
	2	12.00	0.36	-	-	3.36	63.30	19.61	0.53	0.45	0.39
	3	10.69	0.27	0.16	-	3.77	65.13	18.30	0.52	0.45	0.36
	4	11.31	0.29	-	-	4.01	64.67	17.92	0.63	0.48	0.46
	5	16.44	1.28	-	-	3.16	63.16	12.67	1.00	0.49	0.40
	6	12.58	1.04	0.10	-	2.77	69.33	12.80	0.43	0.44	0.37
	7	16.47	0.87	-	-	3.18	62.45	13.86	0.41	0.46	0.46
d3	1	11.03	0.46	0.14	-	3.40	67.78	15.73	0.46	0.44	0.32
	2	11.69	0.24	-	-	3.44	65.20	16.67	0.47	0.46	0.42
	3	9.73	0.35	0.17	-	3.57	67.25	17.36	0.48	0.57	0.37
	4	11.74	0.15	0.44	0.05	3.11	65.88	16.99	0.53	0.57	0.38
EVOO (IOC [18])		7.5–20	3–3.5	-	-	0.5–5	55–83	3.5–21	≤1	≤0.6	≤0.5

d1: 22/11/2017, d2: 19/12/2017, and d3: 19/01/2018. Data are expressed by mean values ±SD of three independent experiments. Values followed by same letters are not significantly different (Duncan's test, $p = 0.05$).

3.2. Total Polyphenols in the Extracts

The distribution of total polyphenols (TP) in olive oil and by-product extracts is represented in (Table 3). A significant variations of TP contents between olive oil extracts as well as between by-products were observed. After vertical centrifugation, TP contents decreased for some olive oil samples and on the contrary increased in a part of olive oil samples. However, an apparent slight decrease was observed for ethyl acetate omww extracts after vertical centrifugation. Among by-products, ethyl acetate omww extracts showed the highest contents. We can say that ethyl acetate was more efficient than methanol in extracting omww polyphenols. For all studied samples, TP contents decreased slightly from olive paste to pomace extracts.

Table 3. Total polyphenols in olive oil, paste, pomace, and omww extracts (expressed as % GAE per extract).

	Samples	Paste	Oonc	Ooc	Pomace	Omww nc EA	Omwwc EA	Omwwnc MeOH	Omwwc MeOH
d1	1	4.5 ± 0.4 [a]	45.5 ± 1.4 [b]	36.8 ± 1.7 [b]	2.2 ± 1.5 [a]	13 ± 4 [a]	13.6 ± 4.4 [a]	2.7 ± 0.4 [a]	8.7 ± 2.9 [a]
	2	1.2 ± 1.2 [a]	35.6 ± 1.8 [b,c]	44.5 ± 3.7 [c]	2.7 ± 2.0 [a]	11.3 ± 3.4 [a,b]	9.7 ± 2.6 [a,b]	3.2 ± 0.8 [a]	3.9 ± 1.7 [a]
	3	2.5 ± 0.4 [a]	44.8 ± 2.5 [b]	27.6 ± 1.3 [b]	2.1 ± 0.8 [a]	8.1 ± 1.7 [a]	6.95 ± 1.4 [a]	3.7 ± 0.6 [a]	3.6 ± 1.1 [a]
	4	3.5 ± 0.8 [a]	36.9 ± 1.6 [b]	35.4 ± 1.7 [b]	1.6 ± 0.3 [a]	13.4 ± 2.3 [a]	11.6 ± 2.3 [a]	2.7 ± 0.4 [a]	4.4 ± 1.4 [a]
	5	3.5 ± 0.6 [a]	37 ± 2 [b]	35.5 ± 1.7 [b]	1.3 ± 0.2 [a]	24.6 ± 6.3 [a]	19.4 ± 4.5 [a]	6.0 ± 3.1 [a]	5.5 ± 1.1 [a]
	6	2.5 ± 0.2 [a]	43 ± 2 [b]	35.7 ± 1.3 [b]	0.7 ± 0.1 [a]	20.7 ± 3.5 [b,c]	16.7 ± 2.8 [a,b]	5.2 ± 1.6 [a,b]	5 ± 1.4 [a,b]
d2	1	2.8 ± 0.4 [a]	37.7 ± 2.0 [b]	30.6 ± 4.2 [b]	-	10.1 ± 5.1 [a]	9.2 ± 2.9 [a]	2.9 ± 0.2 [a]	4.7 ± 0.8 [a]
	2	3.5 ± 0.3 [a]	39.4 ± 1.3 [b,c]	49.8 ± 4.5 [b]	-	29.3 ± 2.9 [a,b,c]	22.5 ± 2.1 [a,b,c]	7.5 ± 1.8 [a,b]	4.8 ± 0.3 [a]
	3	2.1 ± 1.1 [a]	38.7 ± 1.1 [b]	69.4 ± 2.8 [c]	-	-	16.8 ± 2.2 [a,b]	5.3 ± 1.8 [a]	-
	4	2.6 ± 0.8 [a]	31.5 ± 1.1 [b]	68.10 ± 4.05 [c]	2 ± 1.1 [a]	12.7 ± 2.6 [a,b]	10 ± 1.2 [a,b]	7.1 ± 2.3 [a,b]	4.4 ± 1.4 [a,b]
	5	2.2 ± 0.9 [a]	34.21 ± 1.6 [b]	61.8 ± 3.3 [c]	1.5 ± 0.2 [a]	11.5 ± 1.4 [a]	10.4 ± 2.3 [a]	3.8 ± 1.4 [a]	5.44 ± 0.4 [a]
	6	1.02 ± 1.03 [a]	34.3 ± 9.1 [b]	79.09 ± 4.6 [c]	0.06 ± 0.64 [a]	15.1 ± 5.2 [a,b]	12.1 ± 3.7 [a,b]	7.7 ± 2.4 [a,b]	5.3 ± 0.9 [a,b]
	7	-	31.1 ± 9.8 [b,c]	51.46 ± 2.8 [c]	0.3 ± 1.5 [a]	16.4 ± 6.3 [a,b]	-	7.3 ± 2.7 [a,b]	-
d3	1	6.6 ± 0.5 [a]	36 ± 1.6 [b]	49.3 ± 3.1 [b]	1.1 ± 0.1 [a]	10.4 ± 2.9 [a]	7.8 ± 1.4 [a]	7.0 ± 1.4 [a]	3.6 ± 0.6 [a]
	2	2.6 ± 0.3 [a]	47.0 ± 2.1 [b]	45.1 ± 3.2 [b]	0.8 ± 0.1 [a]	4.9 ± 1.6 [a]	5.2 ± 1.1 [a]	2.1 ± 1.1 [a]	4.2 ± 0.5 [a]
	3	6 ± 1 [a]	76.2 ± 3.8 [c]	48.4 ± 1.9 [b]	0.7 ± 0.1 [a]	10.5 ± 0.9 [a]	10 ± 1 [a]	5.6 ± 0.8 [a]	7.3 ± 1.4 [a]
	4	2.2 ± 0.4 [a]	39.4 ± 1.3 [b]	43.6 ± 2.8 [b]	0.4 ± 0.1 [a]	14.6 ± 1.7 [a]	12.1 ± 1.2 [a]	5.6 ± 2.5 [a]	5.1 ± 0.8 [a]

d1: 22/11/2017, d2: 19/12/2017, d3:19/01/2018, oonc: Olive oil before vertical centrifugation, ooc: Olive oil after vertical centrifugation, omwwnc: Olive mill waste water before vertical centrifugation, omwwc: Olive mill waste water after vertical centrifugation, EA: Ethyl acetate extract, and MeOH: Methanolic extract. Data are expressed by mean values ±SD of three independent experiments. [a–c] Values followed by the same letters are not significantly different (Duncan's test, $p = 0.05$).

3.3. Evaluation of the Antioxidant Activity: TEAC Assay

Among the studied samples, the TEAC test was performed on 22 extracts. The latter are the extracts from different matrices (products and by-products) from different collecting dates, and that showed the highest total polyphenol content. TEAC correlates positively to the polyphenol contents [22]. Figure 2 shows the TEAC variation in the extracts of the different samples under study.

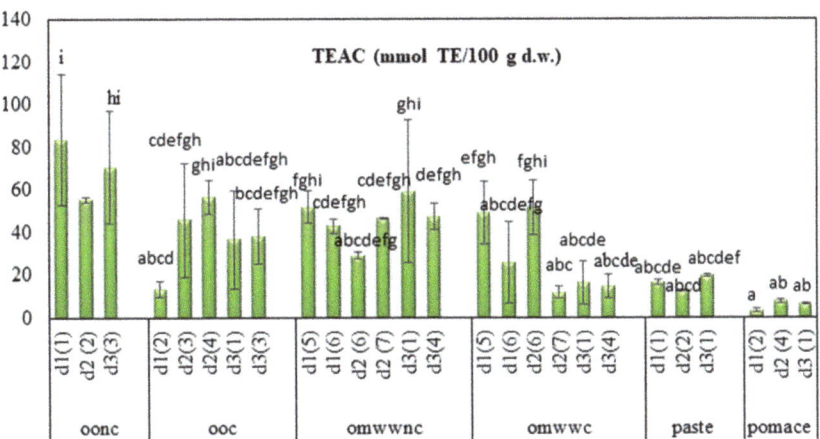

Figure 2. Trolox equivalent antioxidant capacity variation in olive oil, paste, and by-products. d1: 22/11/2017, d2: 19/12/2017, d3: 19/01/2018, oonc: Olive oil before vertical centrifugation, ooc: Olive oil after vertical centrifugation, omwwnc: Olive mill wastewater before vertical centrifugation, and omwwc: Olive mill wastewater after vertical centrifugation. (a-h) The different letters indicate a significant difference (Duncan's test, $p < 0.05$) values are expressed as mean values and standard deviations over three repetitions.

3.4. Phenolic Compound Analysis in Olive Paste, Olive Oil and by-Products

The phenolic compounds were identified using high performance liquid chrmatography coupled to diode-array detector and electrospray ionization mass spectrometry (HPLC-DAD-ESI-MS/MS) analysis. The choice of samples to analyze in this part was based on TEAC activity in different matrices. The objective of this analysis was to assess the behavior of phenolic compounds in the different matrices during olive oil production process. Table 4 shows the identified compounds in olive oil, olive paste, and by-products. Nineteen phenolic compounds could be detected and determined based on available standard compounds, the MS and MS/MS fragments spectra, and the literature [23–30].

Regardless the collection date and vertical centrifugation process, as shown in Table 4 among samples, olive oil extracts showed the highest percentages in oleuropein aglycone (extracts 1, 9, 10, and 11) whereas, the rest of matrices extracts registered the highest percentages in secoiridoid derivative (extracts 2, 3, 5, 6, and 7) as well as in terms of hydroxyttyrosol hexoside dimer (extracts 2, 3, 6, and 7), acyclodihydroelenolic acid hexoside (extract 7), and G13 (extracts 4 and 5). Previously in literature [24] it was cited that most of these compounds are detected in drupe and paste.

In addition, other compounds were also determined such as stachyose which reached 13% in omww (7) extract. The compound (+)−1-Hydroxypinoresinol 1-O-β-D-glucopyranoside was present in omww extract (sample 6). This compounds was found in other researches [25] in wood, leaves, and stems of 'Chemlali' olive cultivar.

p-Coumaroyl-6-oleoside was present only in olive paste extracts (extracts two and three), reaching 14% in olive paste extract three.

Table 4. Polar compounds determined in olive oil, paste, and by-products.

Proposed Compound	M-H]-	MS/MS Fragments	Sample and Percentage	References
Galloyl-HHDP-hexoside	663	-	3 (5.27%)	[23]
Hydroxytyrosol hexoside dimer	631	153; 315	2 (15.00%), 3 (11.09%), 6 (17.48%), 7 (13.85%)	[24]
Stachyose	665	-	4 (2.64%), 7 (13.85%)	[25]
Secoirioid derivative	815	407; 375; 313	2 (63.66%), 3 (39.98%), 5 (50.49%), 6 (35.20%), 7 (37.85%)	[26]
Acyclodihydroelenolic acid hexoside	407	389; 165	4 (12.75%), 7 (34.91%)	[25]
Isonuezhenide	685	523; 453; 421; 299; 223	3 (5.24%), 4 (3.12%)	[27]
Caffeoyl-6-oleoside	551	-	2 (6.61%), 3 (6.75%), 6 (6.56%)	[24]
p-Coumaroyl-6-oleoside	535	491	2 (6.70%), 3 (14.91%)	[24]
(+)-1-Hydroxypinoresinol 1-O-β-D-glucopyranoside	535	-	6 (9.29%)	[25]
Elenolic acid dialdehyde linked to hydroxytyrosol	319	195	1 (10.15%)	[28]
G13	1071	909; 837; 771; 685; 523; 385	2 (8.03%), 3 (7.99%), 4 (33.87%), 5 (22.95%)	[27]
oleuropein aglycone	377	275; 149	1 (54.61%), 8 (33.60%), 9 (17.76%), 10 (59.86%), 11 (37.99%)	[25]
Forsythoside B	755	447	8 (12.30%)	[29]
Leucosceptoside B	781	-	6 (9.63%)	[29]
Secoisolariciresinol	361	-	11 (4.53%)	[30]
Oleuropein hexoside	701	539	1 (6.06%)	[27]

Olive oil samples (1, 8, 9, 10, and 11), paste (2 and 3), pomace (4 and 5), and omww (6 and 7).

4. Discussion

No significant difference was observed among the quality parameters during the three collection dates, except for some samples such as 4C and 6C of 22/11/2018 that showed k_{232} values exceeding 2.5 ($K_{232} = 2.6$). Similarly, samples 2NC and 2C of 19/12/2017 represented a high percentage of free fatty acids (1.2% and 0.9%, respectively). Concerning the peroxide values, which evaluate the hydroperoxide content in olive oil and offer a measure of lipid oxidation, they ranged from 4 meqO$_2$/kg to 18 meqO$_2$/kg for all the studied samples. Peroxide values did not show an apparent variation according to the vertical centrifugation process (Table 1). Regarding free fatty acids, generally, no significant difference was noted between the centrifuged and non-centrifuged olive oils. A slight significant variation in samples collected in January, was found and especially for sample two free fatty acid content showed a decrease from 1.2% before centrifugation to 0.9% after centrifugation. Specific extinction values expressed a slight variation between centrifuged and non-centrifuged oils. Generally, variation obtained in terms of quality indices was observed mostly in samples according to centrifugation process more than the harvesting period. These findings are similar to those reported by other researchers [31] who assessed the variation of quality indices between olive oil obtained from processes of sedimentation and centrifugation with respect to raw olive oil obtained at the decanter exit.

The change in fatty acid composition can be related to the harvest time [32]. It was previously demonstrated that storage conditions, extraction process, and harvesting period might have an effect on the variation of the fatty acid content [32]. The slight variation in the fatty acid contents observed between analyzed samples seems to be also related to the cultivar, which is in accordance with previous researches [3].

According to the data of Table 3, it was found that omww polyphenol-extraction was more efficient with ethyl acetate than with methanol as an extractant solvent. omww comprises different bioactive phenolic compounds that have antimicrobial and phytotoxic effects. This composition is variable and depends on the cultivar, harvesting time, and extraction processes [33]. Its richness in water and nutriment gives to omww a significant value of fertilization. For this reason, it is advised to use this by-product for nutraceutical purposes due to its richness in nutritive components and its lower cost [34], since most of the phenolic compounds are lost lost during oil processing, ending up in wastes instead of oil [35].

Centrifuged and non-centrifuged olive oil samples presented good antioxidant capacities. However, a significant variation was observed in this parameter according to the matrix. The highest value was detected in olive oils followed by omww, paste, and pomace. Moreover, when extracted by ethyl acetate, the polar fraction of omww presented a higher value of TEAC compared to pomace extracts. A slight significant difference was registered between centrifuged and non-centrifuged olive oils and the same behavior was observed for omww (Figure 2). TEAC values for pomace extracts did not exceed 10 mmol TE/100 g DW. Previous studies showed that the most significant influence of radical elimination was resulting from the presence of oleuropein aglycone dialdehyde (3,4-DHPEA-EDA) than other phenolic compounds [24].

The change in phenolic compounds is related to the activity of many enzymes that are released during pressing and malaxation steps [1]. It was previously demonstrated that all glycoside phenols are transformed to their aglycone forms, and the complex phenols are completely hydrolyzed to simple phenolics oleuropein, demethyloleuropein oleoside, and verbascoside [1]. In fact, polyphenol oxidase could be responsible for indirect oxidation of secoiridoids, and β-glucosidase could play a role in the production of phenol-aglycones such as the oleuropein aglycone and its isomers by hydrolysis of oleuropein as explained in literature [36]. The dialdehydic form of elenolic acid linked to hydroxytyrosol 3,4-DHPEA-EDA was detected in olive oil sample C4d2. The richness of olive oil in secoiridoid derivatives is an indicator of degradation pathways for the phenolic oleosides shown in the solid phases [36]. However, some compounds were identified in paste and by-products but not in olive oil such as hydroxytyrosol hexoside dimer, acyclodihydroelenolic acid hexoside, caffeoyl-6-oleoside, G13, and isonuezhenide (Table 4).

The presence of oleoside groups (caffeoyl-6-oleoside and p-coumaroyl-6-oleoside) in paste and by-products (Table 4) results probably from the degradation pathways of simple phenols [1]. The phenolic alcohol hydroxytyrosol hexoside dimer present in paste and by-products gave a base peak at m/z 631 with an MS/MS fragments at m/z 153 and m/z 315 which is in accordance with the results found elsewhere [24]. The presence of this compound in paste and by-products is mainly due to its strong hydrophilic nature and the activity of certain enzymes such as β-glucosidase during the malaxation process that is responsible for the hydrolysis of the glycosides to their respective aglycones [24].

The secoiridoids were present with their derivatives during the different steps of the extraction process specifically, in olive oil, paste, and by-products (Table 4). The transformation of the complex form of secoiridoid to the simple polyphenol form after malaxation is assured by the phenomenon of hydrolysis. So, the secoiridoids present in the paste or more precisely in fruit, are distributed between olive oil and by-product. However, it can be deduced that there is a significant loss of these major phenolic compounds in by-products. The secoiridoids are responsible for the good quality of virgin olive oil. Nevertheless, the extraction process of olive oil, such as the three-phase process, is responsible for the loss of a high amount of certain secoiridoids and their derivatives. On the other hand, galloyl hexahydroxydiphenoyl hexoside was detected in paste and a tetrasaccharide (stachyose) in by-products (Table 4). In our study, the distribution of phenolic compounds in paste, olive oil, and by-products differed significantly during the process of oil extraction.

According to previous works [37–41], the remarkable antioxidant capacity of olive oil, paste, and by-products may encourage their possible valorization. Further researches will be conducted to study in-depth the potential anti-cancer activity of selected extracts as novel cytotoxic agents.

5. Conclusions

The olive oil extraction process provides many valuable by-products thanks to their bioactive compounds. In this study, the matrices entailed in olive oil processing were screened for their quality indices and chemical composition (fatty acids, chlorophylls, carotenoids, and polyphenols). Different distribution of total polyphenols and values of TEAC antioxidant activity in olive oil, paste, and by-products (pomace and omww) extracts were highlighted in this study. Moreover, the distribution of individual phenolic compounds varied significantly according to the matrix. This variation is certainly linked to the transformation of initial phenolic compound in paste after malaxation due to the phenomenon of hydrolysis. Furthermore, we detected a considerable loss of secoiridoids glycosides and their derivatives in by-products. Generally, all samples from the three collecting dates shared similar behaviors for the studied parameters.

Author Contributions: Conceptualization, H.J. and A.T.; Methodology, H.J., M.L.-E. and F.J.Á.-M.; Software, H.J. and M.L.-E.; Validation, E.B.C. and A.T. and I.A.-R.; Formal Analysis, H.J., E.B.C. and A.T.; Investigation, H.J., M.L.-E. and F.J.Á.-M.; Resources, R.M. and E.B.C.; Data Curation, H.J. and F.J.Á.-M.; Writing-Original Draft Preparation, H.J.; writing—review and editing, H.N., I.A.-R. and A.T.; supervision, R.M. and E.B.C.; project administration, R.M. and E.B.C. All authors have read and agreed to the published version of the manuscript.

Funding: This research was funded by the Tunisian Ministry of Higher Education and by project RTI2018-096724-B-21 from the Spanish Ministry of Science, Innovation and Universities.

Conflicts of Interest: The authors declare no conflict of interest.

References

1. Talhaoui, N.; Gómez-Caravaca, A.M.; León, L.; De La Rosa, R.; Fernández-Gutiérrez, A.; Segura-Carretero, A. From olive fruits to olive Oil: Phenolic compound transfer in six different olive cultivars grown under the same agronomical conditions. *Int. J. Mol. Sci.* **2016**, *17*, 337. [CrossRef] [PubMed]
2. Servili, M.; Sordini, B.; Esposto, S.; Urbani, S.; Veneziani, G.; Di Maio, I.; Selvaggini, R.; Taticchi, A. Biological Activities of Phenolic Compounds of Extra Virgin Olive Oil. *Antioxidants* **2014**, 1–23. [CrossRef] [PubMed]
3. Issaoui, M.; Dabbou, S.; Brahmi, F.; Hassine, K.B.; Ellouze, M.H.; Hammami, M. Effect of extraction systems and cultivar on the quality of virgin olive oils. *Int. J. Food Sci. Technol.* **2009**, *44*, 1713–1720. [CrossRef]
4. Chandra, M.; Sathiavelu, S. Waste management in the olive oil industry in the Mediterranean region by composting. *Clean Technol. Environ. Policy* **2009**, 293–298. [CrossRef]
5. Dermeche, S.; Nadour, M.; Larroche, C.; Moulti-Mati, F.; Michaud, P. Olive mill wastes: Biochemical characterizations and valorization strategies. *Process Biochem.* **2013**, *48*, 1532–1552. [CrossRef]
6. Russo, M.; Bonaccorsi, I.L.; Cacciola, F.; Dugo, L.; De Gara, L.; Dugo, P.; Mondello, L. Distribution of bioactives in entire mill chain from the drupe to the oil and wastes. *Nat. Prod. Res.* **2020**, *0*, 1–6. [CrossRef] [PubMed]
7. Roig, A.; Cayuela, M.L.; Sa, M.A. An overview on olive mill wastes and their valorisation methods. *Waste Manag.* **2006**, *26*, 960–969. [CrossRef]
8. Azaizeh, H.; Halahlih, F.; Najami, N.; Brunner, D.; Faulstich, M.; Tafesh, A. Antioxidant activity of phenolic fractions in olive mill wastewater. *Food Chem.* **2012**, *134*, 2226–2234. [CrossRef]
9. Ciriminna, R.; Meneguzzo, F.; Fidalgo, A.; Ilharco, L.M.; Pagliaro, M. Extraction, benefits and valorization of olive polyphenols. *Eur. J. Lipid Sci. Technol.* **2016**, *118*, 503–511. [CrossRef]
10. Frankel, E.; Bakhouche, A.; Lozano-Sánchez, J.; Segura-Carretero, A.; Fernández-Gutiérrez, A. Literature review on production process to obtain extra virgin olive oil enriched in bioactive compounds. Potential use of byproducts as alternative sources of polyphenols. *J. Agric. Food Chem.* **2013**, *61*, 5179–5188. [CrossRef]
11. Ventura, G.; Calvano, C.D.; Abbattista, R.; Bianco, M.; De Ceglie, C.; Losito, I.; Palmisano, F.; Cataldi, T.R.I. Characterization of bioactive and nutraceutical compounds occurring in olive oil processing wastes. *Rapid Commun. Mass Spectrom.* **2019**, *33*, 1670–1681. [CrossRef] [PubMed]
12. El-Abbassi, A.; Kiai, H.; Hafidi, A. Phenolic profile and antioxidant activities of olive mill wastewater. *Food Chem.* **2012**, *132*, 406–412. [CrossRef] [PubMed]
13. Achmon, Y.; Fishman, A. The antioxidant hydroxytyrosol: Biotechnological production challenges and opportunities. *Appl. Microbiol. Biotechnol.* **2014**. [CrossRef] [PubMed]
14. Ramos, P.; Santos, S.A.O.; Guerra, Â.R.; Guerreiro, O.; Felício, L.; Jerónimo, E.; Silvestre, A.J.D.; Neto, C.P.; Duarte, M. Valorization of olive mill residues: Antioxidant and breast cancer antiproliferative activities of hydroxytyrosol-rich extracts derived from olive oil by-products. *Ind. Crops Prod.* **2013**, *46*, 359–368. [CrossRef]
15. Nunzio, M.D.; Picone, G.; Pasini, F.; Caboni, F.; Gianotti, A.; Bordoni, A.; Capozzi, F. Olive oil industry by-products. Effects of a polyphenol-RICH extract on the metabolome and response to inflammation in cultured intestinal cell. *Food Res. Int.* **2018**. [CrossRef]

16. De Marco, E.; Savarese, M.; Paduano, A.; Sacchi, R. Characterization and fractionation of phenolic compounds extracted from olive oil mill wastewaters. *Food Chem.* **2007**, *104*, 858–867. [CrossRef]
17. Abaza, B.L.; Youssef, N.B.; Manai, H.; Haddada, F.M. Chétoui olive leaf extracts: Influence of the solvent type on phenolics and antioxidant activities. *Grasas Aceites* **2011**, *62*, 96–104. [CrossRef]
18. Norme Commerciale Applicable Aux Huiles D'Olive Et Aux Huiles De Grignons D'Olive. *Cons. Oleic. Int.* **2015**, *COI/T.15*, 1–18.
19. De Príncipe, V.; Nunzio, M.D.; Toselli, M.; Verardo, V.; Caboni, F.; Bordoni, A. Counteraction of oxidative damage by pomegranate juice: Influence of the cultivar. *J. Sci. Food Agric.* **2013**. [CrossRef]
20. Tomás-Menor, L.; Barrajón-Catalán, E.; Segura-Carretero, A.; Martí, N.; Saura, D.; Menéndez, J.A.; Joven, J.; Micol, V. The promiscuous and synergic molecular interaction of polyphenols in bactericidal activity: An opportunity to improve the performance of antibiotics? *Phyther. Res.* **2015**, *29*, 466–473. [CrossRef]
21. Talhaoui, N.; Gómez-Caravaca, A.M.; León, L.; De la Rosa, R.; Segura-Carretero, A.; Fernández-Gutiérrez, A. Determination of phenolic compounds of "Sikitita" olive leaves by HPLC-DAD-TOF-MS. Comparison with its parents "Arbequina" and "Picual" olive leaves. *LWT—Food Sci. Technol.* **2014**, *58*, 28–34. [CrossRef]
22. Barrajón-Catalán, E.; Fernández-Arroyo, S.; Saura, D.; Guillén, E.; Fernández-Gutiérrez, A.; Segura-Carretero, A.; Micol, V. Cistaceae aqueous extracts containing ellagitannins show antioxidant and antimicrobial capacity, and cytotoxic activity against human cancer cells. *Food Chem. Toxicol.* **2010**, *48*, 2273–2282. [CrossRef] [PubMed]
23. Fischer, U.A.; Carle, R.; Kammerer, D.R. Identification and quantification of phenolic compounds from pomegranate (*Punica granatum* L.) peel, mesocarp, aril and differently produced juices by HPLC-DAD–ESI/MSn. *Food Chem.* **2011**, *127*, 807–821. [CrossRef] [PubMed]
24. Kanakis, P.; Termentzi, A.; Michel, T.; Gikas, E.; Halabalaki, M.; Skaltsounis, A.L. From olive drupes to olive Oil An HPLC-orbitrap-based qualitative and quantitative exploration of olive key metabolites. *Planta Med.* **2013**, *79*, 1576–1587. [CrossRef] [PubMed]
25. Ammar, S.; Contreras, M.d.M.; Gargouri, B.; Segura-Carretero, A.; Bouaziz, M. RP-HPLC-DAD-ESI-QTOF-MS based metabolic profiling of the potential *Olea europaea* by-product "wood" and its comparison with leaf counterpart. *Phytochem. Anal.* **2017**, *28*, 217–229. [CrossRef] [PubMed]
26. Li, H.; Yao, W.; Liu, Q.; Xu, J.; Bao, B.; Shan, M.; Cao, Y.; Cheng, F.; Ding, A.; Zhang, L. Application of UHPLC-ESI-Q-TOF-MS to identify multiple constituents in processed products of the herbal medicine ligustri lucidi fructus. *Molecules* **2017**, *22*, 689. [CrossRef]
27. Shaoping, F.; Segura Carretero, A.; Arraez Roman, D. Tentative Characterization of Novel Phenolic Compounds in Extra Virgin Olive Oils by Rapid-Resolution Liquid Chromatography Coupled with Mass Spectrometry. *J. Agric. Food Chem.* **2009**, 11140–11147. [CrossRef]
28. Kirmizibekmez, H.; Montoro, P.; Piacente, S.; Pizza, C.; Dönmez, A.; Çalış, I. Identification by HPLC-PAD-MS and quantification by HPLC-PAD of phenylethanoid glycosides of five Phlomis species. *Phytochem. Anal.* **2005**, *16*, 1–6. [CrossRef] [PubMed]
29. Sanz, M.; De Simón, B.F.; Cadahía, E.; Esteruelas, E.; Muñoz, A.M.; Hernández, T.; Estrella, I.; Pinto, E. LC-DAD/ESI-MS/MS study of phenolic compounds in ash (*Fraxinus excelsior* L. and *F. americana* L.) heartwood. Effect of toasting intensity at cooperage. *J. Mass Spectrom.* **2012**, *47*, 905–918. [CrossRef]
30. Cardinali, A.; Pati, S.; Minervini, F.; D'Antuono, I.; Linsalata, V.; Lattanzio, V. Verbascoside, isoverbascoside, and their derivatives recovered from olive mill wastewater as possible food antioxidants. *J. Agric. Food Chem.* **2012**, *60*, 1822–1829. [CrossRef]
31. Altieri, G.; Di Renzo, G.C.; Genovese, F.; Tauriello, A.; D'Auria, M.; Racioppi, R.; Viggiani, L. Olive oil quality improvement using a natural sedimentation plant at industrial scale. *Biosyst. Eng.* **2014**, *122*, 99–114. [CrossRef]
32. Alowaiesh, B.; Singh, Z.; Fang, Z.; Kailis, S.G. Harvest time impacts the fatty acid compositions, phenolic compounds and sensory attributes of Frantoio and Manzanilla olive oil. *Sci. Hortic.* **2018**, *234*, 74–80. [CrossRef]
33. Barbera, A.C.; Maucieri, C.; Cavallaro, V.; Ioppolo, A.; Spagna, G. Effects of spreading olive mill wastewater on soil properties and crops, a review. *Agric. Water Manag.* **2013**, *119*, 43–53. [CrossRef]
34. Sellami, F.; Jarboui, R.; Hachicha, S.; Medhioub, K.; Ammar, E. Co-composting of oil exhausted olive-cake, poultry manure and industrial residues of agro-food activity for soil amendment. *Bioresour. Technol.* **2008**, *99*, 1177–1188. [CrossRef] [PubMed]

35. Jerman Klen, T.; Mozetič Vodopivec, B. The fate of olive fruit phenols during commercial olive oil processing: Traditional press versus continuous two- and three-phase centrifuge. *LWT Food Sci. Technol.* **2012**, *49*, 267–274. [CrossRef]
36. Artajo, L.S.; Romero, M.P.; Suárez, M.; Motilva, M.J. Partition of phenolic compounds during the virgin olive oil industrial extraction process. *Eur. Food Res. Technol.* **2007**, *225*, 617–625. [CrossRef]
37. Reboredo-Rodríguez, P.; González-Barreiro, C.; Cancho-Grande, B.; Forbes-Hernández, T.Y.; Gasparrini, M.; Afrin, S.; Cianciosi, D.; Carrasco-Pancorbo, A.; Simal-Gándara, J.; Giampieri, F.; et al. Characterization of Phenolic Extracts from BRAVA Extra Virgin Olive Oils and Their Cytotoxic Effects on MCF-7 Breast Cancer Cells. *Food Chem. Toxicol.* **2018**, *119*, 73–85. [CrossRef]
38. Barrajón-Catalán, E.; Taamalli, A.; Quirantes-Piné, R.; Roldan-Segura, C.; Arráez-Román, D.; Segura-Carretero, A.; Micol, V.; Zarrouk, M. Differential metabolomic analysis of the potential antiproliferative mechanism of olive leaf extract on the JIMT-1 breast cancer cell line. *J. Pharm. Biomed. Anal.* **2015**, *105*, 156–162. [CrossRef]
39. Bouallagui, Z.; Han, J.; Isoda, H.; Sayadi, S. Hydroxytyrosol rich extract from olive leaves modulates cell cycle progression in MCF-7 human breast cancer cells. *Food Chem. Toxicol.* **2011**, *49*, 179–184. [CrossRef]
40. Taamalli, A.; Arráez-Román, D.; Barrajón-Catalán, E.; Ruiz-Torres, V.; Pérez-Sánchez, A.; Herrero, M.; Ibañez, E.; Micol, V.; Zarrouk, M.; Segura-Carretero, A.; et al. Use of advanced techniques for the extraction of phenolic compounds from Tunisian olive leaves: Phenolic composition and cytotoxicity against human breast cancer cells. *Food Chem. Toxicol.* **2012**, *50*, 1817–1825. [CrossRef]
41. Elamin, M.H.; Daghestani, M.H.; Omer, S.A.; Elobeid, M.A.; Virk, P.; Al-Olayan, E.M.; Hassan, Z.K.; Mohammed, O.B.; Aboussekhra, A. Olive oil oleuropein has anti-breast cancer properties with higher efficiency on ER-negative cells. *Food Chem. Toxicol.* **2013**, *53*, 310–316. [CrossRef] [PubMed]

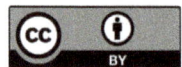

© 2020 by the authors. Licensee MDPI, Basel, Switzerland. This article is an open access article distributed under the terms and conditions of the Creative Commons Attribution (CC BY) license (http://creativecommons.org/licenses/by/4.0/).

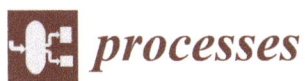

Article

Fatty Acids, Tocopherols, and Phytosterol Composition of Seed Oil and Phenolic Compounds and Antioxidant Activity of Fresh Seeds from Three *Dalbergia* Species Grown in Vietnam

Thi Thuy Nguyen [1,2], Lan Phuong Doan [1,3,*], Thu Huong Trinh Thi [1,3], Hong Ha Tran [3], Quoc Long Pham [3], Hai Ha Pham Thi [4,5], Long Giang Bach [4,5,*], Bertrand Matthäus [6] and Quoc Toan Tran [1,3]

[1] Graduate University of Science and Technology, Vietnam Academy of Science and Technology, Hanoi 100000, Vietnam; nguyenthithuycb@tuaf.edu.vn (T.T.N.); trinhthuhuong2001@gmail.com (T.H.T.T.); tranquoctoan2010@gmail.com (Q.T.T.)
[2] Thai Nguyen University of Agriculture and Forestry, Thai Nguyen 24118, Vietnam
[3] Institute of Natural Products Chemistry, Vietnam Academy of Science and Technology, Hanoi 100000, Vietnam; tranhongha1974@gmail.com (H.H.T.); mar.biochem@fpt.vn (Q.L.P.)
[4] NTT Hi-Tech Institute, Nguyen Tat Thanh University, Ho Chi Minh City 700000, Vietnam; pthha@ntt.edu.vn
[5] Center of Excellence for Biochemistry and Natural Products, Nguyen Tat Thanh University, Ho Chi Minh City 700000, Vietnam
[6] Working Group for Lipid Research, Department of Safety and Quality of Cereals, Max Rubner-Institut, 76131 Karlsruhe, Germany; bertrand.matthaeus@mri.bund.de
* Correspondence: doanlanphuong75@gmail.com (L.P.D.); blgiang@ntt.edu.vn (L.G.B.)

Received: 3 March 2020; Accepted: 21 April 2020; Published: 5 May 2020

Abstract: This research aimed to investigate the chemical composition of seed oils extracted from three Vietnamese *Dalbergia* species (*D. tonkinensis*, *D. mammosa*, and *D. entadoides*). The fatty acid profiles and contents of tocopherols and sterols of the seed oils, and total phenolic compounds extracted from the fresh seeds were characterized using different methods. Among the examined samples, *D. tonkinensis* seed oils showed high contents of linoleic acid (64.7%), whereas in *D. mammosa*, oleic acid (51.2%) was predominant. In addition, α- and γ-tocopherol and β-sitosterol were major ingredients in the seed oils, whereas ferulic acid and rosmarinic acid are usually predominant in the seeds of these species. Regarding sterol composition, the *D. entadoides* seed oil figured for remarkably high content of ∆5,23-stigmastadienol (1735 mg/kg) and ∆7-stigmastenol (1298 mg/kg). In addition, extracts with methanol/water (80:20, *v/v*) of seeds displayed significant in vitro antioxidant activity which was determined by DPPH free radical scavenging assay.

Keywords: *Dalbergia* species; DPPH free radical scavenging assay; fatty acid; phytosterol; tocopherol; total phenolic compound composition

1. Introduction

Plant-derived natural products are known for their enormous health benefits and absence of side effects in humans, and therefore have been extensively studied for practical applications [1–4]. In addition, medicinal plants are considered to be a repository of bioactive compounds with a wide range of therapeutic properties. The research direction involving medicinal plants is also accentuated by the fact that approximately 80% of healthcare in developing countries relies on traditional medicine, making any progress on identification of valuable compounds from plants important and useful [5]. Vietnam possesses an enormous biodiversity with more than 10,000 plant species and a well-established traditional medicine system. Therefore, further advances on the identification of natural compounds with beneficial properties from plants could drive the development of new drugs and open new pathways for more efficient recovery of valuable compounds [6–10].

The *Dalbergia* genus belongs to the family Fabaceae (Leguminosae), which is listed at high confidence and is composed of approximately 300 species [11]. The geographical distribution of the genus spans over various tropical and subtropical regions including Central and South America, Africa, Madagascar, and East and Southern Asia [12–14]. The heartwood and the aromatic oils obtained from species of the genus are commercially valuable materials for furniture, crafts, and treatment of diseases. For example, *Dalbergia odorifera* T. Chen, a well-researched plant with valuable timber, is also known for its abundance of aromatic oils found in the fragrant wood. In culinary use and in traditional medicine, the heartwood of *Dalbergia odorifera* is used as a spice and vulnerary to cure various diseases, including coronary artery disease and arrhythmia, cancer, diabetes, ischemia, necrosis, and blood disorders [15–17]. In addition, the bark decoction of the plant is used for the treatment of dyspepsia and the seed oil is applicable to relieve rheumatism. Such effects are mostly due to various useful bioactivities including anti-inflammatory, antioxidant, antimicrobial, and antiplatelet activity exhibited by phenolic and volatile components in *Dalbergia* species [18–21].

However, the data regarding chemical composition and biological evaluation of seed oil of *Dalbergia* species seem to be lacking. To date, the *Dalbergia* species that have been investigated for seed oil composition include only *D. melanoxylon*, *D. odorifera*, *D. paniculate*, and *D. sissoo* [22–24]. Among them, seed oil of *D. odorifera* has gained the most attention [25–27]. In addition, investigated materials in the aforementioned studies mostly comprised the *Dalbergia* species collected from India and China. Therefore, studies on Vietnamese *Dalbergia* plants and their compounds are limited [28]. One possible reason is the limited availability of *Dalbergia* plant materials in Vietnam due to overexploitation. According to the World Conservation Monitoring Centre (WCMC), the *Dalbergia* genus was categorized as vulnerable globally [29]. However, in Vietnam, the exhaustion of the plant has been increasingly alarming and some species of the genus, such as *Dalbergia tonkinensis* and *Dalbergia mammosa*, have been classified as second-grade state-protected trees [30]. Further knowledge on the chemical composition of seeds of Vietnamese *Dalbergia* species could contribute to the preservation of this huge genetic potential and allow a more sustainable and biobased utilization of the plant in agricultural and medicinal applications.

Therefore, the objective of this study was to evaluate the chemical composition of seed oil extracted from several Vietnamese species of the *Dalbergia* genus. The fatty acid, tocopherol, and phytosterol composition of seed oil, as well as the characterization of the phenolic compounds of seeds from *D. mammosa*, *D. tonkinensis*, and *D. entadoides* species were investigated. Moreover, the in vitro antioxidant activities (DPPH radical scavenging activity) of the three Vietnamese *Dalbergia* seed oils were analyzed. This study contributes to the understanding of the value of seed oils of some species belonging to the genus *Dalbergia* and provides necessary guidelines for future studies on food chemistry and industrial applications.

2. Materials and Methods

2.1. Plant Material

Three *Dalbergia* species (Fabaceae) (Table 1) were collected in southern Vietnam in 2016. Voucher specimens were kept at the Department of Organic Biochemistry, Institute of Natural Products Chemistry, Vietnam Academy of Science and Technology, Hanoi, Vietnam. Samples were identified, assigned herbarium numbers, and then stored at 4 °C for further experiments.

Table 1. List of three Vietnamese *Dalbergia* species.

	Code	Scientific Name	Collecting Place
1	VNMN-B2016.109	*D. entadoides*	Phu Quoc-Kien Giang Province
2	VNMN-B2016.114	*D. mammosa*	Cat Tien-Đong Nai Province
3	VNMN-B2016.1	*D. tonkinensis*	Dau Tieng-Binh Duong Province

2.2. Oil Extraction

Soxhlet extraction was performed to obtain the oils from three *Dalbergia* species using the modified method of ISO 659:2009 [31]. In brief, 10 g of sample material were ground in a ball mill, and then extracted in a Twisselmann apparatus for 6 h with 200 mL of petroleum ether. Afterwards, the solvent was removed by a rotary evaporator at 40 °C and 25 Torr. The oil was dried by a gentle stream of nitrogen and stored at −20 °C until use.

2.3. Analysis of Fatty Acid, Tocopherol, and Sterol Compositions

For the determination of the fatty acid composition, gas chromatography was applied following the method of ISO 5509:2000 [32]. To be specific, 10 mg of oil was dissolved in 1 mL of petroleum ether in a vial, followed by introduction of 25 µL of a methanolic solution of 2 M sodium methoxide and vigorous stirring for 1 min. Next, 20 µL of water was added and after centrifugation, the aqueous solution was removed. Then, 20 µL of 0.1 N HCl was added with methyl orange as the pH indicator. Following a thorough stirring, the lower aqueous phase was discarded, and the upper organic phase was dried by sodium sulphate. A Hewlett-Packard Gas Chromatography Instrument Model 5890 Series II/5989 A80 equipped with a 0.25 mm ZB-1 fused-silica capillary column (30 m × 0.25 µm i.d., Phenomenex, Torrance, CA, USA) was used to analyze the dried product. The carrier gas was helium at a flow rate of 1.0 mL/min.

HPLC analysis was employed to determine tocopherol according to the method of ISO 9936:2006 [33]. A Merck Hitachi low-pressure gradient system was used to analyze the sample containing 250 mg of oil dissolved in 25 mL heptane. The system was equipped with an L-6000 pump, a Merck Hitachi F-1000 fluorescence spectrophotometer (detector wavelengths at 295 nm for excitation, and at 330 nm for emission) and Chemstation integration software. A Spark marathon autosampler (Emmen, The Netherlands) was used to inject 20 µL of the sample onto a Diol phase HPLC column (250 mm × 4.6 mm i.d. Merck, Darmstadt, Germany), which was used at a flow rate of 1.3 mL/min. The mobile phase used was heptane/tert-butyl methyl ether (99 + 1, *v/v*). The results were given as mg vitamin E/100 g oil.

The modified method of DGF-F-III 1 (98) [34] was used to determine the phytosterol composition. First, saponification of the oil sample (250 mg) was conducted with 20 mL of 2 N ethanolic potassium hydroxide solution under reflux. The unsaponifiable components were subjected to purification by an aluminium oxide column (Merck, Darmstadt, Germany) and subsequently, by thin layer chromatography on a basic silica TLC plate (Merck, Darmstadt, Germany). GLC with betulin as the internal standard was used to determine the composition of the sterol fraction re-extracted from the TLC material. To separate the compounds, a SE 54 CB (Macherey-Nagel, Düren, Germany; 50 m long, 0.32 mm ID, 0.25 µm film thickness) was used. Parameters for the GLC included the following: hydrogen as the carrier gas, a split ratio 1:20, injection and detection temperature adjusted to 320 °C, and a temperature program 245 °C to 260 °C of 5 °C/min. For peak identification, either standard compounds (β-sitosterol, campesterol, and stigmasterol) or a mixture of sterols isolated from rapeseed oil (brassicasterol), or a mixture of sterols isolated from sunflower oil (Δ7-avenasterol, Δ7-stigmasterol, and Δ7-campesterol) was used. GC-MS was used to initially identify other sterols. Then, identification was done by comparing the retention time.

The results for fatty acids, tocopherols, and sterols were calculated on the seed oil.

2.4. Determination of Total Phenolic Compounds

Powdered seeds (1.0 g) were extracted with 5 mL methanol/water (80:20 v/v) using ultrasonic treatment (30 min, room temperature). The supernatants were filtered through a Whatman Grade 1 filter paper, and then stored at 4 °C for analysis. The Folin–Ciocalteu method [35] was adopted to determine the concentration of total phenolic compounds and the results were expressed in milligrams of gallic acid (GAE) per gram of sample. A standard curve with gallic acid was prepared from 400 to 1000 mg/L. The amount of total phenolic compounds was calculated using this standard curve. Values presented are means resulting from triplicate experiments.

The HPLC analyses were conducted using a HPLC/DAD system (VWR, Hitachi, Germany), equipped with a reversed phase C18 column (Lichrosphere 100 RP-18e (5 µm, 250 × 4 mm), Merck, Darmstadt, Germany). During the analysis, the column temperature was set to 23 °C. Water/formic acid (99.9:0.1, $v:v$) (solvent A) and acetonitrile/formic acid (99.9:0.1, $v:v$) (solvent B) was used as mobile phase at a flow rate of 1.0 mL/min with the following gradient program: 100% A, 0–5 min; 95% A/5% B, 5–35 min; 65% A/35% B, 35–45 min; 45% A/55% B, 45–55 min; 20% A/80% B, 55–60 min; 20% A/80% B, 60–63 min; and 100% A, 63–70 min. The flow rate was 1 mL/min, and the injection volume was 10 µL. The detection was conducted on a diode array detector L-2455 (Mertck Hitachi, Darmstadt, Germany) at wavelength 280 nm. The software, EZ Chrome Elite, was used for the acquisition and evaluation of the data. Quantification of phenolic compounds was achieved using a known quantity of p-hydroxycinnamic acid as the internal standard with a maximum at 280 nm.

2.5. Determination of Antioxidant Activity with the DPPH Free Radical Scavenging Method

Antiradical activity of extracts obtained with methanol/water (80:20, v/v) was measured by DPPH (2,2-diphenyl-1-picryl hydrazyl) assay and compared to that of ascorbic acid (vitamin C of Sigma, USA). Determination of the DPPH radical scavenging activity was carried out following the modified method of Saeed et al. [35]. First, 0.5 mL of 2,2′-diphenyl-1-picrylhydrazyl (DPPH) solution (50 mg/100 mL) was diluted in 4.5 mL of methanol, followed by the addition of 0.1 mL of extract at various concentrations dissolved in methanol. Then, the mixture underwent vigorous shaking, followed by incubation at RT for 45 min in the dark. A spectrophotometer was used to measure the absorbance at 517 nm against the blank (without any extract). The SC50, defined as the required concentration in which 50% of the initial DPPH radicals was quenched, was calculated from a calibration curve established with different concentrations of extracts.

2.6. Statistical Analyses

The Statistical Package for the Social Sciences (SPSS) software was used to analyze the reliability and validity of the data and to compare the differences among studied values with a significance level of $p < 0.05$. All determinations were carried out in triplicate.

3. Results and Discussion

3.1. Oil Content

Analysis of the total lipid content of all the analyzed species showed only a small amount of oil which ranged from 2.5% for *D. entadoides* and *D. tonkinensis* to 8.2% for *D. mammosa* (Table 2). This is consistent with studies of Augustus and Seiler and Badami et al. who found only small amounts of oil in seeds from two *Dalbergia* species, ranging from 4.8% (*D. sissoo*) to 7.4% (*D. paniculatae*) [22,23].

3.2. Fatty Acid, Tocopherol, and Sterol Compositions

The fatty acid compositions are summarized in Table 2. The oil of *Dalbergia* seeds is characterized by common fatty acids with 16, 18, or 20 carbon atoms. The predominant fatty acids existing in *D. mammosa* and in *D. tonkinensis* are oleic acid (51.2%) and linoleic acid (64.7%), respectively.

D. entadoides species contains comparably high amounts of oleic acid (25.1%) and linoleic acid (23.0%). However, in comparison to the other *Dalbergia species*, *D. entadoides* had a statistically significantly ($p < 0.05$) higher percentage of linolenic acid (7.3%). In another study, seed oil of *D. odorifera*, was reported to contain linoleic acid (60.0%), oleic acid (17.5%), and palmitic acid (16.7%) [27], which is similar to the current composition of *D. tonkinensis*. The fatty acid composition of *D. mammosa* was comparable to that of *D. paniculata* where palmitic acid (17.8%), oleic acid (48.2%), and linoleic acid (22.5%) were found as the main representatives [23]. One noticeable feature of *D. entadoides* seed oil is the relatively high content of behenic acid (22:0) (15.3%) over that of *D. mimosa* (3.4%), *D. tonkinensis* (0.3%), and most plant seeds except for *Arachis hypogaea* in which behenic acid accounts for 27.0% of the total lipid content [36]. The fatty acid composition of *D. tonkinensis* is very similar to that of sunflower oil which is characterized by a high content of linoleic acid, a moderate content of oleic acid, and nearly 82% total unsaturated fatty acids. In addition, there were significant differences ($p < 0.05$) of UFA components of three *Dalbergia* species. The *D. tonkinensis* species had the highest portion of UFA with 81.8%, followed by those of *D. mammosa* and *D. entadoides* with 74.5% and 56.7%, respectively. Similar to the UFA components, the contents of omega 3, omega 6, and omega 9 of the three *Dalbergia* species were distinctly different. The omega 6 content of *D. tonkinensis* accounted for 64.7%, which was about three times higher than those of the other two investigated *Dalbergia* species. *D. mammosa* had the highest proportion of omega 9 (52.5%), which was nearly two times higher than that of *D. entadoides* and approximately five times higher than that of *D. tonkinensis*.

Table 2. Total fat content (%) and fatty acid composition (%) of three *Dalbergia* species.

Fatty Acid Composition	*D. entadoides*	*D. mammosa*	*D. tonkinensis*
Total lipid content *	$2.7^b \pm 0.13$	$8.2^a \pm 0.09$	$2.5^b \pm 0.11$
16:0	$16.9^a \pm 0.04$	$12.0^c \pm 0.02$	$13.2^b \pm 0.02$
16:1($n-7$)	$0.5^a \pm 0.01$	$0.2^b \pm 0.001$	$0.2^b \pm 0.05$
17:0	$0.7^a \pm 0.30$	$0.2^b \pm 0.002$	$0.1^b \pm 0.03$
18:0	$6.5^b \pm 0.02$	$6.6^a \pm 0.01$	$4.5^c \pm 0.04$
18:1($n-9$)	$25.1^b \pm 0.01$	$51.2^a \pm 0.30$	$11.6^c \pm 0.10$
18:1($n-11$)	$0.5^b \pm 0.004$	$0.6^b \pm 0.002$	$3.6^a \pm 0.20$
18:2($n-6$)	$23.0^b \pm 0.02$	$20.1^c \pm 0.01$	$64.7^a \pm 0.05$
18:3($n-3$)	$7.3^a \pm 0.03$	$1.2^c \pm 0.02$	$1.5^b \pm 0.03$
20:0	$1.4^b \pm 0.05$	$1.9^a \pm 0.03$	$0.1^c \pm 0.004$
20:1($n-9$)	$0.5^b \pm 0.002$	$1.3^a \pm 0.04$	$0.1^c \pm 0.002$
22:0	$15.3^a \pm 0.10$	$3.4^b \pm 0.002$	$0.3^c \pm 0.001$
24:0	$2.5^a \pm 0.003$	$1.3^b \pm 0.01$	<LOQ
SFA	$43.3^a \pm 0.01$	$25.5^b \pm 0.04$	$18.2^c \pm 0.04$
UFA	$56.7^c \pm 0.05$	$74.5^b \pm 0.01$	$81.8^a \pm 0.05$
Omega-3 ($n-3$)	$7.3^a \pm 0.02$	$1.2^c \pm 0.03$	$1.5^b \pm 0.01$
Omega-6 ($n-6$)	$23.0^c \pm 0.30$	$20.1^b \pm 0.04$	$64.7^a \pm 0.05$
Omega-9 ($n-9$)	$25.5^b \pm 0.01$	$52.5^a \pm 0.04$	$11.7^c \pm 0.01$

* with regard to fresh seeds. In every row, the values with the same exponent have no statistically significant difference with $\alpha = 5\%$.

3.3. Tocopherol Composition

The total content of tocochromanols in the seed oil varied from 8.5 mg/100 g (*D. entadoides*) to 36.2 mg/100 g (*D. mamosa*) with α- and γ-tocopherol being predominant tocochromanols (Table 3). While γ-tocopherol dominated in *D. mammosa* (20.3 mg/100 g), α-tocopherol was most abundantly found in *D. tokinensis* (20.0 mg/100 g). In comparison to the two other species, *D. entadoides* seed oil contained tocochromanols in a much lower quantity with α- and γ-tocopherol detected in similar amounts (3.8 mg/100 g and 2.7 mg/100 g, respectively). γ-Tocopherol was not found only in *D. tonkinensis*. However, *D. tonkinensis* seed oil contained noticeable amounts of β-tocopherol (2.1 mg/100 g) and δ-tocopherol (1.0 mg/100 g). Tocotrienols were also found in D. entadoides (1.1 mg/100 g (α-tocotrienol)) and D. tonkinensis (2.1 mg/100 g (β-tocotrienol)).

Table 3. Tocopherol compositions (mg/100 g) of three *Dalbergia* species, calculated for the oil extracted from the fresh seeds.

Species	α-T	α-T3	β-T	γ-T	β-T3
D. entadoides	3.8^c ± 0.05	1.1 ± 0.03	0.9^b ± 0.003	2.7^b ± 0.01	<LOQ
D. mammosa	14.9^b ± 0.02	<LOQ	0.3^c ± 0.02	20.3^a ± 0.05	<LOQ
D. tonkinensis	20.9^a ± 0.04	<LOQ	2.1^a ± 0.01	<LOQ	2.1 ± 0.01

Species	P8	γ-T3	δ-T	δ-T3	Sum
D. entadoides	<LOQ	<LOQ	<LOQ	<LOQ	8.5^c ± 0.04
D. mammosa	0.8 ± 0.03	<LOQ	<LOQ	<LOQ	36.2^a ± 0.05
D. tonkinensis	<LOQ	<LOQ	1.0 ± 0.02	<LOQ	26.1^b ± 0.03

* LOQ, limit of quantitation; T, tocopherol; T3, tocotrienol; P8, plastochromanol-8. In every column, the values with the same exponent have no statistically significant difference with α = 5%.

Lianhe et al. described a high total content of tocopherols for seed oil from *D. odorifera* with 511.9 mg/kg [27]. This is much higher than the total amount found in the three *Dalbergia* species of this investigation. The pattern of tocopherols presented by Lianhe et al. for *D. odorifera* seed oil was comparable to the pattern for *D. mammosa* with a higher content of γ-tocopherol (160.8 mg/kg) and a lower amount of α-tocopherol (351.1 mg/kg). In contrast to *D. odorifera* seed, oil from *D. entadoides* and *D. tonkinensis* showed higher amounts of α-tocopherol, and lower amounts or no of γ-tocopherol.

3.4. Sterol Composition

Seed oils of *Dalbergia* species are characterized by the existence of different phytosterols including campesterol, stigmasterol, Δ5,23-stigmastadienol, β-sitosterol, sitostanol, Δ5-avenasterol, and Δ7-stigmastenol in varying amounts (Table 4). The total amount of phytosterols in the seed oils varied between 534.6 mg/kg (*D. tonkinensis*) and 6658 mg/kg (*D. entadoides*) with β-sitosterol being the major constituent in the seed oils of *D. entadoides* (1781 mg/kg) and *D. mammosa* (1878 mg/kg). In seed oil of *D. tonkinensis*, only 156.6 mg/kg of ß-sitosterol were found. Remarkably, *D. entadoides* was abundantly constituted by the high content of Δ5,23-stigmastadienol (1735 mg/kg) and Δ7-stigmastenol (1298 mg/kg), contrasted by the significantly lower amounts in the other species.

Table 4. Sterol compositions (mg/kg) of three *Dalbergia* species, calculated for the oil extracted from the fresh seeds.

Phytosterol	D. entadoides	D. mammosa	D. tonkinensis
Cholesterol	19.9^c ± 0.01	46.7^a ± 0.01	23.6^b ± 0.01
Brassicasterol	38.4^a ± 0.05	7.6^c ± 0.04	14.1^b ± 0.03
24-methylenecholesterol	41.1^a ± 0.01	6.5^c ± 0.01	8.5^a ± 0.01
Campesterol	266.3^a ± 0.02	162.0^b ± 0.01	29.6^c ± 0.01
Campestanol	<LOQ	12.3 ± 0.04	<LOQ
Stigmasterol	334.3^a ± 0.02	334.2^b ± 0.03	50.3^c ± 0.02
Δ7-Campesterol	50.3^a ± 0.04	19.6^b ± 0.01	8.5^c ± 0.04
Δ5,23-Stigmastadienol	1735^a ± 0.01	29.7^c ± 0.04	180.60^b ± 0.03
Chlerosterol	64.3^a ± 0.03	6.7^c ± 0.02	49.5^b ± 0.02
β-Sitosterol	1781^b ± 0.01	1878^a ± 0.01	156.6^c ± 0.01
Sitostanol	347.2^a ± 0.02	72.6^b ± 0.03	<LOQ
Δ5-Avenasterol	152.4^a ± 0.04	127.8^b ± 0.01	13.4^c ± 0.02
Δ5,24-Stigmastadienol	479.8 ± 0.03	<LOQ	<LOQ
Δ7-Stigmastenol	1298^a ± 0.01	68.6^b ± 0.02	<LOQ
Δ7-Avenastenol	84.0^a ± 0.01	14.3^b ± 0.03	<LOQ
Total amount	6658.0^a	2686.7^b	534.6^c

LOQ, limit of quantitation. In every row, the values with the same exponent have no statistically significant difference with α = 5%.

3.5. Content of Total Phenolic Compounds

Extraction with methanol:water (80:20 (v/v)) was more effective for seeds of D. tonkinensis than for seeds of D. entadoides and D. mammosa (Table 5) with respect to the total extractable compounds. To be specific, the amount of total phenolic compounds in seeds of D. tokinensis was three and four times, respectively, higher than those of D. mammosa and D. entadoides seeds. In addition, Folin–Ciocalteau assay showed that most of the compounds extracted from D. tonkinensis did not show the behavior of phenolic compounds. Although the amount of the total extractable compounds in D. tonkinensis was several times higher than those in the two other species, the amounts of total phenolic compounds in seeds of D. entadoides and D. mammosa were higher than that in seeds of D. tonkinensis with the a significant difference of 5%. In comparison to the results of Lianhe et al. [25] who found total phenolic compounds in D. odorifera seeds in the range from 135 to 563.2 mg/g depending on the extraction medium, the present investigation resulted in much lower total amounts of phenolic compounds. One possible reason could be the different solvents used [37]. While the present study used methanol/water (80:20 v/v) as the extraction solvent, Lianhe et al. utilized different kinds of solvents [26], resulting in varied yields due to the strong influence of composition and polarity of the solvent exerting on the yield of extractable and phenolic compounds.

Table 5. Total extractable compounds (EC) (mg/g), total phenolic compounds (PC) (mg/g), and DPPH free radical scavenging activity (SC50) (µg/mL) of extracts of fresh seeds of Dalbergia species obtained by methanol:water (80:20, v:v).

No	Species	EC	PC	DPPH Free Radical Scavenging Activity
1	D. entadoides	87.3[c]	23.0[b]	15.4[c]
2	D. mammosa	144.1[b]	24.8[a]	18.5[b]
3	D. tonkinensis	469.1[a]	19.5[c]	11.9[d]
4	Vitamin C			26.3[a]

In every column, the values with the same exponent have no statistically significant difference with $\alpha = 5\%$.

3.6. Antioxidant Activity with the DPPH Free Radical Scavenging Method

The extracts obtained by extraction of the three oil samples with methanol/water (80:20, v/v) exhibited strong antioxidant activity, as demonstrated by SC50 values ranging from 11.9 to 18.5 µg/mL. Ascorbic acid (Vitamin C), which serves as the standard compound, achieved a SC50 value of 26.32 µg/mL. Among the samples, the extract from D. tonkinensis showed the most promising antioxidant activity (Table 5). Previous studies have investigated antioxidant activity from several species of this genus including D. sissoo, D. odorifera, and D. saxatilis [26,38–40], in which D. odorifera was the most studied plant with antioxidant activity found in bark, roots, seeds, and heartwood [26,39,40].

3.7. Composition of Phenolic Fraction

The amounts of phenolic compounds extracted from fresh seed material of the different Dalbergia species measured by HPLC ranged from below limit of quantification to 34.5 mg/kg (Table 6). As the levels of phenolics were assessed only relatively, with the use of p-coumaric acid as the calibration standard, their actual contents could vary from those reported in Table 6. However, the results effectively illustrate the relative differences in the levels of individual analytes between the analyzed plants. Accordingly, the best source of taxifolin (34.5 mg/kg) and ferulic acid (23.8 mg/kg) was D. entadoides. Rosmarinic acid (27.4 mg/kg) and ferulic acid (21.8 mg/kg) were predominant phenolic acids in D. mammosa. Chlorogenic acid (19.8 mg/kg) and rosmarinic acid (10.6 mg/kg) were abundantly found in D. tonkinensis (Figure 1). Moreover, some other phenolic compounds were relatively abundant, such as naringinin in D. entadoides (6.0 mg/kg), p-coumaric acid in D. mammosa (6.7 mg/kg), and taxifolin in D. tonkinensis (9.8 mg/kg).

Table 6. Composition of phenolic compounds extracted by methanol:water (80:20, v/v) from the fresh seeds of three Dalbergia species (mg/kg).

Phenolic Acid	D. entadoides	D. mammosa	D. tonkinensis
Chlorogenic acid	1.8[b] ± 0.04	0.4[c] ± 0.03	19.8[a] ± 0.02
Gallic acid	0.7[a] ± 0.01	<LOQ	0.7[a] ± 0.03
Caffeic acid	<LOQ	<LOQ	<LOQ
Vanillic acid	2.6[a] ± 0.05	0.4[c] ± 0.04	0.6[b] ± 0.01
Isovanillic acid	<LOQ	<LOQ	2.0 ± 0.04
Vanillin	0.7[a] ± 0.002	<LOQ	0.2[b] ± 0.02
p-Coumaric acid	2.3[b] ± 0.04	6.7[a] ± 0.02	0.6[c] ± 0.05
Ferulic acid	23.8[a] ± 0.4	21.8[b] ± 0.01	0.8[c] ± 0.002
Taxifolin	34.5[a] ± 0.3	3.2[c] ± 0.01	9.8[b] ± 0.4
Rosmarinic acid	0.7[c] ± 0.01	27.4[a] ± 0.3	10.6[b] ± 0.2
Daidzein	2.3[a] ± 0.04	1.9[b] ± 0.04	1.6[c] ± 0.01
Cinnamic acid	0.6[b] ± 0.004	0.7[a] ± 0.001	0.2[c] ± 0.03
Naringinin	6.0[a] ± 0.01	1.2[c] ± 0.03	1.4[b] ± 0.01

LOQ, limit of quantitation. In every row, the values with the same exponent have no statistically significant difference with α = 5%.

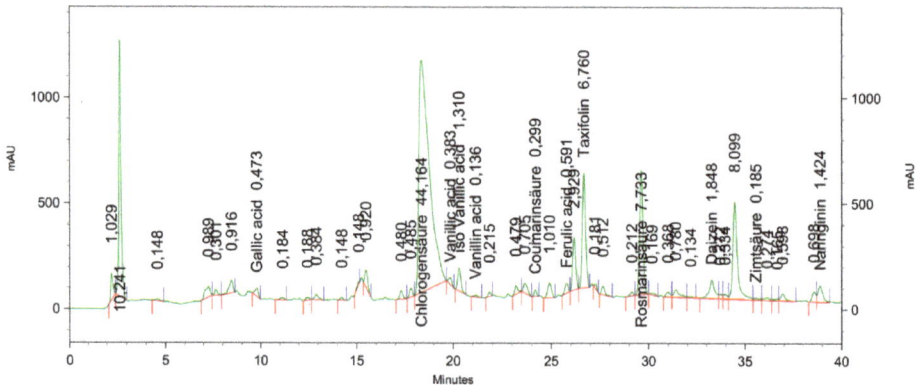

Figure 1. HPLC chromatogram of phenolic compounds of the D. tonkinensis seed.

In comparison to the results from the literature [37], the present work also shows the predominant position of phenolic acids as phenolic compounds found in D. mammosa and D. tonkinensis, while D. entadoides was characterized by a high content of flavonoids (taxifolin). In the other seed materials, significant amounts were also detected. Another flavonoid existing in the three species was naringinin, but the detected levels were low.

Overall, the composition of the phenolic fraction of fresh seeds from three *Dalbergia* species shown in the present work was characterized by multiple types of phenolic acids where rosmarinic acid, chlorogenic acid, and ferulic acid represented the highest amounts in compositions of D. mammosa (27.4 mg/kg), D. tonkinensis (19.8 mg/kg), and D. entadoides (23.8 mg/kg), respectively.

4. Conclusions

This study, for the first time, provides data on the fatty acid, tocopherol, sterol, and phenolic acid compositions of three *Dalbergia* seed oils grown in Vietnam. Among the examined samples, D. tonkinensis and D. mammosa seed oils showed high contents of linoleic acid and oleic acid, respectively. The α- and γ-tocopherols, β-sitosterol, ferulic acid, and rosmarinic acid are usually the major ingredients presented in these species studied. In addition, seed extracts of the *Dalbergia* species in Vietnam, including D. entadoides, D. mammosa, and D. tonkinensis, displayed significant antioxidant potentials with relatively low SC50 values. Consequently, these *Dalbergia* plants should be conserved and the population should be sustained due to their potential as highly nutritional and bioactive oil sources.

Author Contributions: Investigation, L.P.D., T.T.N., T.H.T.T., H.H.T., and H.H.P.T.; Supervision, Q.L.P., L.G.B., B.M., and Q.T.T.; Writing—original draft, L.P.D. All authors have read and agreed to the published version of the manuscript.

Funding: This work was financially supported by the Ministry of Science and Technology, Vietnam (44/2014/HĐ-NĐT).

Conflicts of Interest: The authors declare no conflict of interest.

References

1. Merarchi, M.; Sethi, G.; Shanmugam, M.K.; Fan, L.; Arfuso, F.; Ahn, K.S. Role of Natural Products in Modulating Histone Deacetylases in Cancer. *Molecules* **2019**, *24*, 1047. [CrossRef] [PubMed]
2. Ullah, A.; Munir, S.; Mabkhot, Y.; Badshah, S.L. Bioactivity Profile of the Diterpene Isosteviol and its Derivatives. *Molecules* **2019**, *24*, 678. [CrossRef]
3. Soccio, M.; Laus, M.N.; Flagella, Z.; Pastore, D. Assessment of Antioxidant Capacity and Putative Healthy Effects of Natural Plant Products Using Soybean Lipoxygenase-Based Methods. An Overview. *Molecules* **2018**, *23*, 3244. [CrossRef] [PubMed]
4. Mohamed Eliaser, E.; Hui Ho, J.; Mohd Hashim, N.; Rukayadi, Y.; Lian Ee, G.C.; Abdull Razis, A.F. Phytochemical Constituents and Biological Activities of Melicope lunu-ankenda. *Molecules* **2018**, *23*, 2708. [CrossRef] [PubMed]
5. Aye, M.M.; Aung, H.T.; Sein, M.M.; Armijos, C. A Review on the Phytochemistry, Medicinal Properties and Pharmacological Activities of 15 Selected Myanmar Medicinal Plants. *Molecules* **2019**, *24*, 293. [CrossRef]
6. Nguyen, D.N.V.; Nguyen, T. *An Overview of the Use of Plants and Animals in Traditional Medicine Systems in Viet Nam*; TRAFFIC Southeast Asia, Greater Mekong Programme: Ha Noi, Vietnam, 2008.
7. Nguyen, Q.V.; Nguyen, V.B.; Eun, J.B.; Wang, S.L.; Nguyen, D.H.; Tran, T.N.; Nguyen, A.D. Anti-oxidant and antidiabetic effect of some medicinal plants belong to *Terminalia species* collected in Dak Lak Province, Vietnam. *Res. Chem. Intermed.* **2016**, *42*, 5859–5871. [CrossRef]
8. Nguyen, Q.V.; Nguyen, N.H.; Wang, S.L.; Nguyen, V.B.; Nguyen, A.D. Free radical scavenging and antidiabetic activities of *Euonymus laxiflorus* Champ extract. *Res. Chem. Intermed.* **2017**, *43*, 5615–5624. [CrossRef]
9. Nguyen, V.B.; Nguyen, Q.V.; Nguyen, A.D.; Wang, S.L. Porcine pancreatic α-amylase inhibitors from *Euonymus laxiflorus* Champ. *Res. Chem. Intermed.* **2017**, *43*, 259–269. [CrossRef]
10. Thang, T.D.; Kuo, P.-C.; Hwang, T.-L.; Yang, M.-L.; Ngoc, N.T.B.; Han, T.T.N.; Lin, C.-W.; Wu, T.-S. Triterpenoids and Steroids from *Ganoderma mastoporum* and Their Inhibitory Effects on Superoxide Anion Generation and Elastase Release. *Molecules* **2013**, *18*, 14285–14292. [CrossRef]
11. The Plant List. Available online: http://www.theplantlist.org/tpl1.1/search?q=dalbergia (accessed on 7 May 2019).
12. Sun, S.; Zeng, X.; Zhang, D.; Guo, S. Diverse fungi associated with partial irregular heartwood of *Dalbergia odorifera*. *Sci. Rep.* **2015**, *5*, 8464. [CrossRef]
13. Choi, C.W.; Choi, Y.H.; Cha, M.-R.; Yoo, D.S.; Kim, Y.S.; Yon, G.H.; Hong, K.S.; Kim, Y.H.; Ryu, S.Y. Yeast α-Glucosidase Inhibition by Isoflavones from Plants of Leguminosae as an in Vitro Alternative to Acarbose. *J. Agric. Food Chem.* **2010**, *58*, 9988–9993. [CrossRef] [PubMed]
14. Lee, D.-S.; Jeong, G.-S. Arylbenzofuran isolated from *Dalbergia odorifera* suppresses lipopolysaccharide-induced mouse BV2 microglial cell activation, which protects mouse hippocampal HT22 cells death from neuroinflammation-mediated toxicity. *Eur. J. Pharmacol.* **2014**, *728*, 1–8. [CrossRef] [PubMed]
15. Nguyen, V.B.; Wang, S.-L.; Nhan, N.T.; Nguyen, T.H.; Nguyen, N.P.D.; Nghi, D.H.; Cuong, N.M. New Records of Potent In-Vitro Antidiabetic Properties of *Dalbergia tonkinensis* Heartwood and the Bioactivity-Guided Isolation of Active Compounds. *Molecules* **2018**, *23*, 1589. [CrossRef] [PubMed]
16. Valette, N.; Perrot, T.; Sormani, R.; Gelhaye, E.; Morel-Rouhier, M. Antifungal activities of wood extractives. *Fungal Biol. Rev.* **2017**, *31*, 113–123. [CrossRef]

17. Zhao, X.; Mei, W.; Gong, M.; Zuo, W.; Bai, H.; Dai, H. Antibacterial Activity of the Flavonoids from *Dalbergia odorifera* on *Ralstonia solanacearum*. *Molecules* **2011**, *16*, 9775–9782. [CrossRef] [PubMed]
18. Ninh, T.S.; Masataka, O.; Naoki, H.; Daiki, Y.; Yu, K.; Fumi, T.; Kenichi, H.; Nguyen, M.C.; Yoshiyasu, F. Antimicrobial Activity of the Constituents of *Dalbergia tonkinensis* and Structural-Bioactive Highlights. *Nat. Prod. Commun.* **2018**, *13*, 157–161.
19. Ninh, T.S.; Kenichi, H.; Nguyen, M.C.; Yoshiyasu, F. Two New Carboxyethylflavanones from the Heartwood of *Dalbergia tonkinensis* and Their Antimicrobial Activities. *Nat. Prod. Commun.* **2017**, *12*, 1721–1723.
20. Cuong, N.M.; Nhan, N.T.; Son, N.T.; Nghi, D.H.; Cuong, T.D. Daltonkins A and B, Two New Carboxyethylflavanones from the Heartwood of *Dalbergia tonkinensis*. *Bull. Korean Chem. Soc.* **2017**, *38*, 1511–1514. [CrossRef]
21. Ngu, T.N.; Ninh, T.S.; To, D.C.; Nguyen, P.D.N.; Pham, N.K.; Tran, T.H.; Nguyen, M.C. Further study on chemical constituents from the heartwood of *Dalbergia tonkinensis* collected in Daklak province. *Vietnam J. Sci. Technol.* **2018**, *56*, 252–258.
22. Augustus, G.D.P.S.; Seiler, G.J. Promising oil producing seed species of Western Ghats (Tamil Nadu, India). *Ind. Crop. Prod.* **2001**, *13*, 93–100. [CrossRef]
23. Badami, R.C.; Shivamurthy, S.C.; Joshi, M.S.; Patil, K.B.; Subba Rao, Y.V.; Sastri, G.S.R.; Viswanatha Rao, G.K. Characterisation of fifteen varieties of genotype peanuts for yield, oil content and fatty acid composition. *J. Oil Technol. Assoc. India* **1979**, *11*, 85–87.
24. Kittur, M.H.; Mahajanshetti, C.S.; Lakshminarayana, G. Characteristcs and composition of some convolvulaceae and Leguminosae seeds and the oils. *Fat Sci. Technol.* **1987**, *89*, 269–270.
25. Lianhe, Z.; Li, W.; Guo, X.; Li, X. Chen, Essential oil composition from the seeds of *Dalbergia odorifera* T. Chen grown in Hainan, China. *J. Food, Agric. Environ.* **2011**, *9*, 26–28.
26. Lianhe, Z.; Li, W.; Xing, H.; Zhengxing, C. Antioxidant activities of seed extracts from *Dalbergia odorifera* T. Chen. *Afr. J. Biotechnol.* **2011**, *10*, 11658–11667.
27. Lianhe, Z.; Xing, H.; Li, W.; Zhengxing, C. Physicochemical Properties, Chemical Composition and Antioxidant Activity of *Dalbergia odorifera* T. Chen Seed Oil. *J. Am. Oil Chem. Soc.* **2012**, *89*, 883–890. [CrossRef]
28. Nguyen, V.B.; Nguyen, Q.V.; Nguyen, A.D.; Wang, S.-L. Screening and evaluation of α-glucosidase inhibitors from indigenous medicinal plants in Dak Lak Province, Vietnam. *Res. Chem. Intermed.* **2017**, *43*, 3599–3612. [CrossRef]
29. WCMC. *Dalbergia odorifera*. The IUCN Red List of *Threatened Species*. 1998. Available online: http://www.iucnredlist.org/details/32398/0 (accessed on 8 December 2017).
30. Matthäus, B.; Vosmann, K.; Long, P.Q.; Aitzetmüller, K. Fatty acid and Tocopherol Composition of Vietnamese Oilseeds. *J. Am. Oil Chem. Soc.* **2003**, *80*, 1013–1020. [CrossRef]
31. International Organization for Standardization. *Oil Seeds—Determination of Oil Content*; Standard No. 659:2009; ISO: Geneva, Switzerland, 2009.
32. International Organization for Standardization. *Animal and Vegetable Fats and Oils-Preparation of Methyl Esters of Fatty Acids*; Standard No. 5509:2000; ISO: Geneva, Switzerland, 2000.
33. International Organization for Standardization. *Animal and Vegetable Fats and Oils-Determination of Tocopherol and Tocotrienol Contents by High-Performance Liquid Chromatography*; Standard No. 9936; ISO: Geneva, Switzerland, 2006, 2006.
34. DGF, Deutsche Gesellschaft für Fettwissenschaft. *Deutsche Einheitsmethoden zur Untersuchung von Fetten, Fettprodukten, Tensiden und Verwandten Stoffen*; Wissenschaftliche: Stuttgart, Germany, 2015.
35. Saeed, N.; Khan, M.R.L.; Shabbir, M. Antioxidant activity, total phenolic and total flavonoid contents of whole plant extracts *Torilis leptophylla* L. *BMC Complement. Altern. Med.* **2012**, *16*, 221–233. [CrossRef]
36. Grosso, N.R.; Zygadlo, J.A.; Lamarque, A.L.; Damián, M.; Maestri, C.; Guzmán, A. Proximate, fatty acid and sterol compositions of aboriginal peanut (*Arachis hypogaea* L.) seeds from Bolivia. *J. Sci. Food Agric.* **1997**, *73*, 349–356. [CrossRef]
37. Ganesan, S.; Vadivel, K.; Jayaraman, J. *Sustainable Crop Disease Management Using Natural Products*; CABI: Wallingford, UK, 2015; p. 310.
38. Kumari, A.; Kakkar, P. Screening of antioxidant potential of selected barks of Indian medicinal plants by multiple in vitro assay. *Biomed. Enviro. Sci.* **2008**, *21*, 24–29. [CrossRef]

39. Wang, W.; Weng, X.; Cheng, D. Antioxidant activities of natural phenolic components from *Dalbergia odorifera* T. Chen. *Food Chem.* **2000**, *71*, 45–49. [CrossRef]
40. Hou, J.P.; Wu, H.; Ho, C.T.; Weng, X.C. Antioxidant activity of polyphenolic compounds from *Dalbergia odorifera* T. Chen. *Pak. J. Nutr.* **2011**, *10*, 694–701.

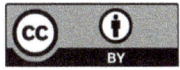 © 2020 by the authors. Licensee MDPI, Basel, Switzerland. This article is an open access article distributed under the terms and conditions of the Creative Commons Attribution (CC BY) license (http://creativecommons.org/licenses/by/4.0/).

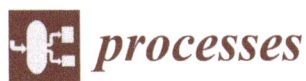

Article

Phytochemical Profile, Antioxidant and Antitumor Activities of Green Grape Juice

Mohamad Nasser [1,2], Hoda Cheikh-Ali [1], Akram Hijazi [1,2,*], Othmane Merah [3,4,*], Abd El-Ameer N. Al-Rekaby [5] and Rana Awada [1,2,*]

1. Doctoral School of Science and Technology, Research Plateform for Environmental Sience (PRASE), Lebanese University, P.O. Box 5, Beirut, Lebanon; mohamed.nasser@ul.edu.lb (M.N.); hodacheikh6@gmail.com (H.C.-A.)
2. Anticancer Therapeutic Approaches Group (ATAC), Rammal Hassan Rammal Research Laboratory, Biology Department, Faculty of Sciences, Lebanese University, P.O. Box 5, Beirut, Lebanon
3. Laboratoire de Chimie Agro-industrielle (LCA), Université de Toulouse, INRA, INPT, 31030 Toulouse, France
4. Département Génie Biologique, IUT A, Université Paul Sabatier, 24 rue d'Embaquès, 32000 Auch, France
5. Department of Biology, College of Science, Al Mustansiriyah University, P.O. Box 14022, Baghdad, Iraq; aghloub@gmail.com
* Correspondence: Akram.Hijazi@ul.edu.lb (A.H.); othmane.merah@ensiacet.fr (O.M.); awada-rana@hotmail.com (R.A.); Tel.: +961-71-905-768 (A.H.); +33-534-323-523 (O.M.); +961-76-004-102 (R.A.)

Received: 26 March 2020; Accepted: 21 April 2020; Published: 26 April 2020

Abstract: (1) Plants, due to their phytochemicals, have long been known for their pharmacological potential and medicinal value. Verjuice, the acidic juice of unripe green grape, is still poorly characterized in terms of its chemical composition and biological activities. (2) In this study, we characterized the chemical composition, antioxidant and antitumor potential of verjuice extract. Folin–Ciocalteu and aluminum chloride reagents were used to identify the total phenol and total flavonoid composition. Various conventional methods were used to quantify the alkaloids and tannins. DPPH (2,2-diphenyl-1-picrylhydrazyl) free radical scavenging assay and Neutral Red assay were used to assess the antioxidant and antitumor activities, respectively. (3) We showed that the verjuice extract contains alkaloids, tannins, and a high quantity of total flavonoids and total phenols. Besides its antioxidant activity, verjuice significantly repressed human pulmonary adenocarcinoma (A549) cells' viability in both dose- and time-dependent manners. Moreover, verjuice extract significantly enhanced the anticancer potential of cisplatin. (4) Altogether, these observations suggest a potential use of verjuice as a natural antitumor remedy.

Keywords: verjuice; phytochemicals; unripe grape juice; pulmonary adenocarcinoma; anti-proliferative; antioxidant

1. Introduction

Besides being a vital source of alimentation, nowadays, plants are being used for cosmetic, food processing, pharmaceutical, and medicinal purposes. Phytochemicals from traditional medicinal herbs have long been known for their therapeutic value in treating a vast array of critical health disorders, including cancer [1]. Nowadays, plant-derived bioactive molecules are used for designing novel remedies [1].

Cancer represents the second leading cause of mortality worldwide and includes many types. Pulmonary cancer, one of the most aggressive human tumors, exists in two forms: NSCLC (Non-Small Cell Lung Cancer) and SCLC (Small Cell Lung Cancer), representing 80–85% and 15–20% of cases, respectively [2]. Distinct strategies, including surgery, chemotherapy, radiation, hormones, and immunotherapy can be employed for lung cancer prevention and treatment. Currently, chemotherapy is the most commonly used strategy. However, its application is challenged with its limited efficacy, toxic side effects, and cancer resistance [3]. Remarkably, medicinal plants have shown potential during pulmonary cancer therapy due to their ability to: (i) increase the sensitizing capacity of conventional agents, (ii) extend patients' survival time, (iii) restrain chemotherapy side effects, and (iv) improve the quality of life of lung cancer patients [4]. In this context, various medicinal plants' extracts as well as plant-derived phytochemicals have exhibited a significant capacity to inhibit lung cancer cell proliferation [5].

Lebanon, due to its geographic location, is characterized by a great variety of plant species known for their therapeutic value. More than ninety wild species encountered in Lebanon are endemics. Therefore, it is of great interest to characterize the biological and therapeutic potential of these endemic plants [6,7]. *Vitis vinifera* L. (the common grape vine) is one of the largest fruit crops worldwide. It is known for its antioxidant potential and ability to protect the cardiovascular system [8,9]. Verjuice (green grape juice or unripe grape juice), which is highly consumed in the Mediterranean region, corresponds to the acidic juice recovered upon mechanically pressing unripe green grape [10]. Although distinct studies have addressed the chemical composition and antioxidant activity of different fruits and seeds of grape [11,12], the chemical composition and biological properties of verjuice are still poorly characterized.

In this study, we aimed at investigating the phytochemical composition of verjuice extract and evaluating its antioxidant effect and anti-proliferative potential against the human pulmonary adenocarcinoma (A549) cell line.

2. Materials and Methods

2.1. Plant Collection and Preparation of the Samples

Unripe green grapes or immature white grapes were obtained in 2017 from Byblos (north-east direction from Beyrouth via Charles Helou station). The juice was collected after pressing the grapes. The main techniques used for green grape juice production were the "Hot press" (HP), "Cold press" (CP), and "Hot Break" (HB) processes [13]. The juice was centrifuged for 10 min (1000 rpm at room temperature). The pellet was discarded, and the supernatant was taken and stored at −80 °C for 48 h. The juice was then lyophilized for 72 h to be converted into powder and then stored in desiccators at room temperature. This powder was used for chemical measurements.

2.2. Qualitative Phytochemical Screening

2.2.1. Total Alkaloid Content (TAC) Determination

Alkaloid content was determined following the method of Harborne [14]. 1 g of dry powder of verjuice extract and 100 mL of 10% acetic acid (in ethanol) were incubated in a covered 250 mL beaker for 4 h. The extract was then filtrated and concentrated. Ammonium hydroxide was added drop by drop until the precipitation was complete. The obtained precipitates were then washed with diluted ammonium hydroxide and filtered with a Whatman filter paper. The residue was then dried (at 40 °C in an oven) and weighted. The alkaloids content was then determined based on the following equation:

$$\% \text{ Alkaloid} = \frac{\text{Final weight of the sample}}{\text{Initial weight of the extract}} \times 100 \quad (1)$$

2.2.2. Estimation of Total Tannins Content (TTC)

Tannins were determined by the Folin–Ciocalteu method [15–17]. The reaction mixture was prepared upon mixing 100 µL of verjuice (10 µL of verjuice in 90 µL of water) extract, 0.5 mL of Folin–Ciocalteu's reagent, 1 mL of Na_2CO_3 (35%), and 8.4 mL of water. Verjuice extract absorbance versus the prepared blank was determined at 765 nm. The blank corresponded to 1 mL water and

1 mL of Na_2CO_3 (35%). Tannin content was expressed as mg Gallic Acid Equivalents (GAE)/g of dry weight extract.

$$\text{Total tannin content} = \frac{GAE * V * D}{m} \qquad (2)$$

2.2.3. Estimation of Total Phenolic Content (TPC)

The method of Folin–Ciocalteu reagent was used to estimate the TPC [17,18]. One milligram (mg) of verjuice powder was dissolved in one milliliter (mL) of distilled water. Polyvinyl pyrrolidone was then added at a ratio of 0.1 mg to 1 mL of distilled water and extract of tannins. From this mixture, 100 µL was added to 0.5 mL of Folin–Ciocalteu's phenol reagent (1/10 dilution in water) (Sigma-Aldrich Co. St Louis, MO, USA). 1.5 mL of a 2% Na_2CO_3 solution was added after 5 min (Fair Lawn, NJ, USA). The mixture was kept in the dark (30 min at room temperature). The absorbance of blue-colored solution of extract was measured at 765 nm upon utilizing a Gene Quant 1300 UV-Vis spectrophotometer (UV–Vis. Cary 4000, Agilent, UK). The extract was prepared in triplicates for each analysis, where the mean value of absorbance was then calculated. The same procedure was applied in the case of the standard solution of gallic acid (Sigma-Aldrich Co. St Louis, MO, USA) and the linear calibration graph was prepared.

The TPC, expressed as mg of gallic acid equivalents per g of extract (mg of GAE/g of extract), was deduced following extrapolation of the calibration curve.

$$\text{Total phenol content} = \frac{GAE * V * D}{m} \qquad (3)$$

where GAE corresponds to the gallic acid equivalents (mg/mL), V represents the volume extract (mL), D represents the dilution factor, and m corresponds to the sample weight (g).

The blank was prepared upon mixing 0.5 mL water-MeOH and 1.5 mL of Na_2CO_3 (2%) (VWR, Fontenay-sous-Bois, France).

2.2.4. Estimation of Total Flavonoid Content (TFC)

The aluminum chloride method [19] was used for the determination of TFC. 1 mL of diluted verjuice extract (5 mg/mL) was mixed with 1 mL of 2% of solution of the methanolic aluminum chloride (Fair Lawn, NJ, USA). The absorbance of verjuice extract versus that of the prepared blank was determined at 415 nm following incubation (1 h at room temperature in the dark). For each analysis, the extract was prepared in triplicate and the mean value of absorbance was then determined in mg per g of Rutin equivalents (RE).

$$\text{Flavonoids content} = \frac{RE * V * D}{W} \qquad (4)$$

where RE corresponds to Rutin equivalents (µg/mL), V represents the total volume of the sample (mL), D corresponds to dilution factor, and W is the sample weight (g).

The blank was prepared upon mixing 1 mL water-MeOH and 1 mL of 2% methanolic aluminum chloride solution.

2.2.5. DPPH_Assay

The antioxidant assay was performed as previously described in the literature [15,18]. Verjuice extract samples of increasing concentrations (1.5, 2.5, 3.5, and 4.5 mg/mL) were prepared. 1 mL of each diluted sample was mixed with 1 mL of the free radical 2,2-diphenyl-1-picrylhydrazyl (DPPH) (0.15 mM in methanol) reagent. The absorbance of each solution was determined at 517 nm by a Gene Quant 1300 UV-Vis spectrophotometer (UV–Vis. Cary 4000, Agilent, UK) following incubation (30 min at room temperature in the dark). For each analysis, samples were prepared in triplicates and the mean value of absorbance was calculated. The DPPH scavenging ability of each sample was calculated using the following the equation:

$$\% \text{ Scavenging activity} = \frac{(Abs\ control - Abs\ sample)}{Abs\ control} \times 100 \qquad (5)$$

The control sample was prepared upon combining 1 mL DPPH with 1 mL of the selected solvent. The blank corresponded to 1 mL of the water-methanol solution. The used positive control was ascorbic acid. The absorbance control was that of DPPH + water-methanol. Sample absorbance corresponded to the absorbance of DPPH radical + sample.

2.3. Cell and Cell Culture

Human lung adenocarcinoma cell line A549 was purchased from the American Type Culture Collection (ATCC, Manassas, VA, USA) and cultivated (at 37 °C under an atmosphere containing 5% CO_2) in DMEM (Dulbecco's Modified Eagle Medium) medium (Sigma Chemical Company, St. Louis, MO, USA) containing 0.1 mg/mL streptomycin, 100 U/mL penicillin, and 10% fetal bovine serum.

2.3.1. Treatment of Cells

A stock solution of lyophilized verjuice extract was prepared at 10 mg/mL in DMEM culture. The stock solution was then diluted to obtain different concentrations that were used for treatments. Cells were plated in a 96-well microtiter plate, at a concentration of 10^5 cells/well. Cell viability was assessed 24, 48, and 72 h after the treatment. Cells were treated with increasing concentrations of either cisplatin (4, 8, 12, and 80 µg/mL) (purchased from Ebewe, Austria) or verjuice extract (1, 2.5, 3, 3.2, 3.4, 3.6, 3.8, and 4 mg/mL). Moreover, A549 cells were simultaneously treated with combinations of verjuice extracts (3.6, 3.8, and 4 mg/mL) and cisplatin (4 µg/mL).

2.3.2. Evaluation of the Anti-Proliferative Activity

Assessment of cell viability was carried out upon applying the Neutral Red assay following a previously described protocol [20,21]. Neutral Red (chromogenic dye) was used as a lysosomal activity indicator in live cells. After 24 h of cultivation in a 96-well microliter plate as described above, cells were exposed to increasing concentrations of verjuice extract and/or cisplatin and re-incubated for 24, 48, and 72 h. Untreated cells were considered as a negative control, whilst ethanol (0.5%, v/v)-treated cells were used as a vehicle control. Following 24, 48, and 72 h, the culture medium was replaced with 100 µL of fresh medium containing 40 µg/mL Neutral Red. Cells were then incubated for 3 h, during which the vital dye can enter the lysosomes of viable and undamaged cells. The media were then discarded, and cells were washed twice (100 µL of 1X PBS). 200 µL of a 50% ethanol–1% acetic acid lysing solution was used to extract the intracellularly accumulated Neutral Red dye. The eluted dye was then characterized in terms of its optical density at 490 nm using a microplate reader. The experiments were performed in triplicates.

2.4. Statistical Analysis

All presented results correspond to mean ± standard deviation (SD). Statistical analyses were carried out by the mean of GraphPad Prism 5 (Graphpad Software Inc., San Diego, CA, USA). A two-way analysis of variance (ANOVA) test was employed to determine the p-values: * $p < 0.05$, ** $p < 0.01$, and *** $p < 0.001$. Duncan's test means comparison test was used to compare the different treatments performed at the $p < 0.05$ probability level.

3. Results and Discussion

3.1. Phytochemical Screening

Given that the pharmacological potential and medicinal value of plants is attributed to their chemical composition, phytochemical analysis was carried out to identify the bioactive compounds present in the verjuice extract. Our results showed that verjuice extract is rich in alkaloids, phenols, flavonoids, and tannins (Table 1). Interestingly, secondary metabolites such as phenols, particularly flavonoids, are well known for their anti-inflammatory and antimicrobial activities as well as their ability to inhibit cholesterol biosynthesis by the liver cells [22,23]. Moreover, phenols and alkaloids usually exert high antioxidant and antibacterial activities [24]. These molecules are well described for their pharmacological potential and are traditionally used to treat different diseases [24].

Table 1. Bioactive compounds in verjuice extract.

Active Compounds	Total Amounts
Total alkaloids content (TAC)	0.057 g (5.7%)
Total phenols content (TPC; mg GAE /mL)	2.82 mg/mL
Total flavonoids content (TFC; mg RE/mL)	2.6 mg/mL
Total tannins content (TTC)	19.9 mg/mL

GAE: Gallic Acid Equivalents; RE: Rutin Equivalents.

Different juices contain an array of secondary metabolites, including phenols, flavonoids, flavanones, tannins, terpenoids, diterpenes, quinones, glycosides, glucides, reducing sugar, and alkaloids. Comparison with other juices showed important differences. Indeed, verjuice contained 1.8, 2.1, and 7.4 times more TPC than grape materne, pomegranate, and pineapple juices, respectively [25,26]. The difference was more marked when considering TFC, in which case, verjuice exhibited 2.2 to 54.1 times more, depending on the species [25,26]. Total tannins comparison highlighted that verjuice presented 73.7, 62.2, and 3.8 times more than pineapple, pomegranate, and grape materne, respectively [25,26].

3.2. Antioxidant Activity of Verjuice

The phytochemical arsenal in verjuice extract suggests potential biological properties for this plant. Therefore, we assessed, in a next step, the antioxidant capacity of the verjuice extract. DPPH free radical scavenging assay was performed to assess the cell-free antioxidant activities of different concentrations of verjuice. The antioxidant activity increased three-fold in a dose-dependent manner between the extreme concentrations of verjuice (Figure 1). This strong antioxidant activity could be explained by the significant phenolic compounds content. In cells, antioxidant molecules prevent the free radicals from causing damage, thus, they are known to reduce chronic diseases like cancer. The observed potent antioxidant capacity highlights potential therapeutic implications of verjuice for protecting cells against oxidative stress.

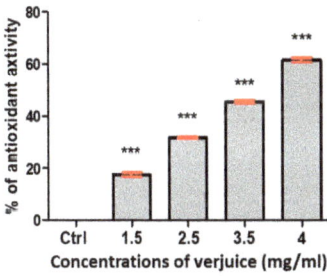

Figure 1. Antioxidant activities of different concentrations of verjuice extract. The samples were prepared in triplicates. The results are expressed as the percentage of control (0 mg/mL verjuice). Each value represents the mean ± standard deviation (SD) of triplicates. *** $p < 0.001$.

3.3. Cytotoxic Effect of Verjuice Extract on A549 Cancer Cells

In order to assess the cytotoxic effect of verjuice extracts on lung cancer cells, the Neutral Red cell viability assay was carried out. A549 cells were treated with distinct concentrations of the verjuice extracts over 24, 48, and 72 h (Figure 2). After 24 h, cells' viability was significantly decreased in a dose-dependent manner. It decreased by 20%, 41%, and 72% in cells treated with verjuice extract at concentrations of 3.2, 3.6, and 4 mg/mL, respectively (Figure 2A). After 48 and 72 h, comparable profiles of dose-dependent decreases in cells' viability were obtained upon treating cells with increasing concentrations of verjuice. This inhibitory effect might be attributed to the high content of phenolic compounds in verjuice. In agreement with our observations, similar results against A549 and H129 cells were reported using grape seed proanthocyanidin extracts [27].

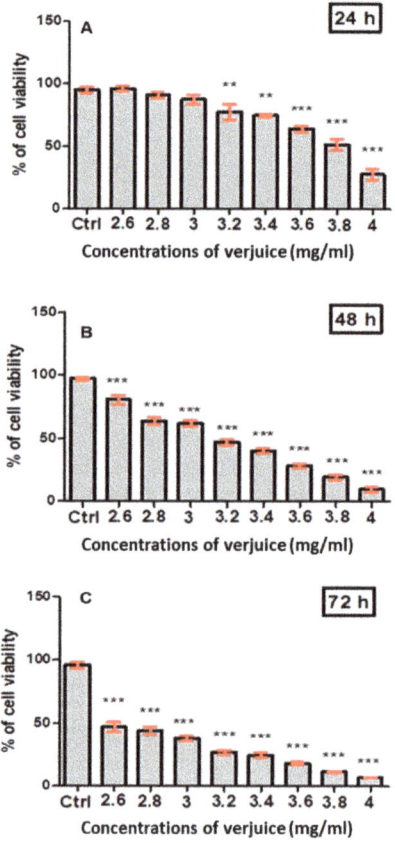

Figure 2. Effect of different concentrations of verjuice on the survival of A549 after (**A**) 24 h, (**B**) 48 h, and (**C**) 72 h of treatment. The results are expressed as the percentage of control cell (0 mg/mL verjuice) viability (Ctrl). Each value represents the mean ± SD of triplicates obtained from five independent experiments. ** $p < 0.01$; *** $p < 0.001$.

3.4. Co-Treatment with Cisplatin and Verjuice Has Superior Inhibitory Effects on A549 Cell Viability

Cisplatin is well known for its cytotoxic effect against different cancer cell lines, including A549 cells. Here, in a first step, we have confirmed, using the Neutral Red assay, the cytotoxic effect of cisplatin on the A459 cells after 24 and 48 h of treatment. As shown in Figure 3, cisplatin reduced cell viability in a dose- and time-dependent manner. For instance, after 24 h of cisplatin treatment, the viability of the cells was reduced by 22%, 46%, 62%, and 78% at 4, 8, 12, and 80 µg/mL, respectively (Figure 3A). On the other hand, after 48 h, cells' viability was reduced by 51%, 72%, 84%, and 90% (Figure 3B).

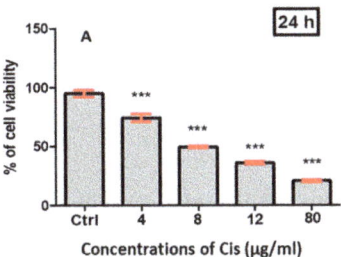

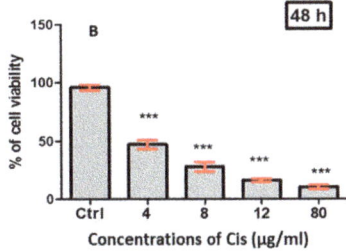

Figure 3. Effect of different concentrations of cisplatin (Cis) on the survival of A549 after (**A**) 24 h and (**B**) 48 h of treatment. The results are expressed as the percentage of control cell (0 mg/mL cisplatin) viability (Ctrl). Each value represents the mean ± SD of triplicates obtained in five independent experiments. *** $p < 0.001$.

In a next step, and in order to determine whether the combination of cisplatin and verjuice may have a greater anticancer effect than cisplatin alone, cells were exposed to a unique low dose of cisplatin 4 µg/mL and different concentrations of verjuice (3.6, 3.8, and 4 mg/mL). The 4 µg/mL dose of cisplatin was chosen based on our above results showing a low level of toxicity at this indicated dose. Interestingly, Figure 4 shows that the verjuice extract significantly enhanced the cisplatin-dependent cytotoxic effect at both time points (24 and 48 h).

Cisplatin, a chemotherapy drug that contains platinum, is used to treat various types of cancer. However, cisplatin has severe side effects such as nephro- and hepato-toxicity [28,29]. One way to increase the efficacy of cisplatin and limit its side effects is the drug combination strategy [30]. Therefore, we studied the potency of verjuice as an anticancer natural product as well as its ability to enhance the anticancer effect of cisplatin. It is noteworthy that this is the first report to study the anticancer potential of verjuice. The major output of this study was that verjuice extract could suppress A549 cells' viability where minor concentrations of this extract could strongly enhance cisplatin's anticancer potential. In this context, various studies have previously reported the importance of the combination of cisplatin and plant-derived natural molecules to increase the anticancer potential of cisplatin [31,32]. Moreover, administration of verjuice was shown to reduce atherosclerotic and fibrinogen lesions in coronary arteries of rabbits [33]. Altogether, these observations suggest that verjuice extracts could increase the efficacy and tolerability of available anticancer chemotherapies.

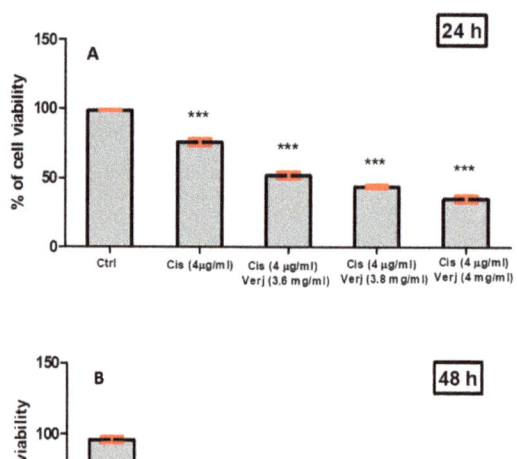

Figure 4. Effect of different concentrations of verjuice (Verj) in combination with cisplatin (Cis) on the survival of A549 cells after (**A**) 24 h and (**B**) 48 h of treatment. The results are expressed as the percentage of control cell (0 mg/mL cisplatin) viability (Ctrl). Each value represents the mean ± SD of triplicates obtained in five independent experiments. *** $p < 0.001$.

The observed anticancer potential of verjuice could be related to its antioxidant capacity. In this context, grape antioxidants have been well reported for their potential anticancer effects. Distinct studies have suggested that high consumption of grape components could be correlated with the low risk of certain cancers, including breast and colon cancers [34]. Various grape antioxidants have been established to elicit cell cycle arrest, trigger apoptosis, and prevent cancer progression in rodent models [35]. Grape antioxidants have also been shown to alter estrogen receptor (ER) levels and are therefore important in the case of breast cancer [34]. Consistently, distinct grape antioxidants (such as resveratrol, quercetin, and catechin), and due to their structural similarity to the steroid hormone estrogen, exhibit both estrogenic and anti-estrogenic effects [36]. On the other hand, feeding grape products in the form of juice (50%) and raisins (10%) strikingly lowered the aberrant crypt foci in male rats. Grapes were also shown to exert a protective effect against chemically induced colon cancer due to their ability to induce Glutathione-S-tranferase enzyme [37]. Remarkably, grape antioxidants could significantly suppress the expression of epidermal growth factor receptor (EGFR), an essential factor accounting for the aggressive growth of cancer cells, in head and neck squamous cell carcinoma (HNSCC) [38]. Grape seed proanthocyanidins have also showed an in vitro potential against oral squamous cell carcinoma (OSCC). Other studies report that phenols extracts increase cell viability in the colon carcinoma cell line [39]. Moreover, grape extract was also shown to be protective against prostate cancer, in which it was shown to inhibit histone acetyltransferases (HATs), leading to decreased androgen-receptor (AR)-mediated transcription and cancer cell growth [40]. Further, one study revealed that grape antioxidants can elicit an antitumor activity due to their immune-potentiating activities via the enhancements of lymphocyte proliferation, natural killer (NK) cell cytotoxic activity, and IFN-γ (Interferon gamma) secretion [41]. By inhibiting genes for the migration of cells, the grape juice acts as an antimetastatic [42] and can be considered as a potential drug for cancer treatments [43,44].

4. Conclusions

Higher levels of phenols, flavonoids, alkaloids, and tannins were reported in the studied unripe grape juice. Besides its antioxidant activity, verjuice extract significantly repressed human pulmonary adenocarcinoma cells' viability and also enhanced the anticancer potential of cisplatin. This is the first report highlighting correction between verjuice composition and its anticancer effects. This study reveals that verjuice contains significant amounts of bioactive molecules and can exert a significant antioxidant potential and prominent inhibitory effect on lung cancer cells' viability. Verjuice could therefore hold therapeutic promise during cancer treatment. Determination of phenolic and alkaloid composition could help to understand if the effects induced by verjuice supply with cisplatin is due to one component of a synergetic impact. Further in vivo studies are needed to ascertain these results.

Author Contributions: Conceptualization, A.H., R.A., and O.M.; Methodology, M.N. and H.C.-A.; Software, A.E.-A.N.A.-R. and O.M.; Validation, R.A., A.H., A.E.-A.N.A.-R., and M.N.; Formal Analysis, M.N. and H.C.-A.; Investigation, M.N., H.C.-A., R.A., and A.H.; Writing—Original Draft Preparation, R.A., M.N., and A.H.; Writing—Review and Editing, O.M., A.E.-A.N.A.-R., R.A., and A.H.; Project Administration and Funding Acquisition, A.H. and O.M. All authors have read and agreed to the published version of the manuscript.

Funding: This study was funded by the Central Administration of the Lebanese University and by the French Foreign Ministry trough the Hubert Curien Project—Cèdre N°42232RE.

Conflicts of Interest: The authors declare that they have no conflicts of interest.

References

1. Sayed Ahmad, B.; Talou, T.; Saad, Z.; Hijazi, A.; Merah, O. The Apiaceae: Ethnomedicinal family as source for industrial uses. *Ind. Crops Prod.* **2017**, *109*, 661–671. [CrossRef]
2. Larsen, J.E.; Minna, J.D. Molecular biology of lung cancer: Clinical implications. *Clin. Chest Med.* **2011**, *32*, 703–740. [CrossRef] [PubMed]
3. Jemal, A.; Siegel, R.; Ward, E.; Murray, T.; Xu, J.; Thun, M.J. Cancer statistics. *CA Cancer J. Clin.* **2007**, *57*, 43–66. [CrossRef] [PubMed]
4. Jeong, S.J.; Koh, W.; Kim, B.; Kim, S.H. Are there new therapeutic options for treating lung cancer based on herbal medicines and their metabolites. *J. Ethnopharmacol* **2011**, *138*, 652–661. [CrossRef]
5. Zhao, T.; Pan, H.; Feng, Y.; Li, H.; Zhao, Y. Petroleum ether extract of *Chenopodium album* L. prevents cell growth and induces apoptosis of human lung cancer cells. *Therap. Med.* **2016**, *12*, 3301–3307. [CrossRef]
6. Nehme, M. *Wild Flowers of Lebanon*; National Council for Scientific Research: Beirut, Lebanon, 1978; p. 238.
7. Post, G.E. *Flora f Syria, Palestine and Sinaio*; American University of Beirut: Beirut, Lebanon, 1932; p. 658.
8. Kaliora, A.C.; Kountouri, A.M.; Karathanos, V.T. Antioxidant properties of raisins (*Vitis vinifera* L.). *J. Med. Food* **2009**, *12*, 1302–1309. [CrossRef]
9. Karthikeyan, K.; Bai, B.R.; Devaraj, S.N. Efficacy of grape seed proanthocyanidins on cardioprotection during isoproterenol-induced myocardial injury in rats. *J. Cardiovas. Pharm.* **2009**, *53*, 109–115. [CrossRef]
10. Setorki, M.; Asgary, S.; Eidi, A.; Haeri Rohani, A. Effects of acute verjuice consumption with a high-cholesterol diet on some biochemical risk factors of atherosclerosis in rabbits. *Med. Sci. Monit.* **2010**, *16*, 124–130.
11. Saad, K. Phytochemical investigation of Fruits and Seeds of Grape (*Vitis vinifera* L.) grown in Iraq. *Int. J. Pharm. Sci. Rev. Res.* **2017**, *42*, 65–66.
12. Alipour, M.; Davoudi, P.; Davoudi, Z. Effects of unripe grape juice (verjuice) on plasma lipid profile, blood pressure, malondialdehyde and total antioxidant capacity in normal, hyperlipidemic and hyperlipidemic with hypertensive human volunteers. *J. Med. Plant Res.* **2012**, *6*, 5677–5683. [CrossRef]
13. Morris, J.R. Factors influencing grape juice quality. *Hort. Technol.* **1998**, *8*, 471–478. [CrossRef]
14. Harborne, A.J. *Phytochemical Methods, A Guide to Modern Techniques of Plant Analysis*; Springer: Berlin/Heidelberg, Germany, 2005; pp. 54–84.
15. Sayed Ahmad, B.; Talou, T.; Saad, Z.; Hijazi, H.; Cerny, M.; Chokr, A.; Kanaan, H.; Merah, O. Fennel seed oil and by-products characterization and their potential applications. *Ind. Crops Prod.* **2018**, *111*, 92–98. [CrossRef]

16. Farhan, H.; Rammal, H.; Hijazi, A.; Daher, A.; Reda, M.; Annan, H.; Chokr, A.; Bassal, A.; Badran, B. Chemical composition and antioxidant activity of a Lebanese plant *Euphorbia macroclada schyzoceras*. *Asian Pac. J. Trop. Biomed.* **2013**, *3*, 542–548. [CrossRef]
17. Makkar, H.P.S. Measurement of Total Phenolics and Tannins Using Folin-Ciocalteu Method. In *Quantification of Tannins in Tree and Shrub Foliage*; Springer: Berlin/Heidelberg, Germany, 2003.
18. Farhan, H.; Rammal, H.; Hijazi, A.; Hamad, H.; Daher, A.; Reda, M.; Badran, B. In vitro antioxidant activity of ethanolic and aqueous extracts from crude *Malva parviflora* L. grown in Lebanon. *Asian J. Pharm. Clin. Res.* **2012**, *5*, 234–238.
19. Quettier-Deleu, C.; Gressier, B.; Vasseur, J.; Dine, T.; Brunet, C.; Luyckx, M.; Cazin, M.; Cazin, J.C.; Bailleul, F.; Trotin, F. Phenolic compounds and antioxidant activities of buckwheat (*Fagopyrum esculentum* Moench) hulls and flour. *J. Ethnopharmacol* **2000**, *72*, 35–42. [CrossRef]
20. Malek, S.N.A.; Lee, G.S.; Hong, S.L.; Yaacob, H.; Wahab, N.A.; Faizal Weber, J.F.; Shah, S.A.A. Phytochemical and cytotoxic investigations of *Curcuma mangga* rhizomes. *Molecules* **2011**, *16*, 4539–4548. [CrossRef]
21. Nasreddine, S.; Salameh, F.; Hassan, K.H.; Daher, A.; Nasser, M.; Rammal, H.; Hijazi, A.; Cheaib, A.; Hadadeh, O.; Fayyad-Kazan, H. Valproic acid induces apoptosis and increases CXCR7 expression in epithelial ovarian cancer cell line SKOV-3. *Eur. Sci. J.* **2015**, *126*, 171–174.
22. Mahato, S.B.; Sen, S. Advances in triterpenoid research, 1990–1994. *Phytochemistry* **1997**, *44*, 1185–1236. [CrossRef]
23. Pietta, P.G. Flavonoids as antioxidants. *J. Nat. Prod.* **2000**, *63*, 1035–1042. [CrossRef]
24. NithyaJayanthi, T.G.; Ragunathan, M.G. Antioxidant activity, total phenol, flavonoid, alkaloid, tannin, and saponin contents of leaf extracts of *Salvinia molesta*. *Asian J. Pharm. Clin. Res.* **2016**, *9*, 185–188.
25. Matute, A.; Tabart, J.; Cheramy-Bien, J.P.; Pirotte, B.; Kevers, C.; Auger, C.; Schini-Kerth, V.; Dommes, J.; Defraigne, J.O.; Pincemail, J. Compared Phenolic Compound Contents of 22 Commercial Fruit and Vegetable Juices: Relationship to Ex-Vivo Vascular Reactivity and Potential in Vivo Projection. *Antioxidants* **2020**, *9*, 92. [CrossRef] [PubMed]
26. Prommajak, T.; Noppol, L.; Rattanapanone, N. Tannins in Fruit Juices and their Removal. *JNS* **2020**, *19*, 76. [CrossRef]
27. Valenzuela, M.; Bastias, L.; Montenegro, I.; Werner, E.; Madrid, A.; Godoy, P.; Parraga, M.; Villena, J. Autumn Royal and Ribier Grape Juice Extracts Reduced Viability and Metastatic Potential of Colon Cancer Cells. *Evid.-Based Complement. Altern. Med.* **2018**, *11*, 1–7. [CrossRef]
28. Jung, Y.; Lippard, S.J. Direct cellular responses to platinum-induced DNA damage. *Chem. Rev.* **2007**, *107*, 1387–1407. [CrossRef] [PubMed]
29. Koyuncu, I.; Kocyigit, A.; Gonel, A.; Arslan, E.; Durgun, M. The Protective Effect of Naringenin-Oxime on Cisplatin-Induced Toxicity in Rats. *Biochem. Res. Int.* **2017**, *6*, 1–9. [CrossRef] [PubMed]
30. Wang, Y.; Lin, B.; Wu, J.; Zhang, H.; Wu, B. Metformin inhibits the proliferation of A549/CDDP cells by activating p38 mitogen-activated protein kinase. *Oncol. Lett.* **2014**, *8*, 1269–1274. [CrossRef]
31. Ramadan, W.S.; Sait, K.H.; Anfinan, N.M. Anticancer activity of aqueous myrrh extract alone and in combination with cisplatin in HeLa cells. *Trop. J. Pharm. Res.* **2017**, *16*, 889–896. [CrossRef]
32. Nasser, M.; Hijazi, A.; Sayed-Ahmad, B.; Jamal Eddine, Z.; Ibrahim, S.; Rammal, H.; Al-Rekaby, A.-E.-A.; Nasser, M. Efficiency of combining pomegranate juice with low-doses of cisplatin and taxotere on A549 human lung adenocarcinoma cells. *Asian Pac. J. Trop. Biomed.* **2018**, *8*, 19–24.
33. Setorki, M.; Nazari, B.; Asgary, S.; Azadbakht, L.; Rafieian-Kopaei, M. Anti-atherosclerotic effects of verjuice on hypocholesterolemic rabbits. *Afr. J. Pharm. Pharm.* **2011**, *5*, 1038–1045.
34. Zhou, K.; Raffoul, J.J. Potential Anticancer Properties of Grape Antioxidants. *J. Oncol.* **2012**. [CrossRef]
35. Aggarwal, B.B.; Bhardwaj, A.; Aggarwal, R.S.; Seeram, N.P.; Shishodia, S.; Takada, Y. Role of resveratrol in prevention and therapy of cancer: Preclinical and clinical studies. *Anticancer Res.* **2004**, *24*, 2783–2840. [PubMed]
36. Schlachterman, A.; Valle, F.; Wall, K.M.; Azios, N.G.; Castillo, L.; Morell, L.; Washington, A.V.; Cubano, L.A.; Dharmawardhane, S.F. Combined resveratrol, quercetin, and catechin treatment reduces breast tumor growth in a nude mouse model. *Transl. Oncol.* **2008**, *1*, 19–27. [CrossRef] [PubMed]
37. Jones, J.; Verghese, M.; Walker, L.T.; Shackelford, L.; Chawan, C.B. Grape Products Reduce Colon Cancer in Azoxymethane-induced Aberrant Crypt Foci in Fisher 344 Rats. *Sci. Alert* **2014**. [CrossRef]

38. Sun, Q.; Prasad, R.; Rosenthal, E.; Katiyar, S.K. Grape seed proanthocyanidins inhibit the invasive potential of head and neck cutaneous squamous cell carcinoma cells by targeting EGFR expression and epithelial-to-mesenchymal transition. *BMC Complement. Altern. Med.* **2011**, *11*, 134. [CrossRef]
39. Di Nunzio, M.; Picone, G.; Pasini, F.; Caboni, M.F.; Gianotti, A.; Bordoni, A.; Capozzi, F. Olive oil industry by-products. Effects of a polyphenol-rich extract on the metabolome and response to inflammation in cultured intestinal cell. *Food Res. Int.* **2018**, *113*, 392–400. [CrossRef]
40. Park, S.Y.; Lee, Y.H.; Choi, K.C.; Seong, A.R.; Choi, H.K.; Lee, O.H.; Hwang, H.J.; Yoon, H.G. Grape seed extract regulates androgen receptor-mediated transcription in prostate cancer cells through potent anti-histone acetyltransferase activity. *J. Med. Food* **2011**, *14*, 9–16. [CrossRef]
41. Zhang, X.Y.; Li, W.G.; Wu, Y.J.; Zheng, T.Z.; Li, W.; Qu, S.Y.; Liu, N.F. Proanthocyanidin from grape seeds potentiates anti-tumor activity of doxorubicin via immunomodulatory mechanism. *Int. Immunopharmacol.* **2005**, *5*, 1247–1257. [CrossRef]
42. Uchino, R.; Madhyastha, R.; Madhyastha, H.; Dhungana, S.; Nakajima, Y.; Omura, S.; Maruyama, M. NFκB-dependent regulation of urokinase plasminogen activator by proanthocyanidin-rich grape seed extract: Effect on invasion by prostate cancer cells. *Blood Coagul. Fibrin.* **2010**, *21*, 528–533. [CrossRef]
43. Cádiz-Gurrea, M.D.L.L.; Borrás-Linares, I.; Lozano-Sánchez, J.; Joven, J.; Fernández- Arroyo, S.; Segura-Carretero, A. Cocoa and grape seed byproducts as a source of antioxidant and anti-inflammatory proanthocyanidins. *Int. J. Mol. Sci.* **2017**, *18*, 376. [CrossRef]
44. Unusan, N. Proanthocyanidins in grape seeds: An updated review of their health benefits and potential uses in the food industry. *J. Funct. Foods* **2020**, *67*, 103861. [CrossRef]

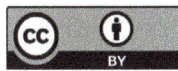

© 2020 by the authors. Licensee MDPI, Basel, Switzerland. This article is an open access article distributed under the terms and conditions of the Creative Commons Attribution (CC BY) license (http://creativecommons.org/licenses/by/4.0/).

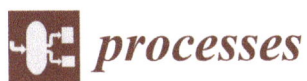

Review

The Significance of Natural Product Derivatives and Traditional Medicine for COVID-19

Dongdong Wang [1,2,*], Jiansheng Huang [3], Andy Wai Kan Yeung [4], Nikolay T. Tzvetkov [5], Jarosław O. Horbańczuk [6], Harald Willschke [7,8], Zhibo Gai [9,10] and Atanas G. Atanasov [6,7,11,12,*]

1. The Second Clinical Medical College, Guizhou University of Traditional Chinese Medicine, Fei Shan Jie 32, Guiyang 550003, China
2. Centre for Metabolism, Obesity and Diabetes Research, McMaster University, 1280 Main St. W., Hamilton, ON L8N 3Z5, Canada
3. Department of Medicine, Vanderbilt University Medical Center, 318 Preston Research Building, 2200 Pierce Avenue, Nashville, TN 37232, USA; jiansheng.huang@vumc.org
4. Oral and Maxillofacial Radiology, Applied Oral Sciences and Community Dental Care, Faculty of Dentistry, The University of Hong Kong, Hong Kong, China; ndyeung@hku.hk
5. Department of Biochemical Pharmacology and Drug Design, Institute of Molecular Biology "Roumen Tsanev", Bulgarian Academy of Sciences, 21 Acad. G. Bonchev Str., 1113 Sofia, Bulgaria; ntzvetkov@gmx.de
6. Department of Biotechnology and Nutrigenomics, Institute of Genetics and Animal Biotechnology of the Polish Academy of Sciences, 05-552 Jastrzębiec, Poland; olav@rocketmail.com
7. Ludwig Boltzmann Institute for Digital Health and Patient Safety, Medical University of Vienna, Spitalgasse 23, 1090 Vienna, Austria; harald.willschke@meduniwien.ac.at
8. Department of Anaesthesia, Intensive Care Medicine and Pain Medicine, Medical University Vienna, Waehringer Guertel 18–20, 1090 Vienna, Austria
9. Experimental Center, Shandong University of Traditional Chinese Medicine, Jinan 250355, China; zhibo.gai@usz.ch
10. Department of Clinical Pharmacology and Toxicology, University Hospital Zurich, University of Zurich, 8006 Zurich, Switzerland
11. Department of Pharmacognosy, University of Vienna, Althanstrasse 14, 1090 Vienna, Austria
12. Institute of Neurobiology, Bulgarian Academy of Sciences, 23 Acad. G. Bonchev Str., 1113 Sofia, Bulgaria
* Correspondence: wangd123@mcmaster.ca (D.W.); atanas.atanasov@univie.ac.at (A.G.A.)

Received: 3 July 2020; Accepted: 30 July 2020; Published: 4 August 2020

Abstract: Coronavirus disease 2019 (COVID-19) is caused by severe acute respiratory syndrome coronavirus 2 (SARS-CoV-2). To date, there have been more than 10 million reported cases, more than 517,000 deaths in 215 countries, areas or territories. There is no effective antiviral medicine to prevent or treat COVID-19. Natural products and traditional medicine products with known safety profiles are a promising source for the discovery of new drug leads. There is increasing number of publications reporting the effect of natural products and traditional medicine products on COVID-19. In our review, we provide an overview of natural products and their derivatives or mimics, as well as traditional medicine products, which were reported to exhibit potential to inhibit SARS-CoV-2 infection in vitro, and to manage COVID-19 in vivo, or in clinical reports or trials. These natural products and traditional medicine products are categorized in several classes: (1) anti-malaria drugs including chloroquine and hydroxychloroquine, (2) antivirals including nucleoside analogs (remdesivir, favipiravir, β-D-N4-hydroxycytidine, ribavirin and among others), lopinavir/ritonavir and arbidol, (3) antibiotics including azithromycin, ivermectin and teicoplanin, (4) anti-protozoal drug, emetine, anti-cancer drug, homoharringtonine, and others, as well as (5) traditional medicine (Lian Hua Qing Wen Capsule, Shuang Huang Lian Oral Liquid, Qingfei Paidu Decoction and Scutellariae Radix). Randomized, double-blind and placebo-controlled large clinical trials are needed to provide solid evidence for the potential effective treatment. Currently, drug repurposing is a promising strategy to quickly find an effective treatment for COVID-19. In addition, carefully combined cocktails need to be examined for preventing a COVID-19 pandemic and the resulting global health concerns.

Keywords: SARS-CoV; coronavirus; traditional Chinese medicine; COVID-19; natural products

1. Introduction

Coronavirus disease 2019 (COVID-19) has, as a causative agent, a new betacoronavirus, severe acute respiratory syndrome coronavirus 2 (SARS-CoV-2/2019-nCoV/CoV-2) [1]. SARS-CoV-2 is a single-stranded, positive-sense, RNA-enveloped virus. It makes use of a densely glycosylated viral structural spike (S) protein to gain entry into host cells by binding to the angiotensin-converting enzyme 2 (ACE2) receptor of host cells [2,3]. Host transmembrane protease serine 2 (TMPRSS2) activates the S protein, and facilitates SARS CoV-2 cell entry [4]. Similar to other coronaviruses, SARS-CoV and Middle East respiratory syndrome (MERS)-CoV, following receptor binding, the virus particles use the non-/endosomal pathway to enter the host cells [5]. Once inside the cell, SARS-CoV-2 then dissemble intracellularly to release their RNA into the cytoplasm for the synthesis of the large replicase polyproteins (such as RNA-dependent RNA polymerase (RdRp) and helicase) and for the replication of viral genomic RNA [5]. The virus structural and accessory proteins are synthesized from subgenomic mRNAs. The helical nucleocapsid, genomic RNA and the other structural proteins form the assembled virions, which are then released from cells [5]. These viral lifecycle steps (virus entry, synthesis of the large replicase polyproteins, replication of genomic RNA, and assembly of virus) provide potential targets for inhibition of SARS-CoV-2 replication [2], as shown in Figure 1.

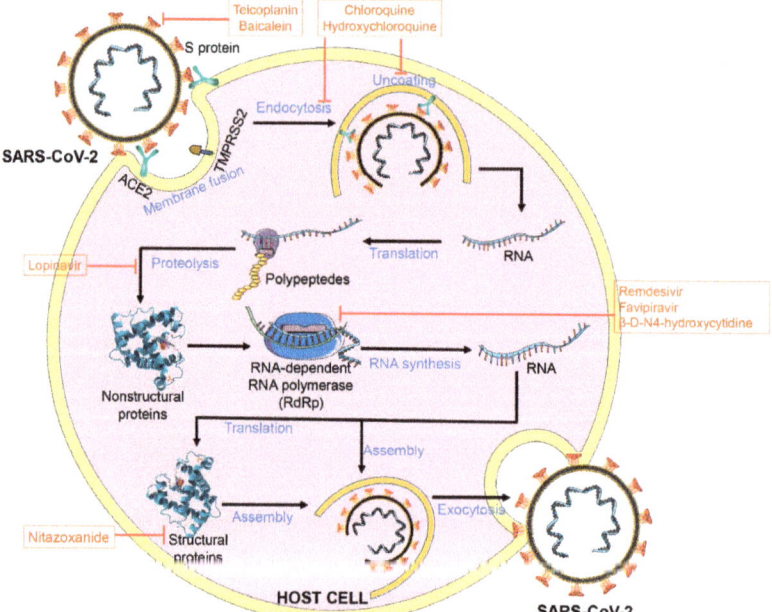

Figure 1. Schematic representation of severe acute respiratory syndrome coronavirus 2 (SARS-CoV-2) replication cycle within host cells. Proposed targets of the examined natural products, their derivatives and mimics are noted. ACE2, angiotensin-converting enzyme 2; S protein, spike protein; TMPRSS2, type 2 transmembrane serine protease, RdRp, RNA-dependent RNA polymerase.

As of July 26th, 2020, there have been more than 15 million reported cases resulting in more than 640 thousand deaths in 216 countries, areas or territories (https://www.who.int/emergencies/diseases/novel-coronavirus-2019). People infected by SARS-CoV-2 have ranged from exhibiting no symptoms, mild, or moderate symptoms to severe illness and death. A recent study has shown that there is a large number of undocumented infections, which boosts the community dissemination of SARS-CoV2 [6]. The most common symptoms of COVID-19 are fever, a cough and tiredness [7]. Recent studies suggest that loss of smell and taste might be a frequent and early symptom of COVID-19 [8,9]. Some patients may have pains, nasal congestion, runny nose, sore throat and/or diarrhea [10]. Around 16.67% patients with COVID-19 become seriously ill, develop pneumonia and develop difficulty breathing. Older people and those with underlying medical problems like hypertension, heart problems or diabetes, are more likely to exhibit cytokine release syndrome (CRS) and develop serious illness [11]. In the early stage, the symptoms of COVID-19 include fever and a cough [12]. The following stage of COVID-19 is the acute pneumonia phase, in which the immune system is affected [12]. The severe stage includes organ dysfunction (e.g., acute respiratory distress syndrome (ARDS), shock, acute kidney injury, and acute cardiac injury) [13]. In total, a 3.4% mortality rate was estimated by the World Health Organization (WHO) as of March 3. There are some available materials published that could be used to treat COVID-19, such as the 7th version of "Chinese Clinical Guidance for COVID-19 Pneumonia Diagnosis and Treatment" (http://kjfy.meetingchina.org/msite/news/show/cn/3337.html) published by the Chinese National Health Commission, and the Treatment Guidelines (https://www.covid19treatmentguidelines.nih.gov/introduction/) from US National Institutes of Health (NIH) [14]. These guides include a deeper contemporary understanding of the clinical manifestations and pathological features of the disease and "the accumulation of experience in diagnosis and treatment" from clinical experts.

Currently, there is no effective vaccine or drug for preventing or managing COVID-19 [15]. Natural products and traditional medicine products are an excellent source for discovery of new drug leads, since they display a great diversity of chemical structural and a various range of biological activities [16–18]. Natural products include compounds from animals, plants, fungi and prokaryote [19,20]. Traditional medicine (or folk medicine) is the sum of the traditional knowledge, skills, and practices based on indigenous theories and experiences, used in the prevention and treatment of diseases, such as traditional Chinese medicine (TCM), ancient Iranian medicine, traditional African medicine, or Islamic medicine [16,21]. There is an increasing number of publications reporting the effect of natural products and traditional medicine products on COVID-19. In our review, we provide an overview of natural products and their derivatives or mimics, as well as traditional medicine products, which were reported to exhibit potential to treat COVID-19 in vitro, in vivo, or in clinical reports or trials.

2. Natural Products and Their Derivatives or Mimics

Currently, clinical management for COVID-19 includes prevention of infection, control measures and supportive health care including oxygen supplement and mechanical ventilation [22]. Effective vaccines against SARS-CoV-2 will also be an important strategy to prevent the second wave of COVID-19, which, however, will require quite a long time (at least 12–18 months) to be developed [23]. A comparative analysis of genome sequences of SARS-Cov-2 with SARS-CoV sequence reveals that the catalytic domains of essential enzymes for viral replication such as RdRp and proteinase are highly conserved between these coronaviruses [23–25]. More importantly, it is plausible that the protein sequence of the drug binding pocket of the enzymes is highly homogeneous [26,27]. Thus, the S protein and enzymes could be very promising drug targets for developing an effective approach for the treatment of COVID-19. Moreover, repurposing approved drugs would be a quick and efficient strategy to manage a COVID-19 pandemic. At present, many antivirals and immunomodulating agents, which belong to natural products, their derivatives or mimics, are already shown to exhibit anti-CoV-2 activity, or are used in treatment of COVID-19 clinically or tested in different clinical trials to evaluate their effects (Table 1). These nature-related medicines from published data and/or recommendations are categorized in several classes: (1) anti-malaria drugs including chloroquine and hydroxychloroquine, (2) antivirals including nucleoside analogs (remdesivir, favipiravir, β-D-N4-hydroxycytidine, ribavirin and among others), lopinavir/ritonavir (LPV/RTV) and arbidol, (3) antibiotics including azithromycin, ivermectin and teicoplanin, as well as (4) anti-protozoal drugs, emetine, anti-cancer drugs, homoharringtonine, and others.

Table 1. Natural products, their derivatives or mimics fighting COVID-19.

Natural Products	Structure	In Vitro and In Vivo Studies	Clinical Studies	Registered Trials
Chloroquine		Inhibits SARS-CoV-2 replication in Vero E6 cells with an half maximal effective concentration (EC50) of 1.13 µM at an MOI of 0.05 [28]	Shortened hospital stay time, improved patient outcome [29], novel coronavirus pneumonia and promoted quick recovery (Dose: 500 mg, orally, twice/day for 10 days) [30], no clinical benefit from use of hydroxychloroquine in hospitalised patients with COVID-19 (https://www.recoverytrial.net/).	ChiCTR: >25 USCTR: >52
Hydroxychloroquine		Inhibits SARS-CoV-2 replication in Vero E6 with an EC50 of 4.51-12.96 µM cells at MOI of 0.01-0.8 [31]	Hydroxychloroquine (~0.46 µg/mL in serum) reduced of the viral carriage in 3-6 days-post inclusion [32]	ChiCTR: >11 USCTR: >148
Remdesivir (GS-5734)		Inhibits CoV-2 replication in Vero E6 cells with an EC50 of 0.77 µM at MOI of 0.05 [28]; Inhibited virus infection in Huh-7 cells [33]; Reduced signs of respiratory disease, pulmonary infiltrates on radiographs and virus titers in bronchoalveolar lavages as early as 12 h after first treatment in a rhesus macaque model [34].	Remdesivir (Day 1: 200 mg daily, Days 2-9: 100 mg daily, administered intravenously) shorten the time of clinical improvement [35], and improved 36 of 53 patients (68%) clinical symptoms [36].	ChiCTR: 0 USCTR: >18
Favipiravir		Inhibits CoV-2 activity with an EC50 of 61.88 µM [28]	Favipiravir (Day 1: 1600 mg twice daily, Days 2-14: 600 mg twice daily) decreased viral clearance time, improved chest imaging [37]; Favipiravir (Day 1: 1600 mg twice daily, Days 2-10: 600 mg twice daily) shortened latencies to relief for both pyrexia and cough [38]	ChiCTR: >8 USCTR: >8

Table 1. *Cont.*

Natural Products	Structure	In Vitro and In Vivo Studies	Clinical Studies	Registered Trials
β-D-N4-hydroxycytidine		Inhibits CoV-2 replication with an EC50 of 0.3 µM in Vero cells, with half maximal inhibitory concentration (IC50) of 0.08 µM in Calu-3 cells, and in HAE cells at 0.01-10 µM [39].	NA	ChiCTR: 0 USCTR: 0
Ribavirin		Does not inhibit viral replication under 100 µM in vitro [33].	NA	ChiCTR: >2 USCTR: >4
Lopinavir/ritonavir (LPV/RTV)		Lopinavir but not ritonavir displayed anti-CoV-2 activity with an IC50 of 26.63 µM in Vero cells [33].	A clinical trial reported no significant benefit of LPV/RTV in hospitalized SARS-CoV-2 patients than standard care [40]; Co-treatment of arbidol and LPV/RTV (arbidol: 200 mg thrice per day orally, and LPV/RTV: 400/100 mg twice per day orally) decreased the percentage of infected patients compared to only LPV/RTV treatment and improved the pneumonia [41].	ChiCTR: >13 USCTR: >33
Arbidol (Umifenovir)		NA	Arbidol (200 mg thrice per day orally) decreased the percentage of infected patients compared to LPV/RTV treatment (400/100 mg twice per day) [42].	ChiCTR: >3 USCTR: >8

Table 1. Cont.

Natural Products	Structure	In Vitro and In Vivo Studies	Clinical Studies	Registered Trials
Galidesivir (BCX4430, Immucillin-A)		Does not inhibit CoV-2 replication under 100 μM in Vero E6 cells [33].	NA	ChiCTR: 0 USCTR: >1
Oseltamivir		Does not inhibit CoV-2 replication under 100 μM in Vero E6 cells [33].	NA	ChiCTR: 0 USCTR: >10
Darunavir		NA	NA	ChiCTR: 0 USCTR: >2
Nitazoxanide		NA	NA	ChiCTR: 0 USCTR: >5

Table 1. *Cont.*

Natural Products	Structure	In Vitro and In Vivo Studies	Clinical Studies	Registered Trials
Azithromycin		Inhibits CoV-2 replication in Vero E6 cells with EC50 of 2.12 µM at an MOI of 0.002 [43].	A combination of hydroxychloroquine (200 mg, orally, thrice/day for 10 days) and azithromycin (Day 1: 500 mg, Days 2-4: 250 mg daily) decreased nasopharyngeal viral loading in patients with relatively mild COVID-19 [44].	ChiCTR: 0 USCTR: >45
Ivermectin		Inhibits CoV-2 replication with IC50 of 2.5 µM in Vero/hSLAM cells at an MOI of 0.1 [45]	NA	ChiCTR: 0 USCTR: >3
Teicoplanin		Prevents the entrance of 2019-nCoV-Spike-pseudoviruses into the cytoplasm in A549 cells, with an IC50 of 1.66 µM, as well as repressed CoV-2 entrance into HEK293T cells and Huh7 cells [46].	NA	ChiCTR: 0 USCTR: 0

Table 1. *Cont.*

Natural Products	Structure	In Vitro and In Vivo Studies	Clinical Studies	Registered Trials
Emetine		Inhibits CoV-2 replication with EC50 of 0.5 µM in Vero E6 cells [33].	NA	ChiCTR: 0 USCTR: 0
Homoharringtonine/Omacetaxine mepesuccinate (Synribo)		Inhibits CoV-2 with EC50 of 2.10 µM in Vero E6 cells [33].	NA	ChiCTR: 0 USCTR: 0

ChiCTR: Chinese Clinical Trial Register, USCTR: US Clinical Trial Register, NA: not applicable.

2.1. Chloroquine and Hydroxychloroquine

Chloroquine is an analog of quinine, which could be extracted from the bark of the Cinchona tree (Cinchona officinalis L.). Chloroquine has been reported to exhibit a curative effect on malaria since the 1600s [47]. Hydroxychloroquine is a derivative synthesized from chloroquine [47], and has a better clinical safety profile compared to chloroquine (during long-term use) and permits a higher daily dose [48]. Chloroquine and hydroxychloroquine have been successfully used to treat malaria, human immunodeficiency virus (HIV), and immune-mediated diseases, among others [47]. Chloroquine is usually dispensed as phosphate, sulfate, and hydrochloride salts.

In vitro studies showed that chloroquine is effective against SARS-CoV [49]. A study, using African green monkey kidney Vero E6 cells infected by SARS-CoV-2, showed that at a multiplicity of infection (MOI) of 0.05, chloroquine was highly effective in reducing SARS-CoV-2 replication with a half-maximal effective concentration (EC50) of 1.13 µM and an 90% effective concentration (EC90) of 6.90 µM [28], which is substantially lower than the plasma concentrations that are reached in human malaria treatment at a dose of 25 mg/kg over 3 days [49]. Chloroquine functioned at both the entry and post-entry stages of the SARS-CoV-2 infection in Vero E6 cells (Figure 1) [28]. The anti-SARS-CoV-2 effect of chloroquine might be caused by increasing endosomal pH and interfering with the glycosylation of cellular receptor of SARS-CoV-2, which is similar with its anti-SARS-CoV activity [28]. Similarly, hydroxychloroquine at different MOIs (0.01, 0.02, 0.2, and 0.8) reduced SARS-CoV-2 replication in Vero E6 cells with EC50 of 4.51, 4.06, 17.31, and 12.96 µM, respectively, higher than that of chloroquine [31]. On the contrary, another study shows that treatment with hydroxychloroquine for 48 h (EC50 = 0.72 µM) was more potent than chloroquine (EC50=5.47 µM) in SARS-CoV-2-infected Vero cells [50]. Further studies suggest that both hydroxychloroquine and chloroquine impaired SARS-CoV-2 transport from early endosomes (EEs) to endolysosomes (ELs), which participate in the release of viral RNA into the cytoplasm [31]. The established physiologically-based pharmacokinetic models (PBPK) suggest that 400 mg (twice/day) of hydroxychloroquine sulfate orally for the first day and 200 mg (twice/day) for the following 4 days could be used to treat COVID-19 [50]. It is also predicted that the potency of chloroquine phosphate increases by three times when 500 mg (twice/day) for 5 days is administered in advance [50].

A published narrative letter showed that chloroquine phosphate promoted a virus negative conversion, inhibited the exacerbation of pneumonia, and shortened the disease course [51]. However, this is an announcement without detailed data to support it. Based on clinical experiences of the experts in this field, it was announced that chloroquine might improve the success rate of treatment, shorten hospital stay time and improve patient outcome [29]. They also suggest that using the chloroquine phosphate tablet, 500 mg twice per day for 10 days could be used to treat COVID-19 patients with mild, moderate and severe pneumonia [29]. Moreover, patients with COVID-19, who received 600 mg of hydroxychloroquine sulfate (~0.46 µg/mL in serum) daily, showed a significant reduction of the viral carriage in 3–6 days-post inclusion compared to control [32]. Co-treatment with hydroxychloroquine and azithromycin was more efficient for virus reduction compared to hydroxychloroquine, suggesting a synergistic effect of the combination of hydroxychloroquine and azithromycin [32]. Another small clinical report showed that the percentages of patients who became SARS-CoV-2 negative in chloroquine (500 mg, orally, twice/day for 10 days) group (n=10) were slightly higher at Day 7, Day 10, and Day 14, compared to LPV/RTV (400/100 mg, orally, twice/day for 10 days) group (n = 12) [30]. Chloroquine also improved novel coronavirus pneumonia and promoted quick recovery compared to the LPV/RTV group [30]. There is no significant difference in T-cell (CD3+, CD4+, CD8+) counts between chloroquine and LPV/RTV groups [30]. These reports are small size (10-20 patients/group) studies without long-term outcome follow-up.

A mechanistic pharmacokinetics/virologic/corrected QT Interval (QTc) model for hydroxychloroquine was created to predict the SARS-CoV-2 decline rate and QTc prolongation [52]. Doses of hydroxychloroquine > 400 mg (twice a day) for ≥5 days were predicted to be effective to decrease viral loading, the number of patients infected with SARS-CoV-2 and treatment term, compared to lower dose (≤400 mg daily). However, doses >600 mg (twice per day) probably prolongs QTc in the model [52]. At present, data about the effect of chloroquine and hydroxychloroquine on COVID-19 are quite limited and inconclusive. High-quality, coordinated, randomized, clinical trials are urgently needed. At least 25 different trials for SARS-CoV-2 were already registered in the Chinese Clinical Trial Register (http://www.chictr.org.cn/searchprojen.aspx) and more than 40 different trials in the US Clinical Trial Register (https://clinicaltrials.gov/) to test chloroquine or hydroxychloroquine for the treatment of COVID-19.

The low cost of chloroquine and hydroxychloroquine would be a major advantage and benefit for all countries, especially middle- and low-income counties in the context of the COVID-19 pandemic. Although side-effects of chloroquine and hydroxychloroquine are generally mild and transitory, chloroquine side effects have been associated with cardiovascular disorders, such as arrhythmias, QT prolongation, and other cardiac toxicity effects [53], which can be life-threatening, especially for critically ill patients and with cardiovascular diseases. The side effects of chloroquine should be considered in clinical trials. Unfortunately, On June 17th, 2020, WHO stopped the hydroxychloroquine (HCQ) arm of the Solidarity Trial to find an effective COVID-19 treatment, since the UK's Recovery trial indicted that there is no clinical benefit from use of hydroxychloroquine in hospitalized patients with COVID-19 (https://www.recoverytrial.net/).

2.2. Remdesivir

Remdesivir is a nucleotide analog, specifically an adenosine derivative, acting as a mimic of naturally occurring nucleosides. It exhibits antiviral activity by being metabolized to an analog of adenosine triphosphate to further inhibit viral RdRp [35]. Remdesivir has broad-spectrum antiviral activity, including against Ebola virus, SARS-CoV, and MERS-CoV [54]. Remdesivir appears very safe for patients, because doses of between 3 mg and 225 mg were well-tolerated without any side effects on liver or kidney in phase 1 clinical trials [55].

A study, using Vero E6 cells infected by SARS-CoV-2, showed that remdesivir was highly effective in reducing SARS-CoV-2 replication with the EC50 of 0.77 µM and the EC90 of 1.76 µM at a MOI of 0.05 [28]. Another study showed that remdesivir exhibited anti-CoV-2 with the EC50 of 23.15 µM and 26.90 µM, respectively, when fitting viral load in logarithm scale (log10TCID50 (50% tissue culture infective dose)/mL and log10 viral RNA copies/mL) [33]. Remdesivir also inhibited virus infection in human liver cell line Huh-7 cells. Remdesivir was initially effective in the early stage of post-entry virus entry (Figure 1) [28]. The molecular mechanism of remdesivir to inhibit SARS-Cov-2 might be by pre-mature termination of viral RNA replication via competing with ATP incorporation into nascent viral RNA chains [28]. This mechanism is consistent with its putative antiviral mechanism as a nucleotide analog. Further study indicated that remdesivir inhibited RdRp from CoV-2 with high potency because RdRp efficiently incorporated the active triphosphate form of remdesivir, and further terminated RNA synthesis [55]. A comparative analysis has shown how remdesivir binds to the binding pocket of RdRp of SARS-CoV-2 [24,56]. Furthermore, in a rhesus macaque model infected by SARS-CoV-2, remdesivir ameliorated the symptoms of respiratory disease, pulmonary infiltrates on radiographs and virus titers in bronchoalveolar lavages as early as 12 h after first treatment [34]. The necropsy results showed that remdesivir decreased lung viral loading and the damage in the lung tissue, which demonstrates the efficacy of remdesivir to potentially manage the COVID-19 pandemic [34].

One clinical report showed that delayed treatment with remdesivir may be effective in treating SARS-CoV-2, unlike other antiviral drugs, which exhibit more effectiveness when applied earlier [57]. In a recent cohort, patients hospitalized for severe COVID-19 received a 10-day course of remdesivir (Day 1: 200 mg daily, Days 2-9: 100 mg daily, administered intravenously) [35]. In total, 36 of 53 patients (68%) had an improvement in the oxygen-support group, including 17 of 30 patients (57%) receiving mechanical ventilation who were extubated during a median follow-up of 18 days. A total of 25 patients (47%) were discharged [35]. However, this study had a lack of placebo-control to show remdesivir's effect, and did not test viral load to confirm the antiviral effects of remdesivir. More than 10 different trials were registered in the US Clinical Trial Register to evaluate its safety and efficacy. The Gilead company has initiated two Phase 3 randomized, open-label, multicenter clinical studies. One randomized, double-blind, placebo-controlled, multicentre trial indicated that remdesivir (n = 158, Day 1: 1200 mg, Day 2-10: 100 mg/day, infusions) was not associated with statistically significant clinical benefits for the severe COVID-19 cases compared to placebo (n = 79) [58]. Remdesivir could shorten the time of clinical improvement, but without statistical significance [58]. It was suggested that the numerical reduction in time to clinical improvement in those treated earlier required confirmation in larger studies [58]. In another cohort of patients with severe Covid-19, treatment with compassionate-use remdesivir improved 36 of 53 patients' (68%) clinical symptoms [36]. It is still early to conclude whether remdesivir is effective in patients with serious COVID-19. On May 1, 2020, The US FDA issued emergency use authorization of remdesivir for potential COVID-19 treatment (https://www.fda.gov/news-events/press-announcements/coronavirus-covid-19-update-fda-issues-emergency-use-authorization-potential-covid-19-treatment).

2.3. Favipiravir

Similar to remdesivir, favipiravir, a nucleoside guanine analog, is pyrazine carboxamide derivative (6-fluoro-3-hydroxy-2-pyrazinecarboxamide). It is well-known as a broad-spectrum antiviral drug by inhibiting the RdRp [59]. Favipiravir displayed anti-SARS-CoV-2 activity with a half maximal inhibitory concentration (IC50) of 61.88 μM in Vero cells and 50% cytotoxic concentration (CC50) >400 μM [28]. However, another study showed that favipiravir did not exhibit anti-SARS-CoV-2 activity in Vero E6 cells under 100 μM [33]. The contradictory results may be caused by using different MOI.

An open-label before-after controlled clinical trial examined the effects of favipiravir plus interferon (IFN)-α by aerosol inhalation (5 million U twice daily) versus LPV/RTV plus IFN-α on COVID-19 [37]. The results showed that favipiravir (n = 35, Day 1: 1600 mg twice daily, Days 2-14: 600 mg twice daily) significantly decreased viral clearance time as compared with the group (n = 45) treated with LPV/RTV (Days 1–14: 400 mg/100 mg twice daily) (median 4 days versus 11 days) [37]. Favipiravir also improved chest imaging compared with LPV/RTV group (91.43% versus 62%) [37]. After adjustment for potential confounders, favipiravir still significantly promoted viral clearance and improved chest imaging [37]. Another prospective, controlled, randomized, open-label multicenter trial was conducted to compare the effect between favipiravir (n = 116, Day 1: 1600 mg twice daily, Days 2-10: 600 mg twice daily) and arbidol (umifenovir) (n = 120, Days 1-10: 600 mg thrice daily) on COVID-19 [38]. This study indicated that favipiravir significantly shortened latencies to relief for both pyrexia and cough compared to arbidol, but did not influence clinical recovery rate on Day 7, as well as the rate of auxiliary oxygen therapy (AOT) or noninvasive mechanical ventilation (NMV) [38]. FUJIFILM Toyama Chemical Co. Ltd. has initiated a Phase 3 clinical trial in Japan to evaluate the safety and efficacy of favipiravir on COVID-19. At least 8 different trials for SARS-CoV-2 were already registered in the Chinese Clinical Trial Register and more than 8 different trials in the US Clinical Trial Register to test the effect of favipiravir on COVID-19.

2.4. β-D-N4-Hydroxycytidine

β-D-N4-hydroxycytidine (NHC, EIDD-1931) is a ribonucleoside analog, specifically a cytidine analog. NHC exhibited broad-spectrum antiviral activity against various RNA viruses, such as Ebola and SARS-CoV [39]. NHC displayed anti-CoV-2 activity with an IC50 of 0.3 μM and CC50 >10 μM in Vero cells, with IC50 of 0.08 μM in human lung epithelial cell line Calu-3 2B4 (Calu-3 cells). It also inhibited CoV-2 proliferation concentration-dependently (0.01-10 μM) in primary human airway epithelial (HAE) cells [39]. Both prophylactic and therapeutic administration of EIDD-2801, an orally bioavailable NHC-prodrug (β-D-N4-hydroxycytidine-5′-isopropyl ester), reduced virus titer, improved pulmonary function, and body weight loss in mice infected with SARS-CoV or MERS-CoV [39]. Unlike remdesivir, this compound is orally active, so it can be administered as a pill. The efficacy of EIDD-2801 needs to be examined in animal and clinical studies.

2.5. Ribavirin

Ribavirin (Tribavirin), a nucleoside ribosyl purine analog, is an antiviral drug. Ribavirin (500 mg twice/thrice per day for less than 10 days) combined with IFN-α was recommended to treat COVID-19 in the Novel Coronavirus Pneumonia Diagnosis and Treatment Plan (the 7th Edition) (http://kjfy.meetingchina.org/msite/news/show/cn/3337.html) edited by the China National Health Commission. However, one study showed that ribavirin did not inhibit viral replication under 100 μM in vitro [33]. There are no in vivo and clinical studies to test the effect of ribavirin on COVID-19. At least two different trials for SARS-CoV-2 were already registered in the Chinese Clinical Trial Register and more than four different trials in the US Clinical Trial Register to test the effect of favipiravir on COVID-19.

2.6. Lopinavir/Ritonavir and Arbidol

Lopinavir (a dicarboxylic acid amide) and ritonavir (an L-valine derivative) are antiretrovirals of the protease inhibitor class. Arbidol, features an indole core, and is an antiviral for influenza infection. An in vitro study indicated that lopinavir but not ritonavir displayed anti-CoV-2 activity with an IC50 of 26.63 μM in Vero cells [33]. A clinical trial reported no significant benefit of LPV/RTV in hospitalized SARS-CoV-2 patients than standard care [40]. A retrospective cohort study showed that the combination treatment of arbidol and LPV/RTV (arbidol: 200 mg thrice per day orally, and LPV/RTV: 400/100 mg twice per day orally; n = 16) significantly decreased the percentage of infected patients compared to only LPV/RTV treatment (400/100 mg twice per day; n = 17) (Day 7: by 75% versus 35%, Day 14: by 94% versus 52.9%) [41]. The combination treatment also improved the pneumonia [41]. These data suggest that the combination treatment of arbidol and LPV/RTV may be better than monotherapy of LPV/RTV. Another clinical report showed that arbidol (arbidol: 200 mg thrice per day orally, n = 16) significantly decreased the percentage of infected patients compared to LPV/RTV treatment (400/100 mg twice per day; n = 34) (Day 14: by 100% versus 55.9%) [42]. The results indicated that arbidol monotherapy may be superior to LPV/RTV in treating COVID-19. However, the sample size in these studies is the major limitation and their results are controversial. High-quality, coordinated, randomized, large clinical trials are urgently needed. At least 13 and 3 different trials were already registered in the Chinese Clinical Trial Register to test LPV/RTV and arbidol in the treatment of COVID-19, respectively. More than 33 and 8 different trials were registered in the US Clinical Trial Register to test LPV/RTV and arbidol in the treatment of COVID-19, respectively. Recently, on July 4th 2020, the WHO discontinued hydroxychloroquine and LPV/RTV treatment arms for COVID-19, since the interim trial results show that hydroxychloroquine and LPV/RTV produce little or no reduction in the mortality of hospitalized COVID-19 patients when compared to standard of care (https://www.who.int/news-room/detail/04-07-2020-who-discontinues-hydroxychloroquine-and-lopinavir-ritonavir-treatment-arms-for-covid-19).

2.7. Other Antiviral Agents

BioCryst Pharmaceuticals have started a clinical trial (NCT03891420) to examine the efficacy of an adenosine analogue galidesivir in patients with COVID-19, although it did not inhibit SARS-CoV-2 replication under 100 μM in Vero E6 cells [33]. In addition, at least 10 different trials for SARS-CoV-2 were already registered on the US Clinical Trial Register to test the influence of a neuraminidase inhibitors oseltamivir on COVID-19, although it showed no apparent antiviral effect against the SARS-CoV-2 in Vero E6 cells at concentrations under 100 μM [33]. The clinical studies (NCT04252274, NCT04303299) about an antiretroviral medication darunavir were initiated for the treatment of COVID-19 recently, although there are no publications reporting its effect on SARS-CoV-2 activity in vitro or in vivo. Nitazoxanide is a broad-spectrum antiviral agent, which exhibited in vitro activity against coronaviruses by inhibiting the expression of the viral nucleocapsid protein [60]. There are no reports about the effect of this compound on SARS-CoV-2 activity. At least five different trials were already registered in the US Clinical Trial Register to test the influence of nitazoxanide on COVID-19. The antiviral drugs baloxavir and nucleoside analogs (tenofovor, or fludarabine phosphate R-1479) showed no apparent antiviral effect against the SARS-CoV-2 in Vero E6 cells at concentrations under 100 μM [33].

2.8. Azithromycin

Azithromycin, a macrolide derivative, is a broad-spectrum macrolide antibiotic. It is used to treat enteric, respiratory, and genitourinary bacterial infections. Azithromycin was not proved to treat viral infections. One paper in preprint service indicated that azithromycin also has anti-SARS-CoV-2 activity with EC50 of 2.12 μM and EC90 of 8.65 μM in Vero E6 cells at MOI of 0.002 [43]. The mechanism of the inhibitory effect of azithromycin on anti-SARS-CoV-2 remains to be further investigated.

Some hospitals combined azithromycin with hydroxychloroquine or chloroquine for treatment of COVID-19 [61]. An open-label non-randomized clinical trial showed that 100% patients with COVID-19 (n = 6) co-treated with hydroxychloroquine and azithromycin had no SARS-CoV-2 infection at day 6 by PCR test, compared to 57.1% patients (n = 14) treated with hydroxychloroquine alone, and 12.5% in a control group (n = 16) [32]. The data suggest that azithromycin enhanced the effect of hydroxychloroquine. A pilot uncontrolled non-comparative observational study showed that a combination of hydroxychloroquine (200 mg, orally, thrice/day for 10 days) and azithromycin (Day 1: 500 mg, Days 2-4: 250 mg daily) significantly decreased nasopharyngeal viral loading in patients (n = 80) with relatively mild COVID-19 [44]. These results further suggest a beneficial effect of co-treatment of hydroxychloroquine and azithromycin on mild COVID-19 [44]. However, high-quality, coordinated, randomized, clinical trials are urgently needed to test the effect of azithromycin and the combination of it with hydroxychloroquine or other antiviral drugs on COVID-19. More than 45 different trials for SARS-CoV-2 were already registered in the US Clinical Trial Register, which are related to the examination of azithromycin in the treatment of COVID-19.

2.9. Ivermectin

Ivermectin is derived from macrocyclic lactone avermectin, which was isolated from the bacterium Streptomyces avermitilis. It is widely used for treating parasite infestation with an excellent safety profile [62]. Ivermectin also displayed inhibitory activity against RNA viral replication [62]. Ivermectin inhibited SARS-CoV-2 replication with IC50 of 2.5 μM in Vero/hSLAM cells at an MOI of 0.1 [45]. However, this concentration is the equivalent of 2190 ng/mL, which is 50-fold the peak concentration in plasma after the single dose of 200 μg/kg that is commonly used [63], which may discourage the following clinical trials. There is no clinical report about ivermectin so far. Around three different trials for SARS-CoV-2 were already registered in the US Clinical Trial Register, which are related to examining of ivermectin in the treatment of COVID-19.

2.10. Teicoplanin

Teicoplanin, a lipoglycopeptide antibiotic, is a complex of related natural products isolated from the fermentation broth of a strain of Actinoplanes teichomyceticus [64]. It consists of five major components (A2-1 through A2-5), one hydrolysis component (A3-1), and four minor components (RS-1 through RS-4) [64]. Teicoplanin has anti-bacterial and anti-SARS-CoV activities [65]. Teicoplanin significantly prevented the entrance of 2019-nCoV-Spike-pseudoviruses into the cytoplasm in A549 cells, with an IC50 of 1.66 μM [46]. The teicoplanin homolog dalbavancin but not vancomycin also inhibited the entry of 2019-nCoV in A549 cells in a dose-dependent manner [46]. Teicoplanin also effectively repressed SARS-CoV-2 entrance into HEK293T cells and Huh7 cells, which also express ACE2 [46]. There are no animal studies or clinical reports investigating the inhibitory effect of teicoplanin on SARS-CoV-2 activity.

2.11. Emetine and Homoharringtonine

Emetine could be extracted from root of a plant Cephaelis ipecacuanha (Brot.) Willd. It has been used as an anti-protozoal drug and an expectorant. It also exhibited antiviral activity, but with potential cardiotoxicity [33]. Emetine inhibited SARS-CoV-2 replication with EC50 of 0.5 µM in Vero E6 cells [33]. Remdesivir (6.25 µM) in combination with emetine (0.195 µM) may achieve 64.9% inhibition in viral yield, suggesting that synergy between remdesivir and emetine [33]. The concentrations of emetine can be almost 300 times higher in the lungs, which indicated that emetine could be much more effective as an anti-coronavirus agent than as an anti-protozoal drug [66]. There are no animal studies, clinical reports or registered clinical trials evaluating the effect of emetine on COVID-19. Homoharringtonine, a cytotoxic plant alkaloid derived from evergreen shrub Cephalotaxus fortune HOOK, has been used to treat chronic myeloid leukemia [33]. Homoharringtonine inhibited SARS-CoV-2 with EC50 of 2.10 µM in Vero E6 cells [33]. There are no studies reporting its effect on SARS-CoV-2 in preclinical in vivo models and clinical trials.

2.12. Others

There are lots of compounds which do not belong to natural products or their derivatives or mimics, but exhibited anti- SARS-CoV-2 activity. We briefly list them here for an overview. Corticosteroids are a class of steroid hormones that are produced in the adrenal cortex or their synthetic analogs. They are involved in various physiological processes, such as regulation of inflammation. They also could suppress lung inflammation in patients with COVID-19 [67]. At least two different trials were already registered in the Chinese Clinical Trial Register and more than 21 different trials in the US Clinical Trial Register to test corticosteroids in the treatment of COVID-19. Humanized antibodies, Tocilizumab and Bevacizumab were also used to treat severe complications related to SARS-CoV-2 [22]. There are more than 29 and 3 clinical trials which were already registered in the US Clinical Trial Register to test tocilizumab and bevacizumab, respectively, in the treatment of COVID-19. An immunomodulating drug, fingolimod, is also tested in several clinical trials registered in US Clinical Trial Register (NCT04280588).

Ibrutinib and acalabrutinib created by scientists are known as Bruton's tyrosine kinase (BTK) inhibitors. They have been used to treat indolent B-cell malignancies and chronic graft versus host disease [68]. A clinical report suggested that ibrutinib may protect against pulmonary injury in SARS-CoV-2 infected patients with Waldenstrom's Macrobulinemia [68]. The authors described that patients (n = 5) with high dose of ibrutinib (420 mg/day) experienced no dyspnea and required no hospitalization compared to a patient (n = 1) with low dose of ibrutinib (140 mg/day), who experienced progressive dyspnea and hypoxia prompting hospitalization [68]. A clinical trial examining the benefit of BTK-inhibitor acalabrutinib was initiated in COVID-19 patients in pulmonary distress (NCT04346199).

Dipyridamole is an antithrombotic agent by inhibiting phosphodiesterase, and then increasing intracellular cAMP/cGMP [69]. Dipyridamole suppressed CoV-2 replication in Vero E6 cells with IC50 of 0.1 µM [69]. In a clinical trial, dipyridamole (50 mg/time, thrice per day orally) treatment (n = 14) decreased D-dimers level, enhanced lymphocyte and platelet recovery in the circulation, and improved clinical outcomes compared to the control group (n = 16) [69]. It is worth noting that all patients in this study received ribavirin, glucocorticoids, and oxygen treatment [69]. High-quality, coordinated, randomized, large clinical trials are urgently needed to confirm the results in this study.

Omeprazole, oxprenolol hydrochloride, clemizole hydrochloride, alprostadil, dolutegravir, sulfadoxine, opipramol dihydrochloride, and quinidine hydrochloride monohydrate have anti-SARS-CoV-2 activity with EC50s of 17.06, 20.22, 23.94, 5.39, 22.04, 35.37, 5.05, and 5.11 µM in Vero E6 cells at an MOI of 0.002 [43]. The effect of these compounds on SARS-CoV-2 activity in preclinical in vivo models and their effects in clinical trials remains to be investigated.

3. Traditional Medicine Products (with Focus on TCM)

Traditional medicine has been used to fight against various diseases, including pandemic diseases, for thousands of years. It has also played an important role in SARS and H1N1 influenza [70]. Recently, some countries, including China, South Korea, Japan and India, have issued traditional medicine treatment guidelines on the prevention and treatment of COVID-19 [71]. Probably the most prominent traditional medicine worldwide is TCM, which has been used for more than five thousand years [16]. In China, more than 85% of SARS-CoV-2 infected patients were receiving TCM treatment [72]. TCM treatment for COVID-19 was based on syndrome differentiation, according to which individual treatment was administered. According to the theory of TCM, the "targeted organ location" of COVID-19 is the lung, and its core pathogenesis is "dampness and plague" caused by external "cold-dampness", which impairs "lung" and "spleen". The "dampness and plague" can transform to "heat" because of dysfunction of "Qi", which is a kind of vital force [73]. Therefore, the main principle of TCM treatment for COVID-19 is to strengthen "Qi" to protect patients from external pathogens, decrease "wind" and discharge "heat", and improve "dampness" [74]. In this part, we reviewed publications regarding the TCM treatment of COVID-19 (Table 2).

Table 2. Traditional medicine products fighting COVID-19 (with focus on traditional Chinese medicine—TCM).

Traditional Medicine	Constituents	In Vitro and In Vivo Studies	Clinical Studies	Registered Clinical Trials
Lian Hua Qing Wen Capsule (LHQWC)	*Forsythiae Fructus* (Chinese name: Lianqiao), *Lonicerae Japonicae Flos* (Jinyinhua), *Ephedrae Herba* (Mahuang), *Armeniacae Semen Amarum* (Kuxingren), *Isatidis Radix* (Banlangen), *Dryopteridis Crassirhizomatis Rhizoma* (Mianmaguanzhong), *Houttuyniae Herba* (Yuxingcao), *Pogostemonis Herba* (Guanghuoxiang), *Rhei Radix et Rhizoma* (Dahuang), *Rhodiolae Crenulatae Radix et Rhizoma* (Hongjingtian), *Glycyrrhizae Radix et Rhizoma* (Gancao), menthol and *Gypsum Fibrosum* (Shigao)	Inhibit SARS-CoV-2 replication in Vero E6 cells (100 TCID50) with an IC50 of 411.2 µg/mL, and reduce mRNA levels of pro-inflammatory cytokines (TNF-α, IL-6, CCL-2/MCP-1 and CXCL-10/IP-10) in Huh-7 cells infected by CoV-2 [75].	NA	ChiCTR: >11 USCTR: 0
Shuang Huang Lian Oral Liquid (SHLOL)	*Lonicerae Japonicae Flos* (Jinyinghua), *Forsythiae Fructus* (Lianqiao) and *Scutellariae Radix* (Huangqin)	NA	The cases had poor response to other medicine (oral moxifloxacin, cefotaxime, arbidol and oseltamivir) but responded well to SHLOL [76].	ChiCTR: >1 USCTR: 0
Qingfei Paidu Decoction (QPD)	*Gypsum Fibrosum* (Shigao), *Cinnamomi Ramulus* (Guizhi), *Ephedrae Herba* (Mahuang), *Glycyrrhizae Radix et Rhizoma* (Gancao), *Pinelliae Rhizoma* (Banxia), *Asteris Radix et Rhizoma* (Ziwan), *Farfarae Flos* (Kuandonghua), *Belamcandae Rhizoma* (Shegan), *Asari Radix et Rhizoma* (Xixin), *Scutellariae Radix* (Huangqin), *Aurantii Fructus Immaturus* (Zhishi), *Dioscoreae Rhizoma* (Shanyao), *Alismatis Rhizoma* (Zexie), *Polyporus* (Zhuling), *Atractylodis Macrocephalae Rhizoma* (Baizhu), *Poria* (Fuling), *Bupleuri Radix* (Chaihu), *Citri Reticulatae Pericarpium* (Chengpi), and *Pogostemonis Herba* (Guanghuoxiang)	NA	The effect of QPD on COVID-19 is inconclusive because there was no control group [77].	ChiCTR: >2 USCTR: 0
Scutellariae Radix	NA	Inhibit activity of a main protease of SARS-CoV-2, 3C-like protease (3CLpro) and CoV-2 replication in Vero cells with an EC50 of 0.74 µg/mL [78].	NA	ChiCTR: >7 USCTR: 0

NA: not applicable.

According to the opinions and frontline experiences of medical experts in China, there are several different herbal formulae which are recommended for COVID-19 treatment in the light of their clinical classification in Chinese Clinical Guidance for COVID-19 Pneumonia Diagnosis and Treatment (7th edition) published by the China National Health Committee [79]. A study in preprint service showed that this guideline-based TCM treatment plus routine treatment (antiviral and antibiotic drugs, nutritional support and mechanical ventilation) may have more beneficial effects compared to only routine treatment on severe COVID-19 [80]. This clinical trial is a small pilot (n = 42), which need further large clinical study to confirm the adjunctive therapeutic effect on COVID-19.

The Lian Hua Qing Wen Capsule (LHQWC), a TCM formula, has been used to treat influenza and exhibited broad-spectrum antiviral effect and immune regulatory activity [75]. LHQWC is constituted by 11 kinds of traditional Chinese herbs, including *Forsythiae Fructus* (Chinese name: Lianqiao, the dried fruit of *Forsythia suspensa* (Thunb.) Vahl), *Lonicerae Japonicae Flos* (Jinyinhua, the dried flowers or flower buds of *Lonicera japonica* Thunb.), *Ephedrae Herba* (Mahuang, the dried herbaceous stem of *Ephedra sinica* Stapf, *Ephedra equisetina* Bge., *Ephedra intermedia* Schrenk et C. A. Mey), *Armeniacae Semen Amarum* (Kuxingren, the dried mature seed of *Prunus armeniaca* L. var. ansu Masim., *Prunus sibirica* L., *Prunus mandshurica* (Maxim.) Koehne or *Prunus armeniaca* L.), *Isatidis Radix* (Banlangen, the dried root of *Isatis indigotica* Fort), *Dryopteridis Crassirhizomatis Rhizoma* (Mianmaguanzhong, the dried rhizome and remnants of leaf stems of *Dtyopteris crassirhiaoma* Nakai), *Houttuyniae Herba* (Yuxingcao, the fresh or dried aerial portion of *Houttuynia cordata* Thunb), *Pogostemonis Herba* (Guanghuoxiang, the dried aerial portion of *Pogostemon cablin* (Blanco) Benth), *Rhei Radix et Rhizoma* (Dahuang, the dried root and rhizome of *Rheum palmatum* L. or *Rheum tanguticum* Maxim. ex Balf, or *Rheum officinale* Baill), *Rhodiolae Crenulatae Radix et Rhizoma* (Hongjingtian, the dried root and rhizome of *Rhodiola crenulata* (Hook. f. et Thoms.) H. Ohba.), and *Glycyrrhizae Radix et Rhizoma* (Gancao, the dried root and rhizome of *Glycyrrhiza uralensis* Fisch), along with menthol and a traditional Chinese mineral medicine *Gypsum Fibrosum* (Shigao). LHQWC significantly inhibited SARS-CoV-2 replication in Vero E6 cells (100 TCID50) with an IC50 of 411.2 μg/mL, and reduced mRNA levels of pro-inflammatory cytokines (TNF-α, IL-6, CCL-2/MCP-1 and CXCL-10/IP-10) in Huh-7 cells infected by CoV-2 [75]. There are no in vivo studies or clinical reports to test the effect of LHQWC on COVID-19. At least 11 different trials were already registered in the Chinese Clinical Trial Register to test the effect of Lian Hua Qing Wen Capsule/Granule on COVID-19.

There is one case report showing the first family case (parents and their daughter) of COVID-19, whereby patients were co-treated by western medicine and Chinese traditional patent medicine Shuang Huang Lian Oral Liquid (SHLOL) [76]. SHLOL, containing extract of three Chinese herbs (*Lonicerae Japonicae Flos* (the dried flowers or flower buds of *Lonicera japonica* Thunb), *Forsythiae Fructus* (the dried fruit of *Forsythia suspensa* (Thunb.) Vahl) and *Scutellariae Radix* (the dried root of *Scutellaria baicalensis* Georgi)), which is usually used to treat cold and cough with fever. These patients were treated using the SHLOL after there were no effects of other treatments (oral moxifloxacin, cefotaxime, arbidol and oseltamivir) [76]. Three cases had poor response to other medicine but responded well to SHLOL [76]. The authors already initiated a clinical trial to examine the effect of SHLOL on COVID-19 (ChiCTR2000029605).

Another case report showed that Qingfei Paidu Decoction (QPD) exhibited a beneficial effect on patients with COVID-19. QPD is consisting of *Gypsum Fibrosum* (Chinese name: Shigao), *Cinnamomi Ramulus* (Guizhi, the dried tender branches of *Cinnamomum cassia* Presl), *Ephedrae Herba* (Mahuang), *Glycyrrhizae Radix et Rhizoma* (Gancao), *Pinelliae Rhizoma* (Banxia, the dried tuberous rhizome of *Pinellia ternate* (Thunb.) Breit), *Asteris Radix et Rhizoma* (Ziwan, the dried root and rhizome of *Aster tataricus* L.), *Farfarae Flos* (Kuandonghua, the dried flower bud of *Tussilago farfara* L.), *Belamcandae Rhizoma* (Shegan, the dried rhizome of *Belamcanda chinensis* (L.) DC.), *Asari Radix et Rhizoma* (Xixin, the dried root and rhizome of *Asarum heterotropoides* Fr. Schmidt var. mandshuricum (Maxim.) Kitag., *Asarum sieboldii* Miq., *Asarum sieboldii* Miq.var. seoulense Nakai), *Scutellariae Radix* (Huangqin), *Aurantii Fructus Immaturus* (Zhishi, the dried young fruit of *Citrus aurantium* L., and its cultivar *Citrus sinensis*

(L.) Osbeck), *Dioscoreae Rhizoma* (Shanyao, the dried rhizome of *Dioscorea opposite* Thunb), *Zingiberis Rhizoma Recens* (Shengjiang, the fresh rhizome of *Zingiber officinale* (Willd.) Rosc), *Armeniacae Semen Amarum* (Kuxingren), *Alismatis Rhizoma* (Zexie, the dried tuberous rhizome of *Alisma orientalis* (Sam.) Juzep), *Polyporus* (Zhuling, the dried sclerotium of *Polyporus umbellatus* (Pers.) Fries), *Atractylodis Macrocephalae Rhizoma* (Baizhu, the dried rhizome of *Atractylodes macrocephala* Koidz), *Poria* (Fuling, the dried sclerotium of *Poria cocos* (Schw.) Wolf), *Bupleuri Radix* (Chaihu, the dried root of *Bupleurum chinense* DC.), *Citri Reticulatae Pericarpium* (Chengpi, the dried mature pericarp of *Citrus reticulate* Blanco and its culticars), and *Pogostemonis Herba* (Guanghuoxiang, the dried aerial portion of *Pogostemon cablin* (Blanco) Benth) [77]. In the treatment of the QPD group ($n = 701$), 130 cases were discharged, and the clinical symptoms of 51 and 268 cases disappeared and improved, respectively [77]. However, the effect of QPD on COVID-19 is inconclusive because there was no control group. There are two clinical trials registered in the Chinese Clinical Trial Register (ChiCTR2000030883, ChiCTR2000030806) to investigate the effect of QPD on COVID-19.

Scutellariae Radix (the dried roots of *Scutellariae baicalensis* Georgi; Chinese name: Huangqin), has been widely used to treat viral infection-related symptoms in China [78]. The ethanol extract of *Scutellariae Radix* inhibited activity of a main protease of SARS-CoV-2, 3C-like protease (3CLpro) and SARS-CoV-2 replication in Vero cells with an EC50 of 0.74 µg/mL [78]. A major component of *Scutellariae Radix*, baicalein, strongly inhibited SARS-CoV-2 3CLpro activity with an IC50 of 0.39 µM [78]. Baicalein inhibited viral replication by docking in the core of the substrate-binding pocket of SARS-CoV-2 3CLpro by interacting with two catalytic residues (the crucial S1/S2 subsites and the oxyanion loop) to prevent the peptide substrate approaching the active site [81]. There are at least seven clinical trials registered in the Chinese Clinical Trial Register to investigate the effect of *Scutellariae Radix* or its components on COVID-19.

In addition, the effects of self-made herbal preparations such as Xin Guan-1 Formula, Xin Guan-2 Formula, Qing Yi-4, and commercially available Tan Re Qing Injection, Xue Bi Jing Injection, Re Du Ning Injection, Shen Qi Fu Zheng Injection, Shen Fu Injection, Xi Yan Ping Injection, Shuang Huang Lian Oral Liquid, Kang Bing Du Granules, Jing Yin Granule, Jin Yin Hua Tang, Ke Su Ting Syrup/Ke Qing Capsule, and Gu Biao Jie Du Ling are examined in the clinical trials registered in the Chinese Clinical Trial Register [72].

Through thousands of years of development, TCM has carved out its own theory and practice. In fact, one classic medicinal book *Shanghan Zabing Lun*, which was compiled by ZHANG Zhongjing around 220 AD, even described how to fight against pandemic diseases. The theory of TCM to treat COVID-19, including concepts like "dampness and plague" and "Qi" among others, are difficult to be understood and accepted by other countries except China, Japan and Korea. Therefore, to verify the potential effect of TCM formulae on COVID-19, high-quality, coordinated, randomized, large clinical trials are needed. In addition, the Chinese medicine formulae are composed of many Chinese herbs which contain complicated chemical compositions. Thus, a systemic evaluation approach needs to be developed to assess diverse traditional Chinese medicine products.

4. Discussion and Conclusions

So far, no specific drug has been discovered for COVID-19 therapy. The whole world is in a rush to find treatments for COVID-19. For this review, many published pre-clinical studies, clinical treatment experience, clinical trials, descriptive reports and case series were summarized that investigated the effect of natural products, their derivatives and mimics, as well as traditional medicine products on COVID-19. Clinical and in vitro antiviral studies indicated that chloroquine, hydroxychloroquine, remdesivir, favipiravir, LPV/RTV and arbidol may exhibit potent therapeutic effects on COVID-19. Randomized, large and placebo-controlled clinical trials were registered to further confirm their effects on COVID-19. It is observed the existence of a synergistic effect of the combination of hydroxychloroquine and azithromycin or nitazoxanide as well as combination of arbidol and LPV/RTV, which also remains to be further investigated in the large clinical studies. There are clinical trials registered to test ribavirin, galidesivir, oseltamivir, darunavir and nitazoxanide in the treatment of COVID-19, although these compounds did not exhibit anti-CoV-2 activity in vitro or there are no related reports. It is reported that β-D-N4-hydroxycytidine, teicoplanin, ivermectin, emetine and homoharringtonine displayed in vitro anti-Cov-2 activity. There are, however, no clinical reports or registered clinical trials to investigate their effect on COVID-19.

It is implicated that some TCM treatments may exhibit beneficial effect on COVID-19. Among the TCM formulae, Lian Hua Qing Wen Capsule, Shuang Huang Lian Oral Liquid, and Qingfei Paidu Decoction were reported to exhibit beneficial effects on COVID-19. Randomized, large and placebo-controlled clinical trials were initiated to investigate their effect. In addition, the ethanol extract of a Chinese herb *Scutellariae Radix* and its main constituent baicalein inhibited SARS-CoV-2 replication in vitro. There are several clinical trials registered to test the effect of this herb or its components on COVID-19. TCM treatment of COVID-19 was based on syndrome differentiation. Mild and severe symptoms were treated by different TCM formulae. Moreover, TCM appeared to regulate human immune function and strengthen the resistance to epidemic diseases before infection [82]. Thus, the effect of TCM formulae on different phases of COVID-19 remains to be investigated, along with an assessment of the prevention effect of pre-treatment with TCM formulae. Although TCM formulae have been used clinically in China for thousands of years, their safety should be also carefully evaluated when treating patients with COVID-19 because formulae contain many complicated chemical compounds, which may affect the efficacy of standard treatment because of herb–drug interaction. The TCM treatment for COVID-19 should be applied under the guidance of TCM practitioners. The mechanism of TCM efficiency on COVID-19 remains to be further dissected. Although it is very difficult to fully understand the molecular mechanism of action of the complicated constituents of TCM formulae, we may consider that TCM might possibly exhibit therapeutic effects by inhibiting the viral replication, blocking the infection, regulating the immune response and decreasing the inflammatory storm [77]. In addition, it is valuable to point out that the studies about TCM treatment on COVID-19 were performed only in China, where the B type of SARS-Cov-2 is the most common type [83]. Since A and C types were found in significant proportions outside China, that is, in Europeans and Americans [83], they may have a different response to TCM treatment.

COVID-19 has now been declared a pandemic and no specific drug could be used for treating it. Therefore, new medicines for the management of COVID-19 are urgently needed. Currently, drug repurposing (such as the ongoing efforts with chloroquine, hydroxychloroquine, remdesivir and so on) is an important strategy to quickly develop an effective treatment for COVID-19, because it will potentially shorten overall drug development timelines and lower development costs [84]. It is of great urgency to also develop new medicines (including searching for new active natural products) to combat this difficult-to-treat new disease at the same time, since repurposed drugs may ultimately not yield a significant clinical benefit [85].

As reviewed in this paper, there is a synergistic effect of the combination of hydroxychloroquine and azithromycin or nitazoxanide as well as combination of arbidol and LPV/RTV on COVID-19. Therefore, carefully combined cocktails may be very effective to treat COVID-19, as was the case for HIV in the 1990s (LPV/RTV) [85]. The synergistic effect could be explained by the different mechanisms of action of these drugs: for example, hydroxychloroquine inhibits SARS-CoV2 replication and azithromycin has anti-inflammatory activities which probably down-regulate cytokine storm in patients with COVID-19. Therefore, it is worthwhile to emphasize the exploration of a logical combination of drugs to manage COVID-19.

Because of the urgency of treating patients with COVID-19, large-scale randomized controlled studies were almost impossible at the beginning when the disease appeared [86]. The published treatment data to date are derived exclusively from observational data, small clinical trials, or poorly designed clinical studies with potential biases in evaluating the effectiveness of treatment for COVID-19. Randomized, double-blind and placebo-controlled large clinical trials are needed to provide reliable evidence for potential effective treatments.

Author Contributions: Resources, D.W.; writing—original draft preparation, D.W, J.O.H., N.T.T.; writing—review and editing, A.G.A., A.W.K.Y., N.T.T., J.O.H., J.H., Z.G., H.W.; All authors have read and agreed to the published version of the manuscript.

Funding: This research was funded by the Cultivation project for clinical medicine of the integrated traditional Chinese and western medicine and Cultivation project for education team of internal medicine of the integrated traditional Chinese and western medicine in the first-term subjects with special support in the first-class universities in Guizhou province (Qin Jiao Gao Fa No. 2017-158), and the Polish KNOW (Leading National Research Centre) Scientific Consortium "Healthy Animal-Safe Food" decision of Ministry of Science and Higher Education No. 05-1/KNOW2/2015.

Conflicts of Interest: The authors declare no conflict of interest. Open Access Funding by the University of Vienna.

References

1. Zhu, N.; Zhang, D.; Wang, W.; Li, X.; Yang, B.; Song, J.; Zhao, X.; Huang, B.; Shi, W.; Lu, R.; et al. A Novel Coronavirus from Patients with Pneumonia in China, 2019. *N. Engl. J. Med.* **2020**, *382*, 727–733. [CrossRef] [PubMed]
2. Sanders, J.M.; Monogue, M.L.; Jodlowski, T.Z.; Cutrell, J.B. Pharmacologic Treatments for Coronavirus Disease 2019 (COVID-19): A Review. *JAMA* **2020**, *323*, 1824–1836. [CrossRef] [PubMed]
3. Wrapp, D.; Wang, N.; Corbett, K.S.; Goldsmith, J.A.; Hsieh, C.L.; Abiona, O.; Graham, B.S.; McLellan, J.S. Cryo-EM structure of the 2019-nCoV spike in the prefusion conformation. *Science* **2020**, *367*, 1260–1263. [CrossRef] [PubMed]
4. Hoffmann, M.; Kleine-Weber, H.; Schroeder, S.; Kruger, N.; Herrler, T.; Erichsen, S.; Schiergens, T.S.; Herrler, G.; Wu, N.H.; Nitsche, A.; et al. SARS-CoV-2 Cell Entry Depends on ACE2 and TMPRSS2 and Is Blocked by a Clinically Proven Protease Inhibitor. *Cell* **2020**, *181*, 271–280.e8. [CrossRef]
5. Zumla, A.; Chan, J.F.; Azhar, E.I.; Hui, D.S.; Yuen, K.Y. Coronaviruses-drug discovery and therapeutic options. *Nat. Rev. Drug Discov.* **2016**, *15*, 327–347. [CrossRef] [PubMed]
6. Li, R.; Pei, S.; Chen, B.; Song, Y.; Zhang, T.; Yang, W.; Shaman, J. Substantial undocumented infection facilitates the rapid dissemination of novel coronavirus (SARS-CoV2). *Science* **2020**, *368*, 489–493. [CrossRef] [PubMed]
7. Guan, W.-J.; Ni, Z.-Y.; Hu, Y.; Liang, W.-H.; Ou, C.-Q.; He, J.-X.; Liu, L.; Shan, H.; Lei, C.-L.; Hui, D.S.C.; et al. Clinical Characteristics of Coronavirus Disease 2019 in China. *N. Engl. J. Med.* **2020**, *382*, 1708–1720. [CrossRef] [PubMed]
8. Cherry, G.; Rocke, J.; Chu, M.; Liu, J.; Lechner, M.; Lund, V.J.; Kumar, B.N. Loss of smell and taste: A new marker of COVID-19? Tracking reduced sense of smell during the coronavirus pandemic using search trends. *Expert Rev. Anti Infect. Ther.* **2020**, 1–6. [CrossRef]
9. Mercante, G.; Ferreli, F.; De Virgilio, A.; Gaino, F.; Di Bari, M.; Colombo, G.; Russo, E.; Costantino, A.; Pirola, F.; Cugini, G.; et al. Prevalence of Taste and Smell Dysfunction in Coronavirus Disease 2019. *JAMA Otolaryngol. Head Neck Surg.* **2020**. [CrossRef]
10. Chen, N.; Zhou, M.; Dong, X.; Qu, J.; Gong, F.; Han, Y.; Qiu, Y.; Wang, J.; Liu, Y.; Wei, Y.; et al. Epidemiological and clinical characteristics of 99 cases of 2019 novel coronavirus pneumonia in Wuhan, China: A descriptive study. *Lancet* **2020**, *395*, 507–513. [CrossRef]
11. Bornstein, S.R.; Dalan, R.; Hopkins, D.; Mingrone, G.; Boehm, B.O. Endocrine and metabolic link to coronavirus infection. *Nat. Rev. Endocrinol.* **2020**, *16*, 297–298. [CrossRef] [PubMed]
12. Fierabracci, A.; Arena, A.; Rossi, P. COVID-19: A Review on Diagnosis, Treatment, and Prophylaxis. *Int. J. Mol. Sci.* **2020**, *21*, 5145. [CrossRef] [PubMed]
13. Wang, D.; Hu, B.; Hu, C.; Zhu, F.; Liu, X.; Zhang, J.; Wang, B.; Xiang, H.; Cheng, Z.; Xiong, Y.; et al. Clinical Characteristics of 138 Hospitalized Patients With 2019 Novel Coronavirus-Infected Pneumonia in Wuhan, China. *JAMA* **2020**, *323*, 1061–1069. [CrossRef] [PubMed]
14. Alhazzani, W.; Moller, M.H.; Arabi, Y.M.; Loeb, M.; Gong, M.N.; Fan, E.; Oczkowski, S.; Levy, M.M.; Derde, L.; Dzierba, A.; et al. Surviving Sepsis Campaign: Guidelines on the Management of Critically Ill Adults with Coronavirus Disease 2019 (COVID-19). *Crit. Care Med.* **2020**, *46*, 854–887. [CrossRef]
15. Holshue, M.L.; DeBolt, C.; Lindquist, S.; Lofy, K.H.; Wiesman, J.; Bruce, H.; Spitters, C.; Ericson, K.; Wilkerson, S.; Tural, A.; et al. First Case of 2019 Novel Coronavirus in the United States. *N. Engl. J. Med* **2020**, *382*, 929–936. [CrossRef]

16. Wang, D.; Hiebl, V.; Xu, T.; Ladurner, A.; Atanasov, A.G.; Heiss, E.H.; Dirsch, V.M. Impact of natural products on the cholesterol transporter ABCA1. *J. Ethnopharmacol.* **2020**, *249*, 112444. [CrossRef]
17. Waltenberger, B.; Mocan, A.; Smejkal, K.; Heiss, E.H.; Atanasov, A.G. Natural Products to Counteract the Epidemic of Cardiovascular and Metabolic Disorders. *Molecules* **2016**, *21*, 807. [CrossRef]
18. El Bairi, K.; Atanasov, A.G.; Amrani, M.; Afqir, S. The arrival of predictive biomarkers for monitoring therapy response to natural compounds in cancer drug discovery. *Biomed. Pharmacother.* **2019**, *109*, 2492–2498. [CrossRef]
19. Wang, D.; Huang, J.; Gui, T.; Yang, Y.; Feng, T.; Tzvetkov, N.T.; Xu, T.; Gai, Z.; Zhou, Y.; Zhang, J.; et al. SR-BI as a target of natural products and its significance in cancer. *Semin. Cancer Biol.* **2020**. [CrossRef]
20. Atanasov, A.G.; Waltenberger, B.; Pferschy-Wenzig, E.M.; Linder, T.; Wawrosch, C.; Uhrin, P.; Temml, V.; Wang, L.; Schwaiger, S.; Heiss, E.H.; et al. Discovery and resupply of pharmacologically active plant-derived natural products: A review. *Biotechnol. Adv.* **2015**, *33*, 1582–1614. [CrossRef]
21. Yeung, A.W.K.; Heinrich, M.; Kijjoa, A.; Tzvetkov, N.T.; Atanasov, A.G. The ethnopharmacological literature: An analysis of the scientific landscape. *J. Ethnopharmacol.* **2020**, *250*, 112414. [CrossRef]
22. El-Aziz, T.M.A.; Stockand, J.D. Recent progress and challenges in drug development against COVID-19 coronavirus (SARS-CoV-2)—An update on the status. *Infect. Genet. Evol.* **2020**, *83*, 104327. [CrossRef]
23. Lu, R.; Zhao, X.; Li, J.; Niu, P.; Yang, B.; Wu, H.; Wang, W.; Song, H.; Huang, B.; Zhu, N.; et al. Genomic characterisation and epidemiology of 2019 novel coronavirus: Implications for virus origins and receptor binding. *Lancet* **2020**, *395*, 565–574. [CrossRef]
24. Huang, J.; Song, W.; Huang, H.; Sun, Q. Pharmacological Therapeutics Targeting RNA-Dependent RNA Polymerase, Proteinase and Spike Protein: From Mechanistic Studies to Clinical Trials for COVID-19. *J. Clin. Med.* **2020**, *9*, 1131. [CrossRef] [PubMed]
25. Yuan, M.; Wu, N.C.; Zhu, X.; Lee, C.D.; So, R.T.Y.; Lv, H.; Mok, C.K.P.; Wilson, I.A. A highly conserved cryptic epitope in the receptor-binding domains of SARS-CoV-2 and SARS-CoV. *Science* **2020**, *368*, 630–633. [CrossRef] [PubMed]
26. Letko, M.; Marzi, A.; Munster, V. Functional assessment of cell entry and receptor usage for SARS-CoV-2 and other lineage B betacoronaviruses. *Nat. Microbiol.* **2020**, *5*, 562–569. [CrossRef] [PubMed]
27. Wu, C.; Liu, Y.; Yang, Y.; Zhang, P.; Zhong, W.; Wang, Y.; Wang, Q.; Xu, Y.; Li, M.; Li, X.; et al. Analysis of therapeutic targets for SARS-CoV-2 and discovery of potential drugs by computational methods. *Acta Pharm. Sin. B* **2020**, *10*, 766–788. [CrossRef]
28. Wang, M.; Cao, R.; Zhang, L.; Yang, X.; Liu, J.; Xu, M.; Shi, Z.; Hu, Z.; Zhong, W.; Xiao, G. Remdesivir and chloroquine effectively inhibit the recently emerged novel coronavirus (2019-nCoV) in vitro. *Cell Res.* **2020**, *30*, 269–271. [CrossRef]
29. Jie, Z.; He, H.; Xi, H.; Zhi, Z. Expert consensus on chloroquine phosphate for the treatment of novel coronavirus pneumonia. *Zhonghua Jie He He Hu Xi Za Zhi* **2020**, *43*, 185–188.
30. Huang, M.; Tang, T.; Pang, P.; Li, M.; Ma, R.; Lu, J.; Shu, J.; You, Y.; Chen, B.; Liang, J.; et al. Treating COVID-19 with Chloroquine. *J. Mol. Cell Biol.* **2020**, *12*, 322–325. [CrossRef]
31. Liu, J.; Cao, R.; Xu, M.; Wang, X.; Zhang, H.; Hu, H.; Li, Y.; Hu, Z.; Zhong, W.; Wang, M. Hydroxychloroquine, a less toxic derivative of chloroquine, is effective in inhibiting SARS-CoV-2 infection in vitro. *Cell Discov.* **2020**, *6*, 16. [CrossRef] [PubMed]
32. Gautret, P.; Lagier, J.-C.; Parola, P.; Hoang, V.T.; Meddeb, L.; Mailhe, M.; Doudier, B.; Courjon, J.; Giordanengo, V.; Vieira, V.E.; et al. Hydroxychloroquine and azithromycin as a treatment of COVID-19: Results of an open-label non-randomized clinical trial. *Int. J. Antimicrob. Agents* **2020**, *56*, 105949. [CrossRef] [PubMed]
33. Choy, K.T.; Wong, A.Y.; Kaewpreedee, P.; Sia, S.F.; Chen, D.; Hui, K.P.Y.; Chu, D.K.W.; Chan, M.C.W.; Cheung, P.P.; Huang, X.; et al. Remdesivir, lopinavir, emetine, and homoharringtonine inhibit SARS-CoV-2 replication in vitro. *Antiviral Res.* **2020**, *178*, 104786. [CrossRef] [PubMed]
34. Williamson, B.N.; Feldmann, F.; Schwarz, B.; Meade-White, K.; Porter, D.P.; Schulz, J.; Doremalen, N.V.; Leighton, I.; Yinda, C.K.; Pérez-Pérez, L.; et al. Clinical benefit of remdesivir in rhesus macaques infected with SARS-CoV-2. *bioRxiv* **2020**. [CrossRef]
35. Grein, J.; Ohmagari, N.; Shin, D.; Diaz, G.; Asperges, E.; Castagna, A.; Feldt, T.; Green, G.; Green, M.L.; Lescure, F.-X.; et al. Compassionate Use of Remdesivir for Patients with Severe Covid-19. *N. Engl. J. Med.* **2020**, *382*, 2327–2336. [CrossRef]

36. Beigel, J.H.; Tomashek, K.M.; Dodd, L.E.; Mehta, A.K.; Zingman, B.S.; Kalil, A.C.; Hohmann, E.; Chu, H.Y.; Luetkemeyer, A.; Kline, S.; et al. Remdesivir for the Treatment of Covid-19—Preliminary Report. *N. Engl. J. Med.* **2020**. [CrossRef]
37. Cai, Q.; Yang, M.; Liu, D.; Chen, J.; Shu, D.; Xia, J.; Liao, X.; Gu, Y.; Cai, Q.; Yang, Y.; et al. Experimental Treatment with Favipiravir for COVID-19: An Open-Label Control Study. *Engineering* **2020**. [CrossRef]
38. Chen, C.; Zhang, Y.; Huang, J.; Yin, P.; Cheng, Z.; Wu, J.; Chen, S.; Zhang, Y.; Chen, B.; Lu, M.; et al. Favipiravir versus Arbidol for COVID-19: A Randomized Clinical Trial. *medRxiv* **2020**. [CrossRef]
39. Sheahan, T.P.; Sims, A.C.; Zhou, S.; Graham, R.L.; Pruijssers, A.J.; Agostini, M.L.; Leist, S.R.; Schafer, A.; Dinnon, K.H., 3rd; Stevens, L.J.; et al. An orally bioavailable broad-spectrum antiviral inhibits SARS-CoV-2 in human airway epithelial cell cultures and multiple coronaviruses in mice. *Sci. Transl. Med.* **2020**, *12*. [CrossRef]
40. Cao, B.; Wang, Y.; Wen, D.; Liu, W.; Wang, J.; Fan, G.; Ruan, L.; Song, B.; Cai, Y.; Wei, M.; et al. A Trial of Lopinavir-Ritonavir in Adults Hospitalized with Severe Covid-19. *N. Engl. J. Med.* **2020**, *382*, 1787–1799. [CrossRef]
41. Deng, L.; Li, C.; Zeng, Q.; Liu, X.; Li, X.; Zhang, H.; Hong, Z.; Xia, J. Arbidol combined with LPV/r versus LPV/r alone against Corona Virus Disease 2019: A retrospective cohort study. *J. Infect.* **2020**, *81*, e1–e5. [CrossRef] [PubMed]
42. Zhu, Z.; Lu, Z.; Xu, T.; Chen, C.; Yang, G.; Zha, T.; Lu, J.; Xue, Y. Arbidol monotherapy is superior to lopinavir/ritonavir in treating COVID-19. *J. Infect.* **2020**, *81*, e21–e23. [CrossRef] [PubMed]
43. Touret, F.; Gilles, M.; Barral, K.; Nougairède, A.; Decroly, E.; de Lamballerie, X.; Coutard, B. In vitro screening of a FDA approved chemical library reveals potential inhibitors of SARS-CoV-2 replication. *bioRxiv* **2020**. [CrossRef]
44. Gautret, P.; Lagier, J.C.; Parola, P.; Hoang, V.T.; Meddeb, L.; Sevestre, J.; Mailhe, M.; Doudier, B.; Aubry, C.; Amrane, S.; et al. Clinical and microbiological effect of a combination of hydroxychloroquine and azithromycin in 80 COVID-19 patients with at least a six-day follow up: A pilot observational study. *Travel Med. Infect. Dis.* **2020**, *34*, 101663. [CrossRef] [PubMed]
45. Caly, L.; Druce, J.D.; Catton, M.G.; Jans, D.A.; Wagstaff, K.M. The FDA-approved drug ivermectin inhibits the replication of SARS-CoV-2 in vitro. *Antiviral Res.* **2020**, *178*, 104787. [CrossRef]
46. Zhang, J.; Ma, X.; Yu, F.; Liu, J.; Zou, F.; Pan, T.; Zhang, H. Teicoplanin potently blocks the cell entry of 2019-nCoV. *bioRxiv* **2020**. [CrossRef]
47. Plantone, D.; Koudriavtseva, T. Current and Future Use of Chloroquine and Hydroxychloroquine in Infectious, Immune, Neoplastic, and Neurological Diseases: A Mini-Review. *Clin. Drug Investig.* **2018**, *38*, 653–671. [CrossRef]
48. Marmor, M.F.; Kellner, U.; Lai, T.Y.; Melles, R.B.; Mieler, W.F.; American Academy of, O. Recommendations on Screening for Chloroquine and Hydroxychloroquine Retinopathy (2016 Revision). *Ophthalmology* **2016**, *123*, 1386–1394. [CrossRef]
49. Savarino, A.; Boelaert, J.R.; Cassone, A.; Majori, G.; Cauda, R. Effects of chloroquine on viral infections: An old drug against today's diseases? *Lancet Infect. Dis.* **2003**, *3*, 722–727. [CrossRef]
50. Yao, X.; Ye, F.; Zhang, M.; Cui, C.; Huang, B.; Niu, P.; Liu, X.; Zhao, L.; Dong, E.; Song, C.; et al. In Vitro Antiviral Activity and Projection of Optimized Dosing Design of Hydroxychloroquine for the Treatment of Severe Acute Respiratory Syndrome Coronavirus 2 (SARS-CoV-2). *Clin. Infect. Dis.* **2020**, *71*, 732–739. [CrossRef]
51. Gao, J.; Tian, Z.; Yang, X. Breakthrough: Chloroquine phosphate has shown apparent efficacy in treatment of COVID-19 associated pneumonia in clinical studies. *Biosci. Trends* **2020**, *14*, 72–73. [CrossRef] [PubMed]
52. Garcia-Cremades, M.; Solans, B.P.; Hughes, E.; Ernest, J.P.; Wallender, E.; Aweeka, F.; Luetkemeyer, A.; Savic, R.M. Optimizing hydroxychloroquine dosing for patients with COVID-19: An integrative modeling approach for effective drug repurposing. *Clin. Pharmacol. Ther.* **2020**, *108*, 253–263. [CrossRef] [PubMed]
53. Touret, F.; de Lamballerie, X. Of chloroquine and COVID-19. *Antiviral Res.* **2020**, *177*, 104762. [CrossRef] [PubMed]
54. Mulangu, S.; Dodd, L.E.; Davey, R.T., Jr.; Tshiani Mbaya, O.; Proschan, M.; Mukadi, D.; Lusakibanza Manzo, M.; Nzolo, D.; Tshomba Oloma, A.; Ibanda, A.; et al. A Randomized, Controlled Trial of Ebola Virus Disease Therapeutics. *N. Engl. J. Med.* **2019**, *381*, 2293–2303. [CrossRef] [PubMed]

55. Gordon, C.J.; Tchesnokov, E.P.; Woolner, E.; Perry, J.K.; Feng, J.Y.; Porter, D.P.; Gotte, M. Remdesivir is a direct-acting antiviral that inhibits RNA-dependent RNA polymerase from severe acute respiratory syndrome coronavirus 2 with high potency. *J. Biol. Chem.* **2020**, *295*, 6785–6797. [CrossRef] [PubMed]
56. Gao, Y.; Yan, L.; Huang, Y.; Liu, F.; Zhao, Y.; Cao, L.; Wang, T.; Sun, Q.; Ming, Z.; Zhang, L.; et al. Structure of RNA-dependent RNA polymerase from 2019-nCoV, a major antiviral drug target. *bioRxiv* **2020**. [CrossRef]
57. Hillaker, E.; Belfer, J.J.; Bondici, A.; Murad, H.; Dumkow, L.E. Delayed Initiation of Remdesivir in a COVID-19 Positive Patient. *Pharmacotherapy* **2020**, *40*, 592–598. [CrossRef]
58. Wang, Y.; Zhang, D.; Du, G.; Du, R.; Zhao, J.; Jin, Y.; Fu, S.; Gao, L.; Cheng, Z.; Lu, Q.; et al. Remdesivir in adults with severe COVID-19: A randomised, double-blind, placebo-controlled, multicentre trial. *Lancet* **2020**, *395*, 1569–1578. [CrossRef]
59. Tu, Y.F.; Chien, C.S.; Yarmishyn, A.A.; Lin, Y.Y.; Luo, Y.H.; Lin, Y.T.; Lai, W.Y.; Yang, D.M.; Chou, S.J.; Yang, Y.P.; et al. A Review of SARS-CoV-2 and the Ongoing Clinical Trials. *Int. J. Mol. Sci.* **2020**, *21*, 2657. [CrossRef]
60. Rossignol, J.F. Nitazoxanide, a new drug candidate for the treatment of Middle East respiratory syndrome coronavirus. *J. Infect. Public Health* **2016**, *9*, 227–230. [CrossRef]
61. Damle, B.; Vourvahis, M.; Wang, E.; Leaney, J.; Corrigan, B. Clinical Pharmacology Perspectives on the Antiviral Activity of Azithromycin and Use in COVID-19. *Clin. Pharmacol. Ther.* **2020**, *108*, 201–211. [CrossRef] [PubMed]
62. Chaccour, C.; Hammann, F.; Ramon-Garcia, S.; Rabinovich, N.R. Ivermectin and Novel Coronavirus Disease (COVID-19): Keeping Rigor in Times of Urgency. *Am. J. Trop. Med. Hyg.* 2020. [CrossRef]
63. Chaccour, C.; Hammann, F.; Rabinovich, N.R. Ivermectin to reduce malaria transmission I. Pharmacokinetic and pharmacodynamic considerations regarding efficacy and safety. *Malar. J.* **2017**, *16*, 161. [CrossRef] [PubMed]
64. Bernareggi, A.; Borghi, A.; Borgonovi, M.; Cavenaghi, L.; Ferrari, P.; Vekey, K.; Zanol, M.; Zerilli, L.F. Teicoplanin metabolism in humans. *Antimicrob. Agents Chemother.* **1992**, *36*, 1744–1749. [CrossRef] [PubMed]
65. Baron, S.A.; Devaux, C.; Colson, P.; Raoult, D.; Rolain, J.M. Teicoplanin: An alternative drug for the treatment of COVID-19? *Int. J. Antimicrob. Agents* **2020**, 105944. [CrossRef]
66. Bleasel, M.D.; Peterson, G.M. Emetine, Ipecac, Ipecac Alkaloids and Analogues as Potential Antiviral Agents for Coronaviruses. *Pharmaceuticals* **2020**, *13*, 51. [CrossRef]
67. Huang, C.; Wang, Y.; Li, X.; Ren, L.; Zhao, J.; Hu, Y.; Zhang, L.; Fan, G.; Xu, J.; Gu, X.; et al. Clinical features of patients infected with 2019 novel coronavirus in Wuhan, China. *Lancet* **2020**, *395*, 497–506. [CrossRef]
68. Treon, S.P.; Castillo, J.; Skarbnik, A.P.; Soumerai, J.D.; Ghobrial, I.M.; Guerrera, M.L.; Meid, K.E.; Yang, G. The BTK-inhibitor ibrutinib may protect against pulmonary injury in COVID-19 infected patients. *Blood* **2020**, *135*, 1912–1915. [CrossRef]
69. Liu, X.; Li, Z.; Liu, S.; Sun, J.; Chen, Z.; Jiang, M.; Zhang, Q.; Wei, Y.; Wang, X.; Huang, Y.Y.; et al. Potential therapeutic effects of dipyridamole in the severely ill patients with COVID-19. *Acta Pharm. Sin. B* 2020. [CrossRef]
70. Luo, H.; Tang, Q.-L.; Shang, Y.-X.; Liang, S.-B.; Yang, M.; Robinson, N.; Liu, J.-P. Can Chinese Medicine Be Used for Prevention of Corona Virus Disease 2019 (COVID-19)? A Review of Historical Classics, Research Evidence and Current Prevention Programs. *Chin. J. Integr. Med.* **2020**, *26*, 243–250. [CrossRef]
71. Ang, L.; Lee, H.W.; Choi, J.Y.; Zhang, J.; Soo Lee, M. Herbal medicine and pattern identification for treating COVID-19: A rapid review of guidelines. *Integr. Med. Res.* **2020**, *9*, 100407. [CrossRef] [PubMed]
72. Yang, Y.; Islam, M.S.; Wang, J.; Li, Y.; Chen, X. Traditional Chinese Medicine in the Treatment of Patients Infected with 2019-New Coronavirus (SARS-CoV-2): A Review and Perspective. *Int. J. Biol. Sci.* **2020**, *16*, 1708–1717. [CrossRef] [PubMed]
73. Chan, K.W.; Wong, V.T.; Tang, S.C.W. COVID-19: An Update on the Epidemiological, Clinical, Preventive and Therapeutic Evidence and Guidelines of Integrative Chinese-Western Medicine for the Management of 2019 Novel Coronavirus Disease. *Am. J. Chin. Med.* **2020**, *48*, 737–762. [CrossRef] [PubMed]
74. Ren, X.; Shao, X.X.; Li, X.X.; Jia, X.H.; Song, T.; Zhou, W.Y.; Wang, P.; Li, Y.; Wang, X.L.; Cui, Q.H.; et al. Identifying potential treatments of COVID-19 from Traditional Chinese Medicine (TCM) by using a data-driven approach. *J. Ethnopharmacol.* **2020**, *258*, 112932. [CrossRef]

75. Runfeng, L.; Yunlong, H.; Jicheng, H.; Weiqi, P.; Qinhai, M.; Yongxia, S.; Chufang, L.; Jin, Z.; Zhenhua, J.; Haiming, J.; et al. Lianhuaqingwen exerts anti-viral and anti-inflammatory activity against novel coronavirus (SARS-CoV-2). *Pharmacol. Res.* **2020**, *156*, 104761. [CrossRef]
76. Ni, L.; Zhou, L.; Zhou, M.; Zhao, J.; Wang, D.W. Combination of western medicine and Chinese traditional patent medicine in treating a family case of COVID-19 in Wuhan. *Front. Med.* **2020**, *14*, 210–214. [CrossRef]
77. Ren, J.L.; Zhang, A.H.; Wang, X.J. Traditional Chinese medicine for COVID-19 treatment. *Pharmacol. Res.* **2020**, *155*, 104743. [CrossRef]
78. Liu, H.; Ye, F.; Sun, Q.; Liang, H.; Li, C.; Lu, R.; Huang, B.; Tan, W.; Lai, L. Scutellaria baicalensis extract and baicalein inhibit replication of SARS-CoV-2 and its 3C-like protease in vitro. *bioRxiv* **2020**. [CrossRef]
79. Ho, L.T.F.; Chan, K.K.H.; Chung, V.C.H.; Leung, T.H. Highlights of traditional Chinese medicine frontline expert advice in the China national guideline for COVID-19. *Eur. J. Integr. Med.* **2020**, *36*, 101116. [CrossRef]
80. Ye, Y.-A. Guideline-based Chinese herbal medicine treatment plus standard care for severe coronavirus disease 2019 (G-CHAMPS): Evidence from China. *medRxiv* **2020**. [CrossRef]
81. Su, H.; Yao, S.; Zhao, W.; Li, M.; Liu, J.; Shang, W.; Xie, H.; Ke, C.; Gao, M.; Yu, K.; et al. Discovery of baicalin and baicalein as novel, natural product inhibitors of SARS-CoV-2 3CL protease in vitro. *bioRxiv* **2020**. [CrossRef]
82. Lu, C.C.; Chen, M.Y.; Chang, Y.L. Potential therapeutic agents against COVID-19: What we know so far. *J. Chin. Med. Assoc.* **2020**. [CrossRef] [PubMed]
83. Forster, P.; Forster, L.; Renfrew, C.; Forster, M. Phylogenetic network analysis of SARS-CoV-2 genomes. *Proc. Natl. Acad. Sci. USA* **2020**, *117*, 9241–9243. [CrossRef] [PubMed]
84. Pushpakom, S.; Iorio, F.; Eyers, P.A.; Escott, K.J.; Hopper, S.; Wells, A.; Doig, A.; Guilliams, T.; Latimer, J.; McNamee, C.; et al. Drug repurposing: Progress, challenges and recommendations. *Nat. Rev. Drug Discov.* **2019**, *18*, 41–58. [CrossRef]
85. Senanayake, S.L. Drug repurposing strategies for COVID-19. *Future Drug Discov.* **2020**, *2*. [CrossRef]
86. Zhang, K. Is traditional Chinese medicine useful in the treatment of COVID-19? *Am. J. Emerg. Med.* **2020**. [CrossRef]

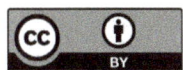

© 2020 by the authors. Licensee MDPI, Basel, Switzerland. This article is an open access article distributed under the terms and conditions of the Creative Commons Attribution (CC BY) license (http://creativecommons.org/licenses/by/4.0/).

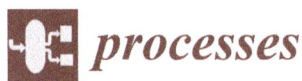

Review

Conventional and Emerging Extraction Processes of Flavonoids

Mónica L. Chávez-González [1,*], Leonardo Sepúlveda [1], Deepak Kumar Verma [2], Hugo A. Luna-García [1], Luis V. Rodríguez-Durán [3], Anna Ilina [1] and Cristobal N. Aguilar [1,*]

[1] Bioprocesses and Bioproducts Research Group, Food Research Department, School of Chemistry, Universidad Autónoma de Coahuila, 25280 Saltillo, Mexico; leonardo_sepulveda@uadec.edu.mx (L.S.); hugoluna@uadec.edu.mx (H.A.L.-G.); annailina@uadec.edu.mx (A.I.)

[2] Agricultural and Food Engineering Department, Indian Institute of Technology Kharagpur, Kharagpur 721302, India; deepak.verma@agfe.iitkgp.ernet.in

[3] Department of Biochemical Engineering, Unidad Académica Multidisciplinaria Mante, Universidad Autónoma de Tamaulipas, 89840 Ciudad Mante, Mexico; luis.duran@docentes.uat.edu.mx

* Correspondence: monicachavez@uadec.edu.mx (M.L.C.-G.); cristobal.aguilar@uadec.edu.mx (C.N.A.); Tel.: +52-844-416-1238 (M.L.C.-G.)

Received: 14 January 2020; Accepted: 24 February 2020; Published: 7 April 2020

Abstract: Flavonoids are a group of plant constituents called phenolic compounds and correspond to the nonenergy part of the human diet. Flavonoids are found in vegetables, seeds, fruits, and beverages such as wine and beer. Over 7000 flavonoids have been identified and they have been considered substances with a beneficial action on human health, particularly of multiple positive effects because of their antioxidant and free radical scavenging action. Although several studies indicate that some flavonoids have provident actions, they occur only at high doses, confirming in most investigations the existence of anti-inflammatory effects, antiviral or anti-allergic, and their protective role against cardiovascular disease, cancer, and various pathologies. Flavonoids are generally removed by chemical methods using solvents and traditional processes, which besides being expensive, involve long periods of time and affect the bioactivity of such compounds. Recently, efforts to develop biotechnological strategies to reduce or eliminate the use of toxic solvents have been reported, reducing processing time and maintaining the bioactivity of the compounds. In this paper, we review, analyze, and discuss methodologies for biotechnological recovery/extraction of flavonoids from agro-industrial residues, describing the advances and challenges in the topic.

Keywords: flavonoids; extraction methods; biotransformation; human health

---

1. Introduction

Flavonoids are natural pigments present in the plant or microbial sources and correspond to a specific group of chemical constituents called phenolic compounds [1,2]. They are found in vegetables, seeds, fruit, and various fruits and alcoholic beverages [3]. Flavonoids have important positive effects on human health especially due to their antioxidant and free radical scavenging. Although several studies have shown that some flavonoids have a pro-oxidant effect, they only occur at high doses, most of which confirm the existence of anti-inflammatory effects, antiviral or anti-allergic, and their protective role against cardiovascular disease, cancer, and various pathologies [2,4].

Flavonoids protect the human body from damage caused by oxidizing agents such as ultraviolet rays, environmental pollution, food chemicals, etc. The human organism cannot produce these chemicals in a protective manner, so they must be obtained by means of feed or as supplements. These compounds have been discovered by Nobel Prize winner Szent-György, who in 1930 isolated a substance, citrine, which regulates the permeability of the capillaries from the lemon peels. Flavonoids were first identified as vitamin P (because of the ability to increase capillary permeability) and vitamin C2 (because some flavonoids had similar properties to vitamin C) [1]. However, the fact that flavonoids were vitamins could not be confirmed, and both names remain around 1950. Flavonoids contain in their chemical structure a variable number of phenolic hydroxyl groups and excellent properties of iron chelation and other transition metals, which give them a high antioxidant capacity; therefore, they play an essential role in the protection against oxidative damage and have therapeutic effects in a wide range of conditions, including heart disease ischemic, or atherosclerosis cancer [5–7]. Antifree radical properties of flavonoids are primarily aimed at hydroxyl and superoxide radicals, highly reactive species involved in the onset of lipid chain peroxidation and described their ability to modify eicosanoid synthesis (with antiprostanoid and anti-inflammatory reactions) to prevent platelet aggregation (antithrombotic effects) and to protect low-density lipoproteins from oxidation [8,9].

In addition to its known antioxidant effects, flavonoids have other properties, including stimulation of communication through gap junctions, effects on the regulation of cell growth and induction of enzymes, detoxification such as dependent monooxygenase Cytochrome P-450, among others. [10]. However, most of the biological properties of flavonoids are strongly determined by the mode of extraction for their recovery. Efforts have recently been reported to develop biotechnological strategies to reduce or eliminate the use of toxic solvents, reduce processing time, and maintain the bioactivity of the compounds. This paper examines, analyzes, and discusses the biotechnological methodologies and the recovery/extraction of flavonoids from agro-industrial residues, describing the advances and challenges in the field.

2. Flavonoids

Flavonoids are a type of polyphenolic compound, its chemical structure is varied but the general skeleton structure is composed of 15 carbones (C_6-C_3-C_6), which are grouped in two aromatic rings (A and B) connected by a 3-carbon bridge that gives rise to an oxygenated heterocycle (C) [11–15] (Figure 1). Flavonoids are derivatives of 1, 3-diphenylpropan-1-one and their biosynthetic pathway is the condensation of three malonyl-CoA molecules with one p-coumaroyl-CoA molecule to the intermediate chalcone [16,17]. Flavonoids are water-soluble pigments present in the plant kingdom as secondary plant metabolites [2,18,19], which can be found specifically in the cytosol and stored in the plant cell vacuole [12,17].

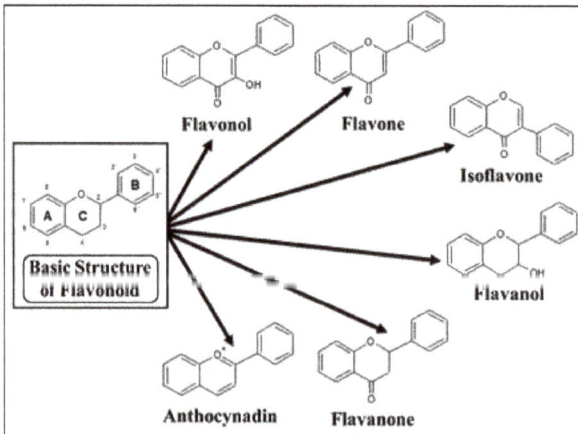

Figure 1. Basic chemical structures of flavonoids and their different class.

Flavonoids are classified according to differences in the structure of the heterocyclic C ring; these differences may be caused by the oxidation state and the degree of unsaturation of the heterocyclic ring (or the lack thereof in the case of chalcones). It has been estimated that the number of identified flavonoids exceeds 7000 and that the number of flavonoids continues to increase due to their important biological activities [17]. Variations in the basic structure of flavonoids give rise to six different classes of this group of compounds: Isoflavones, flavanone, flavanone, flavan-3-ol, flavonol, and anthocyanidin, each of which has particular characteristics [18,20].

2.1. Flavanones

Flavanones (dihydroflavones) have a structure that differs in the lack of a double bond (C_2-C_3) in the C-ring of the flavonoid structure. This type of flavonoid can be found in aromatic plants (such as mint), tomatoes, citrus (especially grapefruit) [12]. Flavanones can be found in nature as forms of aglycones and glycosides, some examples of such compounds are naringenin, hesperetin, and eriodictyol [21].

2.2. Flavonols

Flavonols are called 3-hydroxyflavones and are the most commonly found flavonoids in the plant kingdom [22]. A double bond between C_2 and C_3 and a hydroxyl group is included in their structures [13]. Some of the most important phytochemical compounds that represent this group are as follows: Myricetin, quercetin, isorhamnetin, and kaempferol [12,22,23]. They can be found in a variety of colors (from white to yellow). In nature, flavonols can be found in two forms: Glycosides and aglycone (quercetin and kaempferol) [12].

2.3. Flavones

Flavones can be found in all parts of the plants, above-and belowground, in vegetative and generative organs; stem, leaves, buds, bark, heartwood, thorns, roots, rhizomes, flowers, farina, fruit, seeds, and also in root and leaf exudates or resin. They result from the introduction of a double bond between C_2 and C_3 by the abstraction of two hydrogen atoms [16,18]. Flavones are present in all major land-plant lineages. The plant species that contain flavones belong to over 70 different families in the plant kingdom [16].

2.4. Anthocyanins

Anthocyanins are primarily found in nature in glycosidic form. This type of flavonoid is responsible for plant pigment (such as blue, red, pink, and purple) by the formation of weak covalent bonding complexes with other organic compounds [23,24]. More than 500 anthocyanins have been reported and are the product of methoxylation, hydroxylation, and glycosylation patterns in the B ring. The most representative compounds of this subclass of flavonoids are pelargonidin, cyanidin, and delphinidin [12].

2.5. Flavanols

Flavanols (flavan-3-ols) are also called catechins, which have a typical flavonoid structure but have different hydroxylation patterns of rings A and B and asymmetrical carbon stereochemistry of ring C (C_2 and C_3) [25,26]. The catechins are classified into two groups; free catechins and esterified catechins [27], and constitute the most complex class of flavonoids due to their size, monomers (catechin), or polymeric forms (condensed tannins) [21]. They can be found as the main ingredient in green tea [12].

2.6. Isoflavones

Another type of flavonoids, isoflavones are commonly referred to as phytoestrogens due to their considerable estrogen activity. They are characterized by the fusion of their ring B with the C_3 position of the ring C [21,28–30]. They are an important group in a variety of fields, such as medicine, cosmetics, and nutrition. These flavonoids can be found in plants of the Leguminosae family (soybeans, alfalfa sprouts, and red clover leaves) [30,31].

3. Isolation and Extraction Methods

There is a general methodology consisting of three stages for the isolation, extraction, and identification of phytochemicals from natural sources. Pretreatment or preparation of a sample is the first step in which the centrifuge, filtration, or drying process and others can be used. In the second stage, the extraction, isolation, and purification of flavonoid compounds from different plant samples are most notably. In this step, phytochemicals are extracted using processes such as soxhlet, maceration, water infusion, supercritical fluid extraction, solid microphase extraction, microwave extraction, ultrasound, autohydrolysis, etc. In the last step, the purified and extracted extracts are normally used for further study by chromatography techniques, usually involving the identification, quantification, and recovery of flavonoid compounds.

Details of each method, such as conventional and emerging methods used by a number of researchers for flavonoid extraction, are given in the following sections:

3.1. Conventional Methods

Flavonoid extraction and recovery have been booming over recent years because of population trends in healthier lifestyles and the integration of antioxidants into the diet. Therefore, several methods for extracting flavonoids to increase the extraction yields of these major bioactive compounds have been implemented.

Various extractive methods have been proposed, including maceration, percolation, hydro-distillation, boiling, reflux, soaking, and soxhlet [32]. Soxhlet was the most commonly used method for the extraction of flavonoids due to its simplicity and ease of maintenance, low cost, and lower solvent content compared to other methods such as soaking, boiling, or maceration [14,33,34]. Various solvents such as ethanol, methanol, benzene, chloroform, ethyl acetate, etc. have been tested in this extraction method to compare the effect on extraction yields [15,32].

In general, liquid–liquid or solid–liquid extraction is the most widely used process for the extraction of flavonoids. Although maceration and water infusion are conventional extraction processes, they are still used today [35,36]. These methodologies have adopted the use of solvents such as ethanol, methanol, acetone and not just water for the extraction of bioactive compounds [14,37,38]. These conventional extraction methods are characterized by the use of large amounts of solvent, lower extraction yields, and long extraction times compared to other methods. It has been reported that when extraction methodologies involve heat treatments, degradation in the chemical structures of the extracted flavonoids can result in a reduction in bioactivity [39].

Parameters such as time, particle size, type of solvents, mass to volume ratio, temperature, etc. have been evaluated in conventional extraction methods of flavonoid (Table 1) [40–42]. The nature of the extracting agent (solvent) will affect the type of flavonoid extracted and will directly influence the biological activity of the recovered compounds. Of the solvents tested, ethanol and methanol are the most widely used for the extraction of flavonoids due to higher yields achieved in the recovery of flavonoids [13,14].

Table 1. Summary of studies of isolation and extraction of flavonoids from different plant sources.

Type	Substrate	Solvent	Temperature (°C)	Time	Analysis	Yields	Bioactivities/ Bioactives	References
ASE	*Impatiens glandulifera* (roots)	Methanol (80%)	80	30 min	LC-MS	257.34 µg PAC/g of dw	Phenolic acid content	[45]
ASE	*Impatiens glandulifera* (flowers)	Methanol (80%)	80	30 min	LC-MS	188.86 µg PAC/g of dw	Phenolic acid content	[45]
ASE	Broccoli	Acetone/water/ acetic acid (70:29,5:0.5 $v/v/v$)	70–80	5 min	-	3377 ± 62 mg GAE/100 g edp	AoA	[46]
ASE	Cabbage common	Acetone/water/ acetic acid (70:29,5:0.5 $v/v/v$)	70–80	5 min	-	2037 ± 31 mg GAE/100 g edp	AoA	[46]
ASE	Cabbage red	Acetone/water/ acetic acid (70:29,5:0.5 $v/v/v$)	70–80	5 min	-	2547 ± 18 mg GAE/100 g edp	AoA	[46]
ASE	*Cauliflower*	Acetone/water/ acetic acid (70:29,5:0.5 $v/v/v$)	70–80	5 min	-	274 mg GAE/100 g edp	AoA	[46]
ASE	*Lepidium sativum*	Ethanol (96%)	50	5 min	GC-MS	58 mg RuE/g dm of flavonoid content	AmA and CtA	[47]
ASE	*Impatiens glandulifera* (leaves)	Methanol (80%)	80	30 min	LC-MS	244.73 µg PAC/g of dw	Phenolic acid content	[45]
HWE	Pine (*Pinus rigida* × *taeda* and *Pinus koraiensis*) bark	Boiling water	100	1 h	-	111–862 mg CAE/g dw	AoA	[48]
Maceration	Broccoli	Acetone/water (70:30 v/v)	4	24 h	LC-MS	82.2 ± 8.9 mg GAE/100 g edp	AoA	[49]
Maceration	Cauliflower	Acetone/water (70:30 v/v)	4	24 h	LC-MS	27.8 ± 71.5 mg GAE/100 g edp	AoA	[49]
Maceration	Chinese cabbage	Acetone/water (70:30 v/v)	4	24 h	LC-MS	118.9 ± 712.5 mg GAE/100 g edp	AoA	[49]
Maceration	White cabbage	Acetone/water (70:30 v/v)	4	24 h	LC-MS	15.37 ± 2.1 mg GAE/100 g edp	AoA	[49]
Maceration	Broccoli	Acetone/water (80:20 v/v)	Room temperature	8 min	-	80.87 ± 1.2 mg GAE/100 g edp	AoA and ApA	[50]
Maceration	Cabbage	Acetone/water (80:20 v/v)	Room temperature	8 min	-	36.77 ± 6.9 mg GAE/100 g edp	AoA and ApA	[50]
Maceration	Broccoli	Methanol/water (80/20 v/v)	Room temperature	-	-	34.571.0 mg GAE/100 g edp	AoA	[51]
Maceration	*Solanum scabrum* leaves	Acetone	-	72 h	-	34.2 g GAE/100g	AoA	[52]
Maceration	*Lepidium sativum*	Ethanol (96%)	50	24 h	GC-MS	25 mg RuE/g dw	AmA and CtA	[47]
Maceration	Banana	Water	-	-	-	8.51 µg QuE/g dw	AoA	[42]
Maceration	Pitanga	Ethanol (75%) and Hexane	25	4 h	-	232.2 mg GAE/g and 12.4 mg GAE/g dw, respectively	AoA and AbA	[53]
Maceration	*Artocarpus heterophyllus* wastes	Ethanol (70%) and ethanol pure	25	72 h	LC-MS	871.4 mg QuF/g dw	AoA	[44]
Maceration	Kinnow mandarin	Methanol (80%)	-	-	LC-MS	28.40 mg GAF/g dw	AoA and AmA	[41]
Maceration	Apple tree wood residues	50% Ethanol	55	2 h	LC-PdAD	43.2 mg GAE/g dw	Food, pharmaceutical and cosmetic applications	[54]
Maceration	*Pinus radiata* bark	Acetone:water 70:30 v/v	40	180 min	-	412 ± 0 mg CAE/g	ArA	[55]
Maceration	*Quercus* (*Q. robur* L.) bark	Water	25	120 min	-	3.7 ± 0.6 mg GAE/g	AoA and AbA	[56]
Maceration	Chokeberry (*Aronia melanocarpa*)	50% Ethanol. Ratio 1:20	Ambient temperature	60 min	LC-MS	27.7 mg GAE/g dw	Extraction of bioactive compounds	[35]

Table 1. Cont.

Type	Substrate	Solvent	Temperature (°C)	Time	Analysis	Yields	Bioactivities/Bioactives	References
Percolation	Artocarpus heterophyllus wastes	Ethanol (70%)	25	1 h	LC-MS	511.6 mg QuE/g dw	AoA	[44]
Reflux	Portulaca oleracea L.	Ethanol–water (70:30, v/v)	-	150 min	-	6.8 mg RuE/g	Flavonoid content	[57]
RSlSE	Tomatoes	Ethanol (60%)	Room temperature	15 h	HPLC	602.91 mg GAE/100 g dw (TPC)	AoA	[58]
SDE	Dried leaves of basil (Ocimum basilicum L.), and epazote (Chenopodium ambrosioides L.).	Water	-	30 min	GC-MS	0.47 y 0.39% yield of EO from basil and epazote	Essential oil extraction	[59]
SlE	Vitis vinifera waste	Methanol or with ethanol	25	19 h	HPLC	67.88 mg GAE/g dw	ArA	[60]
Soxhlet	Portulaca oleracea L.	Ethanol–water (70:30, v/v)	-	300 min	-	7.0 mg RuE/g	Flavonoid content	[57]
Soxhlet	Buddleia officinalis Maxim	Ethanol (95%)	-	2 h	-	62.56 mg CAE/g dw	AoA	[61]
Soxhlet	Morus nigra (dried)	Petroleum ether	50	3 h	-	58.94% of flavonoid yield	AoA	[62]
Soxhlet	Fresh leaves of Vernoniaamygdalina	Water	100	8 h	GC-MS	-	AoA	[63]
Soxhlet	Vernonia cinerea leaves	Ethanol (60%)	-	2 h	LC–Q-TOF-MS	26.22 mg QuE/g dw	AoA	[32]
Soxhlet	Artocarpus heterophyllus wastes	Ethanol (70% and pure)	Boiling point	5 h	LC-MS	381.4 mg QuE/g dw	AoA	[44]
Soxhlet	Impatiens glandulifera (leaves)	Chloroform, 80% Methanol and pure Methanol	-	72 h	LC-ESI-MS	286.39 mg PAC/g dw	AoA	[45]
Soxhlet	Impatiens glandulifera (roots)	Chloroform, 80% Methanol and pure Methanol	-	72 h	LC-MS	281.82 mg PAC/g dw	AoA	[45]
Soxhlet	Impatiens glandulifera (flowers)	Chloroform, 80% Methanol and pure Methanol	-	72 h	LC-MS	188.07 mg PAC/g dw	AoA	[45]
Soxhlet	Pinus radiata bark	Acetone:water 70:30 v/v	82	60, 120, 180, and 360 min	-	622 ± 40 mg CAE/g	ArA	[55]
Soxhlet	Spearmint (Mentha spicata L.)	Methanol	40	6 h	HPLC	0.144 mg CAE/g dw	Flavonoid extraction	[64]
Soxhlet	Knotwood (Populus tremula)	Methanol	-	48 h	LC-MS	11.5 mg/g	Flavonoid extraction	[65]

Abbreviations: AbA: Antibacterial activity; AmA: Antimicrobial activity; AoA: Antioxidant activity; ApA: Antiproliferative activities; ArA: Antiradical activity; ASE: Accelerated solvent extraction; CAE: Catechin equivalents; CtA: Cytotoxicity activity; dm: Dry matter; dw: Dry weight; edp: Edible portion; ESI: Electrospray ion source; GAE: Gallic acid equivalents; GC-MS: Gas chromatography mass spectrometer; HPLC: High performance liquid chromatography; HWE: Hot water extraction; LC: Liquid chromatography; LC-MS: Liquid chromatography mass spectrometer; MS: Mass spectrometer; PAC: Phenolic acid content; PDAD: Photodiode array detector; Q-TOF: Quadrupole-time of flight; QuE: Quercetin equivalents; RSlSE: Rotary solid–liquid solvent extraction as Traditional Method; RuE: Rutin equivalents; SDE: Steam distillation extraction; SlE: Solid–liquid extraction; TPC: Total phenolic content.

The high demand for antioxidants gave way to the search for methodological alternatives that would increase the yield of flavonoid extraction and reduce process costs. In addition, it has been found that the methodologies implemented are cleaner and environmentally friendly.

3.2. Emerging and Advanced Methods

Two of the most widely used techniques for the extraction of flavonoids are emerging microwave (MAE) and ultrasound-assisted extraction (UAE) technologies. Table 2 shows some of the published works on the extraction of flavonoids using these emerging methods.

Table 2. Studies on emerging methods of isolation and extraction of flavonoids from different plant sources.

Substrate	Extraction Conditions			Analysis	Bioactive	Bioactivity	References
	Solvent	Temperature (°C)	Time				
(A) *Microwave-Assisted Extraction*							
Fresh leaves of *Vernonia amygdalina*	Water	100	7 min	GC-MS	87.05 mg QuE/g total flavonoid content	AoA	[63]
Black rice (*Oryza* sativa cv. *Poireton*) husk	Ethanol 40%–70% (relation m/v (1:20, 1:35, 1:50)	40–60	20–60 s	HPLC	Gallic acid, *p*-coumaric acid, ferulic acid, quercetin, salicylic acid, quimic acid, apigenin, syringic acid, chlorogenic acid, catechin	AoA	[66]
Apple tree wood residues	Ethanol (60%)	100	20 min	HPLC-PdAD	47.7 mg GAE/g dw	Pharmaceutical and cosmetic applications	[54]
Moringa oleifera leaves	Water, ethanol:water, and etanol	50–180	3–20 min	HPLC–ESI-Q-TOF–MS	Quercetin sambubioside/ Quercetin-3-vicianoside, kaempferol diglycoside, multiflorin B, kaempferol-3-O-glucosidde, vitexin, quercetin-3-O-glucosidde, quercetin malonylglucoside, quercetin hydroxyl methylglutaroyl, glycoside, quercetin triacetylgalactoside, quercetin acetyl glycoside, isorhamnetin-3-O-glucoside, quercetin, kaempferol	AoA	[67]
Coriander (*Coriandrum sativum* L.) seeds	Ethanol (52%)		35 min	-	382.32 mg GAE/100 g dw	AoA	[68]
Quercus (*Q. robur* L) bark	Water	100	120 min	HPLC-PdAD-ESI-MS/MS	16.50 ± 0.07 mg GAE/dw	AoA	[69]
Canola seed cake	Ethanol (10%)	70	20 min	-	-	Polyphenols extraction	[70]
Tomatoes	Ethanol	Room temperature	10 min	HPLC	646.40 mg GAE/100 g dw (TPC)	AoA	[58]
Pinus radiata bark	acetone:water 70;30 v/v	-	3 min	-	479 ± 49 mg CAE/g dw	ArA	[55]
Grape skins	40% methanol	100	5 min	HPLC	1.858 mL AntE/g of MEC/MoS	Anthocyanins extraction	[71]
Uncaria sinensis	Ultra pure water	100	20 min	LC-MS	44 mg EpiCAE/100 g	Quality of medicinal herbs	[72]
Buddleia officinalis Maxim	Ethanol (65%–100%)	40–78	10–30 min	-	75.33 mg CAE/g dw	AoA	[61]

Table 2. *Cont.*

Substrate	Extraction Conditions			Analysis	Bioactive	Bioactivity	References
	Solvent	Temperature (°C)	Time				
(A) *Microwave-Assisted Extraction*							
Citrus unshiu	Ethanol (70%)	140	8 min	HPLC-PdAD	47.7 mg HspE/g of MEC/MoS	TpP	[73]
Defatted residue of yellow horn	Etanol (40%)	50	7 min, 3 extraction cycles	-	11.62% (triterpene saponins) MEAC × 100/MoS	Food and pharmaceutical industries	[74]
Peanut skins	Ethanol (30%)	-	30 s	HPLC and LC-MS–MS	144 mg PAC/g of MEC/MoS	AoA	[75]
Pigeonpea (*Cajanus cajan*) leaves	Ethanol (80%)	65	1 min (2 min total), 2 extraction cycles	RP-HPLC-PdAD	18.8 mg AAE/g and 3.5 mg PinE/g of MEC/MoS	TpP	[76]
Portulaca oleracea L.	Ethanol–water (70:30, v/v)	50	9 min	–	7.1 mg RuE/g	Flavonoid content	[57]
Purple corn	15 M HCl: 95% ethanol in 15:85 ratio	55	19 min	LC-MS	1.851 mg AntE/g of MEC/MoS	Anthocyanin extraction	[77]
Radix puerariae	Ethanol (70%)	-	6 min	-	8.37 mg RuE/g	Flavonoid content	[78]
Sea buckthorn (*Hippophae rhamnoides*) food by-products	Water	20–100	15 min	HPLC	Flavonol isorhamnetin 3O-rutinoside	AoA	[79]
Tea residues (oolong)	Water	230	2 min	GC-MS	144.0 mg GAE/g dw	AoA	[80]
Tea residues (green)	Water	230	2 min	GC-MS	87.2 mg GAE/g dw	AoA	[80]
Vitis vinifera seed	Methanol	110	60 min	HPLC	86.2 mg GAE/g and 46.8 mg CAE/g dw	ArA	[60]
Alpinia zerumbet (Pers.) Burtt et Smith leaves	Ethanol (70%)	60–70	3s	HPLC	11% w/w	Flavonoid extraction	[81]
Bark of *Phyllanthus emblica* L.	Aqueous ethanol (75%)	45	25 min	-	19.78 %	AoA	[82]
Citrus mandarin peels	Methanol (66%)	1–120	49 s	HPLC	3779.37 µg PAC/g of MEC/MoS	Phenolic acids extraction	[83]
Milk thistle seed	Ethanol (82%)	112	60 min	-	56.67 mg SilE/g of MEC/MoS	Silymarin extraction	[84]
Morus alba L. leaves	Ethanol (60%)	100	5 min	-	2.4% flavonoid	AfA	[85]
Onion (*Allium cepa* L.)	Methanol (80%)	2–100	Up to 60 min	HPLC	330.46 mg of flavonol content	Food application	[86]
Herba epimedii	Ethanol	-	-	HPLC	921 peak Area of total flavonoids	Flavonoid extraction	[87]
Myrica rubra leaves	-	60	20 min	HPLC	-	Polyphenol extraction	[88]
Radix astragali	Ethanol (90%)	110	50 min	HPLC	1.190 mg flavonoids/g	Flavonoid extraction	[89]
Radix astragali roots	Ethanol (90%)	110	25 min (50 min total), 2 extraction cycles	-	1.19 mg/g (flavonoids) of MEC/MoS	Flavonoid extraction	[89]

Table 2. Cont.

Substrate	Extraction Conditions			Analysis	Bioactive	Bioactivity	References
	Solvent	Temperature (°C)	Time				
(A) Microwave-Assisted Extraction							
Platycladus orientalis leaves	Methanol (80%)	-	5 min	-	1.72% (flavonoids) MEAC × 100/MoS	Flavonoid extraction	[90]
Epimedium koreamum Nakai	Ethanol (40%)	-	15 min	LC-ESI-MS	280 m AU/min	Flavonoid extraction	[91]
Olive leaves	Ethanol (80%)	-	8 min	HPLC- PdAD	95% (oleuropein) MEAC × 100/MTACcS	Biophenols extraction	[92]
Acanthopanax senticosusleaves	Ethanol (50%)	-	10 min	ESI-MS	-	Flavonoid extraction	[93]
Eucommia ulmodies oliv.	Methanol:water:acetic acid (20:80:1.0, v/v)	-	30–40 s	HPLC	75.6%–83.2% (geniposidic acid) and 77.4%–86.3% (chlorogenic acid) of MEAC × 100/MTACcS	TpP	[94]
Capsicum fruit	Acetone	-	15 min	GC-MS	0.48 mg CpE/g fw	Food aditives	[95]
(B) Ultrasound-Assisted Extraction							
Dysphania ambrosioides (L)	Ethanol (57% w/w)	57	60 min	-	1.09% of flavonoids equivalents of rutin	Flavonoid extraction	[96]
Lepidium sativum seeds	Ethanol	50	24 h	GC-MS	97 mg GAE/g dm	AmA and CtA	[47]
Fruit of rugose rose (Rosa rugose Thumb)	Ethanol (50%)	50	40 min	-	31.88 mg /g dw	AoA	[97]
Impatiens glandulifera (flowers)	Methanol (80 %)	30	60 min	LC-MS	216.03 µg/g dw	AoA	[45]
Impatiens glandulifera (leaves)	Methanol (80 %)	30	60 min	LC-MS	291.55 µg/g dw	AoA	[45]
Impatiens glandulifera (roots)	Methanol (80 %)	30	60 min	LC-MS	286.04 µg/g dw	AoA	[45]
Kinnow mandarin	Ethanol (80%)	35, 45, 55	40–70 min	HPLC	28.40 mg GAE/g extract	AoA and AmA	[41]
Nephelium lappaceum L. fruit peel	Solid–liquid ratio 1:18.6 g/mL		50	20 min	10.26 ± 0.69 mg AntE/100 g; 552.64 ± 1.57 mg GAE/100 g; 104 ± 1.13 mg RuE/100 g	Flavonoid extraction	[98]
Curry leaf (Murraya koenigii L.)	Methanol 80% 55.9% 145.49 W	55.9	-	UHP-LC	0.482 mg CAE/g dw; 0.517 mg NrgE/g dw; 0.394 mg QuE/g dw	Pharmaceutical application	[99]
Portulaca oleracea L	Ethanol 39.01%	55.25	15 min	-	16.25 mg RuE/g dw	-	[100]
Pinus radiata bark	acetone:water 70:30 v/v	-	3-12 min	-	388 ± 7 mg CAE/g bark	ArA	[55]
Morus laevigata W. M. alba L. and M. nigra L	Methanol (80%)	-	-	HPLC	3.89 to 11.79 µmoL GAE/100 g	AoA	[101]
Portulaca oleracea L.	Ethanol–water (70:30, v/v)	25	60 min	-	6.7 mg RuE/g	Flavonoid content	[57]
Vitis vinifera seed	Methanol	25	60 min	HPLC	55.9 mg GAE/g and 39.5 mg CAE/g dw	ArA	[60]

Table 2. Cont.

Substrate	Extraction Conditions			Analysis	Bioactive	Bioactivity	References
	Solvent	Temperature (°C)	Time				
(C) Supercritical Fluid Extraction							
Dried bilberry fruits (*V. myrtillus* L.)	CO_2 + Ethanol (10%)	-	30 min	HPLC-PdAD-ESI-MS/MS	0.52 mg AntE/g dw	AoA	[102]
Spearmint (*Mentha spicata* L.)	Absolute ethanol (EtOH) Flow rate: 3 g/min Pressure: 200 bar	60	60 min	HPLC	0.140 mg CAE/g dw	Bioactive flavonoid extraction	[64]
Pueraria lobata	Ethanol Flow rate: 3 g/min Pressure: 20.04 MPa	50.24	90 min	-	16.95 ± 0.43 mg flavonoid/g dw	Flavonoid extraction	[103]
Ganoderma atrum	CO_2 + ethanol Flow rate: 30 L/h (80 g sample) Pressure: 25 MPa	55	3 h	-	1.52% (triterpenoid saponins) MEAC × 100/MoS	Triterpenoid saponins extraction	[104]
Lepidium sativum	CO_2 + ethanol (96 %)	50	70 min	GC-MS MALDI-TOF-MS	58 mg RuE/g dm (Total flavonoid)	AmA and CtA	[47]

Abbreviations: AAE: Ajaninstilbene acid equivalents; AfA: Antifatigue activity; AmA: Antimicrobial activity; AntE: Anthocyanins equivalents; AoA: Antioxidant activity; ArA: Antiradical activity; CAE: Catechin equivalents; CpE: Capsaicin equivalents; CtA: Cytotoxicity activity; dm: Dry matter; dw: Dry weight; EpiCAE: Epicatechin equivalents; ESI: Electrospray ion source; GAE: Gallic acid equivalents; GC-MS: Gas chromatography mass spectrometer; HPLC: High performance liquid chromatography; HspE: Hesperidin equivalents; LC: Liquid chromatography; LC-MS: Liquid chromatography mass spectrometer; MAE: Microwave assisted extraction; MALDI: Matrix-assisted laser desorption ionization; MEAC: Mass of extracted active compound; MEC: Mass of extracted compound; MoS: Mass of sample; MS: Mass spectrometer; MTACcS: Mass of total active compound content in the sample; NrgE: Narengine equivalents; PAC: Phenolic acid content; PdAD: Photodiode array detector; PinE: Pinostrobin equivalents; Q-TOF: Quadrupole-time of flight; QuE: Quercetin equivalents; RP: Reversed-phase; RuE: Rutin equivalents; SilE: Silymarin equivalents; TOF: Time of flight; TPC: Total phenolic content; TpP: Therapeutic potential; UHP: Ultra high performance.

3.2.1. Microwave-Assisted Extraction

Microwave is an electromagnetic spectrum of radiation ranging from 300 MHz (radio radiation) to 300 GHz (infrared radiation). This heating technique uses microwave energy and is based on the direct effect of microwaves on dipole polarization and ion conduction molecules [105–107] (Figure 2). The extraction of flavonoids may be affected by a large number of parameters, among the most important of which are: Time, temperature, plant material-solvent ratio, solvent concentration, solvent polarity, irradiation, frequency of intensity, and microwave power [63,106,108–110].

It has been reported that MAE allows for a significant reduction in the extraction times of a wide variety of compounds, also reduces the volumes of solvents used, and it has been shown that the extraction yields of bioactive compounds are superior to conventional methods such as maceration, Soxhlet, or heat reflux [66,106,112,113]. Reduction of extraction times and the use of solvents are employed to improve the cost of extraction [39].

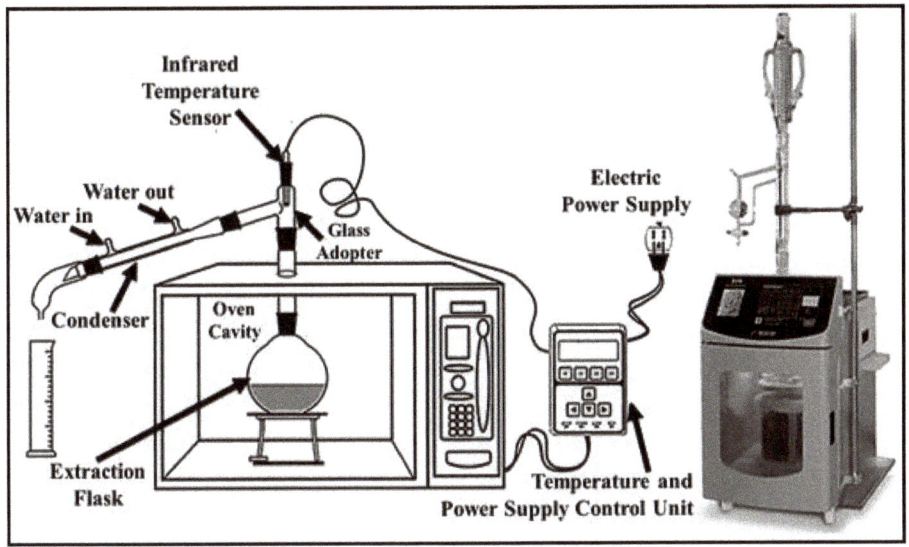

Figure 2. Schematic setup of microwave-assisted extraction (MAE) [111].

The choice of solvent is not only important in this methodology; the dielectric properties of the solvent must be taken into account [106]. The most commonly used solvents for MAE are ethanol and methanol, both of which have shown the best extraction yields, although water has also shown positive effects [66,68,107]. The efficacy of MAE will also depend on the type of flavonoid to be recovered. For example, the polarity of the flavonoid will be a very important parameter to consider; the type of solvent used will be the polarity of the desired recovery. Moreover, the solvent used in the extraction process may have an effect on the bioactivity of the recovered flavonoids [66]. Apolar solvents such as dichloromethane, ethyl acetate, diethyl ether, chloroform are commonly used for the extraction of isoflavones, flavones, and methylated flavones due to their apolar nature. In contrast, solvents such as ethanol or methanol are used to extract polar flavonoids such as flavonoid glycosides and aglycones (Table 2A).

3.2.2. Ultrasound-Assisted Extraction

Ultrasound-assisted extraction is a technique that is used to rupture the plant material and extract the bioactive compounds with applications in industries such as food and pharmaceuticals [108]. This technique is based on the phenomenon of acoustic cavitation, which consists of the formation of bubbles and the subsequent rupture, which causes the release of bioactive compounds, and this rupture depends on the extraction conditions [97,114] (Figure 3).

The cavitation effect produced by this methodology not only enables the destruction of the cell walls of the plant material but also promotes the reduction of the particle size that benefits the solvent–substrate interaction [97]. There are many variables that can have an effect on flavonoid extractive processes and therefore on the number of experiments; in order to optimize a particular process, experimental matrices are usually used to perform the optimization process in order to determine the conditions that favor the recovery of the maximum flavonoid content. Most of the published works have opted to use the surface response methodology to achieve this objective [63].

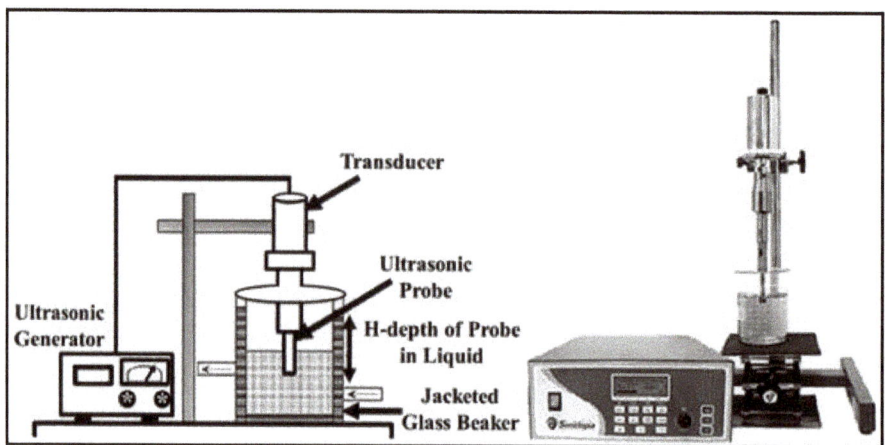

Figure 3. Schematic setup of ultrasound-assisted extraction (UAE) [111].

The UAE increased the yield of bioactive compounds and the yield of flavonoids were shown to be variable depending on the method of extraction, as well as on the type of plant material (Table 2B). Mainly phenolic compounds and flavonoids, as well as the reduction of extraction times, and another of the advantages of this methodology is that it improves the biological properties of the extracts [115]. The extraction of bioactive compounds depends on a variety of factors, such as the frequency used and usually between 20 kHz and 100 MHz [116], solvent selection, solvent concentration, solid–solvent ratio, temperature, and time extraction (Table 2B).

Among the flavonoid compounds that have been extracted and recovered using this methodology are the following: Rutin, narcissin, nicotiflorin, epicatechin, epicatechin gallate, catechin, procyanidin B_2, apiofuranosyl(1‴→2″)-β-D-glucopyranosyl] rhamnocitrin, quercetin-3-O-rhamnoglucoside, quercetin-3-O-β-D-glucopyranoside, myricetin-5′-O-β-D-glucopyranoside, 4′-O-(3‴-O-dihydrophaseoyl-β-D-glucopyranosyl) rhamnocitrin, formononetin-7-O-glucoside, myricomplanoside, kaempferol-3-O-glucosylrutinoside, complantoside A, quercetin-3-O-acylglycoside, etc. [117–119].

3.2.3. Supercritical Fluid Extraction

Any substance at a temperature and pressure above its thermodynamic critical point is a supercritical fluid. Under these conditions, the properties of the fluids generate a high diffusivity and low viscosity of the solvents used to improve the process of transfer of the matter [120]. Due to this, the SFE methodology (Figure 4) has reported flavonoid extraction yields much higher than those used in other techniques [121].

The most commonly used solvent in this extraction method is carbon dioxide (CO_2) due to its numerous advantages, such as that it is flammable, nontoxic, cheap, and very easy to remove due to its volatility [123,124]. It is a strong solvent for supercritical extraction with all these features.

Certain advantages of this extraction methodology are low temperatures that maintain the integrity of the products, high volatility of the solvents which keep the waste low, the extraction is carried out without phase changes, easy separation of volatile and nonvolatile compounds. However, they present some limitations such as the difficult equilibrium between solute and solvent, may require other separation processes, high pressures hinder the continuous addition of solids to the extract, operating costs are high, equipment is low, maintenance cost is high, etc. [125,126].

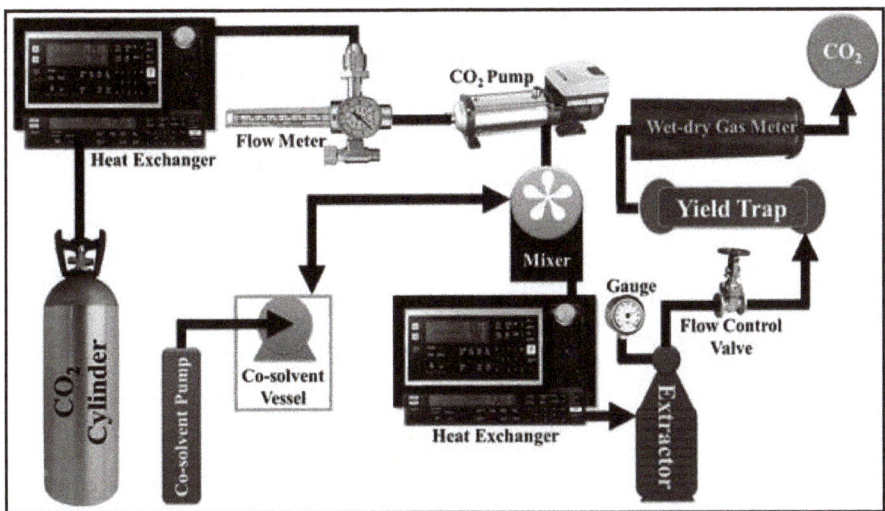

Figure 4. Schematic setup of supercritical fluid extraction (SFE) [122].

Temperature is one of the most important factors in the process. In this methodology, the use of reduced temperatures is intended to keep the product as stable as possible. In one study, for example, the valorization of agro-industrial residues (expellers) from the extraction of soybean oil by pressing was analyzed. Extractions were carried out at 40 MPa and at 35 or 40 °C using CO_2 as a solvent. Moreover, the expellers were impregnated with ethanol. The best results showed the flavonoids content of 65.0 and 31.3 QE/100 gdm [127]. On the other hand, flavonoids were extracted from *Odontonema strictum* leaves with supercritical carbon dioxide and ethanol. The effect of temperature (55–65 °C) on the total flavonoid content was optimized. The total flavonoid content and flavonoid recovery vary respectively from 99.33 to 247.78 mg/g of dried extract and 10.68–18.92 mg/g of dried leaves powder [128]. In another study, supercritical CO_2 extraction with/without ethanol from *Citrus unshiu* peels was examined at a temperature of 59.85 °C and a pressure of 30 MPa. The best results obtained were that the extracts, including nobiletin, increased the concentration of ethanol in supercritical CO_2 and increased the time of extraction. On the other hand, the role of pressure in these methods is very important and depends on the solvent used. For example, an effective method of extracting *Medicago sativa* using enzyme-assisted supercritical fluid was developed in another study. The design of the Box-Behnken was chosen to optimize the extraction process parameters, including pressure (100–300 bar). Optimal extraction parameters for total polyphenol content were: 68 °C, 205 bar, and 15.5% for temperature, pressure and co-solvent content, respectively. This methodology provides effective enzyme-assisted supercritical fluid extraction for the enhanced release of polyphenol compounds [129]. Supercritical fluids are a more efficient, safer, and environmentally friendly method for extracting and recovering flavonoids for the purpose of bioactive compounds study (Table 2C).

3.2.4. Enzyme and Microorganism-Assisted Extraction

There are several different techniques for the extraction of flavonoids, including conventional solid–liquid extraction, pressurized fluid extraction, pressurized hot water extraction. Supercritical fluid extraction, MAE, UAE, and pulsed electrical field extraction are among the most sustainable alternatives to these traditional methods [130]. The process of extraction of flavonoids is usually performed using organic solvents mixed with or without water. The extraction can be controlled by different parameters, such as the selection of extraction procedures, as well as the flow rate used for extraction, solvent and temperature, pressure and time. In addition, other techniques have yielded similar results; these techniques involve the use of microorganism-and enzyme-assisted extractions.

Enzyme-assisted extraction is a promising alternative to conventional extraction methods where a high amount of solvent is used. The advantages of this method are regioselectivity and specificity of enzyme action, their ability to catalyze reactions in aqueous solutions under mild conditions [131]. Furthermore, the application of enzyme is an environmentally friendly method for the extraction of flavonoids due to a decrease in solvent quantity in order to reduce extraction times and increase extraction yield and quality of flavonoids. Enzymes and microorganisms may also be used for pretreatment in different agro-industrial and food industries.

Enzymes obtained from fungi, bacteria, vegetable extracts and animal organs, such as pectinases, different glucanases, hemicellulases, cellulases, etc., in mixtures or alone, break down the cell wall by hydrolysis of biopolymeric components to increase the permeability of the cell wall and also increase the yield of flavonoids and other physiologically active extractants [132,133].

Hydrolytic enzymes can break down the cell wall of polysaccharides to improve intracellular release. Cellulose is hydrolyzed by four classes of enzymes: Endo-and exoglucanases, cellobiohydrolases, and β-glucosidases. The main chain of hemicellulose can be hydrolyzed by endooxylanases, endomannanases, β-xylosidases, and β-mannanases. Degradation of the backbone of pectin requires a number of enzymes such as pectin lyases, pectate lyases, endo- and exo-polygalacturonases, endo- and exo-rhamnogalacturonases and rhamnogalacturan lyases. In addition, to hydrolyze the side chains of polysaccharides, by-product enzymes (such as arabinases, galactosidases and feruloyl, esterases) are needed [134].

Several authors have utilized enzymatic treatments with commercial preparations for the extraction of flavonoids from plant material (Table 3). These commercial enzymes usually have one or more main hydrolytic activities and a number of side activities. Commercial pectinases have been used for enzyme-assisted extraction of black currant phenols (*Ribes nigrum*) juice press residues [135]. Mixtures of pectinases and cellulases have been used for the extraction of polyphenols from grape pomace [136,137]. A combination of enzymatic hydrolysis and ultrasonic-assisted extraction was used for the extraction of flavonoids from pigeon pea (*Cajanus cajan*) leaves [138], celery (*Apium graveolens*) leaves [139], shepherd's purse (*Capsella bursa-pastoris*) pulp [140], and mulberry (*Morus nigra*) must [141]. A set of combinations of different extraction methods (*viz.* enzymatic hydrolysis, ultrasonic, and microwave-assisted extraction) that were used for the recovery of flavonoids from *Nitraria tangutorun* juice by-product [142].

Special attention must be paid to the presence of undesirable enzyme activities during the enzyme-assisted extraction of flavonoids. These activities may be caused by endogenous enzymes of plant material or by side activities of commercial preparations. Polyphenol oxidases may induce coupled oxidative browning reactions; β-glucosidases, β-galactosidases, and α-L-arabinosidases may hydrolyze native glycosylated anthocyanins and cause unstable aglycons [135]. For example, Kammerer et al. (2005) [136] observed a low yield of anthocyanin recovery (2.9%) during enzyme-assisted extraction of polyphenols from grape pomace (Vitis vinifera) at the pilot plant level. This low yield was associated with the action of endogenous enzymes. In subsequent research, thermal inactivation of endogenous enzymes prior to aqueous extraction and enzyme treatment allowed 63.4% of anthocyanins to be recovered from grape pomace [137].

Landbo and Meyer (2001) [135] found that two commercial pectinases had a negative effect on the recovery of anthocyanins during enzyme-assisted extraction of phenolic compounds from black currant (*Ribes nigrum*) pomace. This negative effect was associated with the presence of glycosidase activities in enzyme preparations. On the other hand, Xu et al. (2013b) [145] used the activity of glycosylase present in commercial enzyme preparations to improve the extraction of bioactive compounds from two medicinal plants (*Glycyrrhizae radix* and *Scutellariae radix*). Bifunctional enzymes were used for the simultaneous degradation of the cell wall and deglycosylation of native flavonoid glycosides.

Table 3. Studies on enzyme assisted isolation and extraction of flavonoids from different plant sources.

Source	Enzyme (s)	Compound (s)	Reference
Ginkgo biloba leaves	Cellulase	Flavonols	[143]
Grape (*Vitis vinifera*) skins	Oenological preparation (pectinase + cellulase + hemicellulase)	Anthocyanins, flavonol glycosides, and flavan-3-ols	[144]
Mulberry (*Morus nigra*) must	Pectinase	Anthocyanins and nonanthocyanin flavonoids	[141]
Nitraria tangutorum juice by-products	Cellulase	Anthocyanins and nonanthocyanin flavonoids	[142]
Shepherd's purse (*Capsella bursa-pastoris*) pulp	Pectinase and cellulase	Flavonoids	[140]
Glycyrrhizae radix	Cellulase	Liquiritigenin and isoliquiritigenin	[145]
Celery (*Apium graveolens*) leaves	Pectinase	Luteolin and apigenin	[139]
Scutellariae radix	Naringinase	Bacalein and wogonin	[146]
Grape (*Vitis vinifera*) pomace	Pectinase and cellulase	Anthocyanins and nonanthocyanin flavonoids	[137]
Pigeonpea (*Cajanus cajan*) leaves	Pectinase	Luteolin and apigenin	[138]
Grape (*Vitis vinifera*) pomace	Pectinase and cellulase	Anthocyanins and nonanthocyanin flavonoids	[136]
Black currant (*Ribes nigrum*) pomace	Pectinase	Anthocyanins	[135]

Chen et al. (2011) [146] developed a method for enzyme-assisted extraction of flavonoids from Ginkgo biloba leaves in which the enzyme was used not only for cell wall degradation but also to increase the solubility of target compounds. They used commercial *Penicillium decumbens* cellulase with high transglycosylation activity. The presence of maltose *P. decumbens* cellulase transglycosylated flavonol aglycones in more polar glucosides with higher solubility in polar solvents improves the extraction yield.

The parameters to be taken into account for increasing the extraction yield of flavonoids are treatment time, pH, and temperature, as well as the enzyme quantity in relation to the concentration of the substrate. Various studies reported the optimization of these parameters [143,144].

There are also disadvantages of enzymatic methods, which have been reported in many reports: To date, the enzyme tested has not been able to achieve complete plant cell wall hydrolysis due to the major difficulties of scale-up enzyme-assisted extraction at industrial level and the relatively high cost of biocatalyst for large volumes of raw materials [132]. The use of microorganisms as enzyme producers may replace the use of food-grade enzymes in the extraction of flavonoids. However, their growth and activity are sensitive to changes in environmental conditions (temperature, percentage of dissolved oxygen, agitation rate, design of reactors, and availability of nutrients) [147].

4. Transformation of Flavonoids

4.1. Microbial Biotransformation

Biotransformation of flavonoids to increase the biological activity of the recovered compounds is a trend. Biotransformation is a process in which the chemical structure of the compounds is modified by the use of microorganisms. The objective of biotransformation is to produce fine chemical compounds (high added value) that are difficult to produce by chemical synthesis under low-severity reaction conditions. These processes have good production yields and the recovery of flavonoids. The main biotransformations reported in flavonoids are as follows: Dehydroxylation, dehydrogenation, hydrogenation, glycosylation, O-methylation, O-demethylation, deglycosylation, cyclization, sulfation, and carbonyl reduction [148]. This section discusses some biotransformation studies on flavonoids using filamentous fungi and bacteria.

Filamentous fungi and 20 strains of *Streptomyces* for the production of flavonoids were evaluated and two derivatives of quercetin were obtained from *Beauveria bassiana* ATCC7159 in the bioconversion of quercetin. Furthermore, the bioconversion of rutin was obtained by *Cunninghamella echinulata* ATCC 9244 rutin sulfate, rutin glucuronide, and rutin methylation. This biotechnology method was appropriate to produce biologically-active flavonoids [149]. In another study, the biodegradation of isoflavones into 4'-fluoroisoflavone were evaluated by *Aspergillus niger* and *Cunninghamella elegans* strains and obtained more than 20 metabolites. *A. niger* was the microbial strain that has the most ability to degrade isoflavones which could be used as bioactive compounds [150]. Furthermore, the biotransformation of icariin, epimedin C, epimedoside A, epimedin A, and epimedin B were evaluated from the *Epimedium koreanum* plant using *Cunninghamella blakesleana*. This process generated flavonoids that posed potential applications in the pharmaceutical and food industries [151].

A new method was developed to produce genistein from roots of pigeon pea (*Cajanus cajan*) using immobilized strains of *Aspergillus oryzae* and *Monacus anka*. This biotransformation method was a good alternative to the production of genistein from plants with food industry potential [152]. Different filamentous fungi used in solid-state fermentation were evaluated for the biotransformation of phenolic compounds in cauliflower leaves. *A. sojae* strain was best suited to high yields of flavonoids, including kaempferol-derived metabolites. This bioprocess was proposed as an alternative for the development of the concept of bio-refinery and the use of agricultural by-products [153]. In another study, a process of biotransformation of phenolic compounds from citrus waste using solid-state fermentation by *Peacilomyces variotii* was developed, where remarkable production of naringenin and hesperetin was achieved and the antioxidant capacity increased to 73%. These compounds are of high added value that can be used in the food sector [154].

Moreover, a strategy for the biodegradation pathway from tyrosine to the production of fisetin using *Escherichia coli* has been developed. The production of this flavonoid is of great interest because it has different biological properties for human health, such as antiviral and anticancer [155]. In another study, the biotransformation of soy isoflavones in *ortho*-hydroxyisoflavones was evaluated using CYP105D7 from *Streptomyces avermitilis* MA4680 and expressed in *Pichia pastoris*. This study provides evidence of the great potential of the use of genetic microorganisms for the production of isoflavonoids for food industry applications [156]. Puerarin catalyzed by Bacillus cereus NT02 was evaluated for its biotransformation. The results showed that puerarin phosphorylation innovations in medicinal chemistry have particular importance [157].

4.2. Enzyme-Catalyzed Transformation

Flavonoids are characterized by their low solubility and stability in aqueous and lipid phases. For instance, aglycones are less soluble than their derivatives. Aglycones are readily absorbed by passive diffusion through biological membranes, while flavonoid glucosides can be introduced into cells by means of a sodium-dependent glucose transporter 1. Therefore, deglycosylation is important for the assimilation of dietary flavonoids [158]. They may be modified chemically, enzymatically, or chemo-enzymatically to enhance these properties.

Glycosylation and acylation are the most important transformations of flavonoids catalyzed by enzymes. Glycosylation allowed flavonoids to enhance their hydrophilic character by adding sugars, while acylation makes them more hydrophobic due to the combination of fatty acids. Chemical acylation is not regioselective [159] and results in the modification of phenolic groups responsible for the antioxidant activity of flavonoids [158]. The enzyme groups used for flavonoid transformation are presented in Table 4.

Table 4. Flavonoids transformation catalyzed by different enzymes.

Enzymes Type		Transformation	Reference
Esterases	Esterases (carboxyl esterases)	Reaction similar to lipases, but with short-chain fatty acids and difference in the interfacial activation. Low practical applications in enzymatic transformation of flavonoids with a short aliphatic chain length such as acetate, propionate, and butyrate.	[160]
Isomerase	Chalcone isomerase (CHI)	Cyclization of chalcone to form flavanone, transformation of chalcone and 6′-deoxychalcone into (2S)-naringerin and (2S)-5-deoxyflavanone. Soybean CHIs do not require the 4′-hydroxy moiety on the substrate for high enzyme activity.	[161]
Laccase	Laccase from *Myceliophthora*	Synthesis of a flavonoid polymer and high molecular fraction of extracted flavonoids from rutin as substrate in the mixture of methanol and buffer. Oxidation of catechin in the presence of gelatin and synthesize the gelatin-catechin conjugate.	[162,163]
Lipase	*Candida antarctica* lipase B	Acetylation only on the primary 6′-OH of the isoquercitrin glucose and the secondary 4′-OH of the rutin rhamnose were expected to be acetylated.	[164]
	Pseudomonas cepacea lipase	Acetylation occurred only on 3′-OH, 5′-OH, and 7-OH hydroxyls.	
Pectinase and Cellulase	Commercial Cellulases from *Trichoderma viride*	Transglucosylation activity toward (+)-catechin and (−)-epigallocatechin gallate (EGCG) using dextrin as a glucosyl donor. EGCG glucosides were functionally superior to EGCG as food additives.	[146,165,166]
	Pectinolytic and Cellulolytic Enzymes	Hydrolysis of main- and side-chain of polysaccharides, and glycosidase activities.	
Peroxidase	Chloroperoxidase	Halogenation of naringenin and hersperetin, at C-6 and C-8 with chloride and bromide ions.	[167,168]
	Horseradish peroxidase	Conjugation of green-tea catechin with amine substituted octahedral silsesquioxane.	
Protease	Alkaline protease from *Bacillus subtilis*	Synthesis of 3″-O-substituted vinyl rutin esters in pyridine.	[169–171]
	Novozym 435	Synthesis of 4″-O-substituted vinyl rutin esters in tert-butanol.	
	Proteases	Hydrolytic and synthetic functions. Enzymatic transformations of flavonoids were affected by the type, origin and concentration of enzymes, nature of flavonoids, donor and optimal conditions (temperature, substrates, and solvent).	
	Subtilisin (serine protease)	Flavonoid ester synthesis, the selective rutin acylation in organic solvents with excellent selectivity. The structure of the sugar moiety affected the regioselectivity.	

Table 4. *Cont.*

Enzymes Type		Transformation	Reference
Transferase	Glycosyltransferases (GTs)	Glycosylation of on one or more of five hydroxyl groups of flavonol quercetin, as well as formation of hesperetin-7-glucoside. Some natural GTs is characterized by low specificity and other by the stringent specificity for glycosylation patterns. Positions, number, and length of the sugar moieties are significant factors for yield reaction.	[95,172–175]
	Prenyltransferase (from *Morus nigra*)	Exclusive prenylation of chalcones (1, 2, 3, bearing two hydroxyl groups (C-2′, C-4′) on ring A) with a 2′, 4′ dihydroxy substitution and the isoflavone genistein. The position of substituents in ring B appeared to be critical for the prenylation.	
	Prenyltransferase (NovQ):	Transferring of a dimethylallyl group to the B-ring of flavonoids. Genistein and naringenin and yielded two products with a dimethylallyl group at C-3′ or O-4′.	

Lipase (Table 4) catalyzed flavonoids acylation with phenolic acids leads to increased solubility, stability, and antioxidant activity of flavonoids in different media [176]. In addition, the presence of electron-donating or withdrawing substituents in the aromatic ring of flavonoids appears to be essential for their activity in the central nervous system as anxiolytic, anticonvulsant, and sedative and skeletal muscle relaxant drugs.

Chemical modifications are complex and laborious work that requires specific conditions. Therefore, enzyme modification can be a very promising alternative technique in this way. It is a well-known enzymatic halogenation of organic compounds by means of chloroperoxidase (EC 1.11.1.10). Chloroperoxidase from *Caldariomyces fumago* (Table 4) and whole microbial cells were applied to halogenate the flavones, naringenin, and hesperetin, at C-6 and C-8 in the presence of chloride and bromide ions [168]. Biomodified compounds have shown similar properties compared to derivatives obtained by chemical modification using highly aggressive agents such as molecular halogens and hypohalous acid.

The use of different enzymes (Table 4) has been studied in order to find the most potent biocatalyst for the selective transformation of flavonoids (acylation, deacylation, etc.). Applications of thermostable enzymes have been reported [166]. Enzyme immobilization has been performed to increase enzyme stability, facilitate enzyme reuse, and product insulation [177].

The regioselective synthesis of phloridzin-6′-O-cinnamate has been carried out using *Candida antarctic* lipase B immobilized with a macroporous acrylic resin [178,179]. Different enzymes have been used in immobilized forms to reduce the cost of enzymatic modifications of structural flavonoids due to their advantages such as easy isolation and re-use, increased enzyme stability, and regioselectivity in nonaqueous media [164].

Oxidative and conjugative biocatalyzed transformations of flavonoids may be performed in the presence of different microorganisms (*Bacillus* sp., *Aspergillus* sp., *Saccharomyces cerevisiae, E. coli*) [132]. Biotransformations performed by microorganisms consist of very complex mechanisms, including cyclization reactions, condensation, dehydroxylation, hydroxylation, O-dealkylation, alkylation, dehydrogenation, halogenation, double-bond reduction, carbonyl reduction, glycosylation, sulfation, dimerization, or various types of ring degradation. They were described earlier [132,180,181].

5. Human Health and Biological Properties

There is a strong link between a high intake of flavonoids and low cardiovascular disease, neurodegeneration, and cancer in the population in which a food that includes high levels of these phytochemicals is included in a daily diet [18,22,182]. These properties are based on protein interaction (enzyme, factor transcription, and receptor transcription) [22]. The use of herbs with a high content of flavonoids has been used as part of traditional remedies to treat various diseases that improve the immune system, as shown by antioxidants, anti-inflammatory, anti-allergenic, and antithrombotic drugs (Figure 5) [19,183,184]. There are some reports indicating the pro-oxidant activity of flavonoids [185]. Flavonoids generally act to protect plants from UV-B radiation and have the potential to reduce oxidative damage, act as photoreceptors, and have the power to attract flower pigment pollinators and protect against pathogen attack [19,23,186].

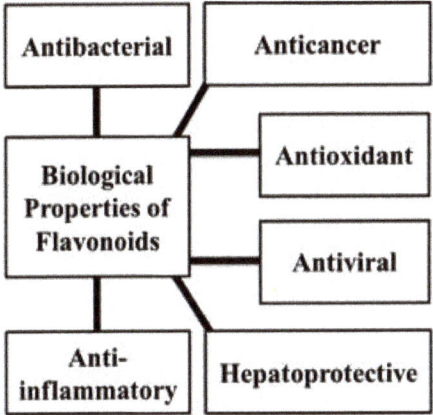

Figure 5. Different biological properties of plant flavonoids for human health and disease.

In particular, isoflavones have shown a variety of effects on human health, especially in women's health, such as the prevention and reduction of climate symptoms (such as hot flushes). The control of diseases such as diabetes, osteoporosis, and breast cancer has also been reported to be associated with the consumption of food rich in isoflavones [28,30,31]. In addition, even for prostate cancer isoflavones have shown their chemical-prevention effect [29].

6. Concluding Remarks

Flavonoids are a category of compounds with diverse biological activities that are of interest to various industrial areas, such as food, health pharmaceuticals, and cosmetics. Due to consumers demands today for products that benefit their quality of life substantially. Several extraction methods for the recovery of these flavonoids have been proposed for its wide range of applications. Today, microwave, ultrasound, and supercritical fluid technologies are among the most used methods of flavonoid extraction by most researchers worldwide. In addition, the use of biotechnological alternatives has attracted the attention of research to finding cleaner and more efficient ways to recover flavonoids. These methodologies have been distinguished from conventional methods by a marked increase in extraction yields and the displacement of organic solvents by "green" solvents, as well as a significant decrease in extraction times. Most studies have reported the extraction of flavonoids from vegetable sources such as fruits, seeds, roots or by-products of food, and/or beverage processing such as peels. Although progress has been made in this area, it is necessary to redefine the extractive techniques, since the majority is focused on increasing the yield of total flavonoids, leaving aside the purity of the extracts. The acquisition of extracts and/or purer flavonoid compounds would allow us to know more precisely the biological activities and thus to understand the mechanisms of action and the effects on their consumption, allowing for greater diversification of their applications and generating more knowledge in this area.

Author Contributions: Conceptualization, M.L.C.-G. and C.N.A.; literature survey, organization, and critical analysis of data, M.L.C.-G., L.S., H.A.L.-G., L.V.R.-D., A.I., and C.N.A.; initial writing, M.L.C.-G.; revisions and proofreading, M.L.C.-G., D.K.V., L.V.R.-D., and C.N.A.; funding acquisition, M.L.C-G. and C.N.A. All authors have read and agreed to the published version of the manuscript.

Funding: This research received no external funding.

Conflicts of Interest: The authors declare no conflict of interest.

References

1. Guo, L.; Gao, L.; Ma, X.; Guo, F.; Ruan, H.; Bao, Y.; Wang, Y. Functional analysis of flavonoid 3′-hydroxylase and flavonoid 3′,5′-hydroxylases from tea plant (*Camellia sinensis*), involved in the B-ring hydroxylation of flavonoids. *Gene* **2019**, *717*, 144046. [CrossRef]
2. Raffa, D.; Maggio, B.; Raimondi, M.V.; Plescia, F.; Daidone, G. Recent discoveries of cancer flavonoids. *EJMC* **2017**, *142*, 213–228.
3. Aherne, S.A.; O'Brien, N.M. Dietary flavonols: Chemistry, food content, and metabolism. *Nutrition* **2002**, *18*, 75–81. [CrossRef]
4. Amri, F.S.; Hossain, M.A. Comparison of total phenols, flavonoids and antioxidant potential of local and imported ripe bananas. *EJBAS* **2018**, *5*, 245–251. [CrossRef]
5. Miao, M.; Cao, L.; Xu, K.; Xin, W.; Zheng, Y. Intervention action of total flavonoids from root of Ilex pubescens in cerebral ischemic tolerance with blood stasis. *Saudi J. Biol. Sci.* **2017**, *24*, 729–736. [CrossRef]
6. Moon, K.M.; Lee, B.; Cho, W.K.; Lee, B.S.; Kim, C.K.; Ma, J.Y. Swertiajaponin as an anti-browning and antioxidant flavonoid. *Food Chem.* **2018**, *252*, 207–214. [CrossRef]
7. Diwan, V.; Brown, L.; Gobe, G.C. The flavonoid rutin improves kidney and heart structure and function in an adenine-induced rat model of chronic kidney disease. *J. Funct. Foods* **2017**, *33*, 85–93. [CrossRef]
8. Geleijnse, J.M.; Launer, L.J.; Van der Kuip, D.A.; Hofman, A.; Witteman, J.C. Inverse association of tea and flavonoid intakes with incident myocardial infarction: The Rotterdam study. *AJCN* **2002**, *75*, 880–886. [CrossRef]
9. Spagnuolo, C.; Moccia, S.; Ruso, G.L. Anti-inflammatory effects of flavonoids in neurodegenerative disorders. *EJMC* **2018**, *153*, 105–115. [CrossRef]
10. Stahl, W.; Ale-Agha, N.; Polidori, M.C. Non-antioxidant properties of carotenoids. *JBC* **2002**, *383*, 553–558. [CrossRef]
11. Xu, M.S.; Chen, S.; Wang, W.Q.; Liu, S.Q. Employing bifunctional enzymes for enhanced extraction of bioactives from plants: Flavonoids as an example. *J. Agric. Food Chem.* **2013**, *61*, 7941–7948. [CrossRef]
12. Zuiter, A.S.; Zarqa, J. Proanthocyanidin: Chemistry and biology: From phenolic compounds to proanthocyanidins. In *Reference Module in Chemistry, Molecular Sciences and Chemical Engineering*; Reedijk, J., Ed.; Elsevier: Amsterdam, The Netherlands, 2014; pp. 1–29.
13. Karabin, M.; Hudcova, T.; Jelinek, L.; Dostalek, P. Biotransformation and biological activities of hop flavonoids. *Biotech. Adv.* **2015**, *33*, 1063–1090. [CrossRef]
14. Sharma, V.; Janmeda, P. Extraction, isolation and identification of flavonoid from *Euphorbia neriifolia* leaves. *AJC* **2017**, *10*, 509–514. [CrossRef]
15. Arora, S.; Itankar, P. Extraction, isolation and identification of flavonoid from *Chenopodium album* aerial parts. *JTCM* **2018**, *8*, 476–482. [CrossRef]
16. Martens, S.; Mithöfer, A. Flavones and flavone synthases. *Phytochemistry* **2005**, *66*, 2399–2407. [CrossRef]
17. De Villiers, A.; Venter, P.; Pasch, H. Recent advances and trends in the liquid-chromatography-mass spectrometry analysis of flavonoids. *J. Chromatogr. A* **2016**, *1430*, 16–78. [CrossRef]
18. Olagaray, K.E.; Bradford, B.J. Plant flavonoids to improve productivity of ruminants—A review. *Anim. Feed Sci. Tech.* **2019**, *251*, 21–36. [CrossRef]

19. Ververidis, F.; Trantas, E.; Douglas, C.; Vollmer, G.; Kretzschmar, G.; Panopoulos, N. Biotechnology of flavonoids and other phenylpropanoid-derived natural products. Part I: Chemical diversity, impacts on plant biology and human health. *Biotechnol. J.* **2007**, *2*, 1214–1234. [CrossRef]
20. Kale, A.; Gawande, S.; Kotwal, S. Cancer phytotherapeutics: Role for flavonoids at the cellular level. *Phytother. Res.* **2008**, *22*, 567–577. [CrossRef]
21. Cassidy, A.; Kay, C. Phytochemicals: Classification and occurrence. In *Encyclopedia of Human Nutrition*; Caballero, B., Ed.; Elsevier: Amsterdam, The Netherlands, 2013; pp. 39–46.
22. Rybarczyk-Plonska, A.; Wold, A.B.; Bengtsson, G.B.; Borge, G.I.A.; Hansen, M.K.; Hagen, S.F. Flavonols in broccoli (*Brassica oleracea* L. var. *italica*) flower buds as affected by postharvest temperature and radiation treatments. *Postharvest Biol. Technol.* **2016**, *116*, 105–114. [CrossRef]
23. Cui, B.; Hu, Z.; Zhang, Y.; Hu, J.; Yin, W.; Feng, Y.; Xie, Q.; Chen, G. Anthocyanins and flavonols are responsible for purple color of *Lablab purpureus* (L.) sweet pods. *Plant Physiol. Biochem.* **2016**, *103*, 183–190. [CrossRef] [PubMed]
24. Xu, Y.; Simon, J.E.; Ferruzzi, M.G.; Ho, L.; Pasinetti, G.M.; Wu, Q. Quantification of anthocyanidins in the grapes and grape juice products with acid assisted hydrolysis using LC/MS. *JFF* **2012**, *4*, 710–717. [CrossRef]
25. Oliveira, J.; Mateus, N.; de Freitas, V. Flavanols: Catechins and proanthocyanidins. In *Natural Products*; Ramawat, K.G., Mérillon, J.M., Eds.; Springer: Berlin/Heidelberg, Germany, 2013; pp. 1753–1801.
26. Pons, Z.; Margalef, M.; Bravo, F.I.; Arola-Arnal, A.; Muguerza, B. Grape seed flavanols decrease blood pressure *via* Sirt-1 and confer a vasoprotective pattern in rats. *JFF* **2016**, *24*, 164–172. [CrossRef]
27. Vuong, Q.V.; Golding, J.B.; Nguyen, M.; Roach, P.D. Extraction and isolation of catechins from tea. *JSS* **2010**, *33*, 3415–3428. [CrossRef] [PubMed]
28. Zhao, C.C.; Kim, P.H.; Eun, J.B. Influence of high-intensity ultrasound application on the physicochemical properties, isoflavones composition and antioxidant activity of tofu whey. *LWT-Food Sci. Technol.* **2020**, *117*, 108618. [CrossRef]
29. Duru, K.C.; Kovaleva, E.; Danilova, I.; Belousova, A. Production and assessment of novel probiotic fermented oat flour enriched with isoflavones. *LWT-Food Sci. Technol.* **2019**, *117*, 108618. [CrossRef]
30. Nemitz, M.C.; Argenta, D.F.; Koester, L.S.; Bassani, V.L.; von Poser, G.L.; Teixeira, H.F. The international scenario of patents concerning isoflavones. *Trends Food Sci. Technol.* **2016**, *49*, 85–95. [CrossRef]
31. Ganzera, M. Supercritical fluid chromatography for the separation of isoflavones. *J. Pharm. Biomed. Anal.* **2015**, *107*, 364–369. [CrossRef]
32. Alara, O.R.; Abdurahman, N.H.; Ukaegbu, C.I. Soxhlet extraction pf phenolic compounds from *Vernonia cinereal* leaves and its antioxidant activity. *J. Appl. Res. Med. Aromat. Plants* **2018**, *11*, 12–17.
33. Sati, P.; Dhyani, P.; Bhatt, I.D.; Pandey, A. Ginkgo biloba flavonoid glycosides in antimicrobial perspective with reference to extraction method. *JTCM* **2019**, *9*, 15–23. [CrossRef]
34. Mackela, I.; Andriekus, T.; Venskutonis, P.R. Biorefinning of buckwheat (*Fagopyru, esculentum*) hulls by using supercritical fluid, Soxhlet, pressurized liquid and enzyme-assisted extraction methods. *JFE* **2017**, *213*, 38–46. [CrossRef]
35. Cujic, N.; Svikin, K.; Jankovic, T.; Pljevljakusic, D.; Zdunic, G.; Ibric, S. Optimization of polyphenols extraction from dried chokeberry using maceration as traditional technique. *Food Chem.* **2016**, *194*, 135–142. [CrossRef]
36. Pereira, S.V.; Reis, R.A.S.P.; Garbuio, D.C.; de Freitas, L.A.P. Dynamic maceration of *Matricaria chamomilla* inflorescences: Optimal conditions for flavonoids and antioxidant activity. *Rev. Bras. Farmacogn.* **2018**, *28*, 111–117. [CrossRef]
37. Agustin-Salazar, S.; Medina-Juárez, L.A.; Soto-Valdez, H.; Manzanares-López, F.; Gámez-Meza, N. Influence of the solvent system on the composition of phenolic substances and antioxidant capacity of extracts of grape (*Vitis vinifera* L.) marc. *AJGWR* **2014**, *R20*, 208–213. [CrossRef]
38. Albuquerque, B.R.; Prieto, M.A.; Vazquez, J.A.; Barreirio, M.F.; Barros, L.; Ferreira, I.C.F.R. Recovery of bioactive compounds form Arbutus unedo L. fruits: Comparative optimization study of maceration/microwave/ultrasound extraction techniques. *Food Res. Int.* **2018**, *109*, 455–471. [CrossRef]
39. Farzaneth, V.; Carvalho, I.S. Modelling of Microwave Assisted Extraction (MAE) of Anthocyanins (TMA). *JARMAP* **2017**, *6*, 92–100.
40. Ye, C.L.; Liu, X.G. Extraction of flavonoids from *Tetrastigma hemsleyanum* diels et gilg and their antioxidant activity. *JFPP* **2015**, *39*, 2197–2205.

41. Safdar, M.N.; Kausar, T.; Jabbar, S.; Mumtaz, A.; Ahad, K.; Saddozai, A.A. Extraction and quantification of polyphenols from kinnow (*Citrus reticulate* L.) peel using ultrasound and maceration techniques. *JFDA* **2017**, *25*, 488–500. [CrossRef]
42. Bergeron, C.; Gafner, S.; Clausen, E.; Carrier, D.J. Comparison of the Chemical Composition of Extracts from Scutellaria lateriflora Using Accelerated Solvent Extraction and Supercritical Fluid Extraction versus Standard Hot Water or 70% Ethanol Extraction. *J. Agric. Food Chem.* **2005**, *53*, 3076–3080. [CrossRef]
43. Yu, M.; Wang, B.; Qi, Z.; Xin, G.; Li, Q. Response Surface method was used to optimize the ultrasonic assisted extraction of flavonoids from *Crinum asiaticum*. *Saudi J. Biol. Sci.* **2019**, *26*, 2079–2084. [CrossRef]
44. Daud, M.N.H.; Fatanah, D.N.; Abdullah, N.; Ahmad, R. Evaluation of antioxidant potential of *Artocarpus heterophyllus* L. J33 variety fruit waste from different extraction methods and identification of phenolic constituents by LCMS. *Food Chem.* **2017**, *232*, 621–632. [CrossRef] [PubMed]
45. Szewczyk, K.; Olech, M. Optimization of extraction method for LC-MS based determination of phenolic acid profiles in different Impatiens species. *Phytochem. Lett.* **2017**, *20*, 322–330. [CrossRef]
46. Wu, X.; Beecher, G.R.; Holden, J.M.; Haytowitz, D.B.; Gebhardt, S.E.; Prior, R.L. Lipophilic and Hydrophilic Antioxidant Capacities of Common Foods in The United States. *J. Agric. Food Chem.* **2004**, *52*, 4026–4037. [CrossRef]
47. Rafińska, K.; Pomastowski, P.; Rudnicka, J.; Krakowska, A.; Maruska, A.; Narkute, M.; Buszewski, B. Effect of solvent and extraction technique on composition and biological activity of Lepidium sativum extracts. *Food Chem.* **2019**, *289*, 16–25. [CrossRef] [PubMed]
48. Ku, C.S.; Jang, J.P.; Mun, S.P. Exploitation of polyphenol-rich pine barks for potent antioxidant activity. *J. Wood Sci.* **2007**, *53*, 524–528. [CrossRef]
49. Bahorun, T.; Luximon-Ramma, A.; Crozier, A.; Aruoma, O.I. Total phenol, flavonoid, proanthocyanidin and vitamin C levels and antioxidant activities of Mauritian vegetables. *J. Sci. Food Agric.* **2004**, *84*, 1553–1561. [CrossRef]
50. Chu, Y.-F.; Sun, J.; Wu, X.; Liu, R.H. Antioxidant and Antiproliferative Activities of Common Vegetables. *J. Agric. Food Chem.* **2002**, *50*, 6910–6916. [CrossRef]
51. Zhang, D.; Hamauzu, Y. Phenolics, ascorbic acid, carotenoids and antioxidant activity of broccoli and their changes during conventional and microwave cooking. *Food Chem.* **2004**, *88*, 503–509. [CrossRef]
52. Anokwuru, C.P.; Anyasor, G.N.; Ajibaye, O.; Fakoya, O.; Okebugwu, P. Effect of extraction solvents on phenolic, flavonoid and antioxidant activities of three nigerian medicinal plants. *Nat. Sci.* **2011**, *9*, 53–61.
53. Vieitez, I.; Maceiras, L.; Jachmanián, I.; Alborés, S. Antioxidant and antibacterial activity of different extracts from herbs obtained by maceration or supercritical technology. *JSF* **2018**, *133*, 58–64. [CrossRef]
54. Moreira, M.M.; Barroso, M.F.; Boeykens, A.; Withouck, H.; Morais, S.; Delerue-Matos, C. Valorization of apple tree wood residues by polyphenols extraction: Comparison between conventional and microwave-assisted extraction. *Ind. Crop. Prod.* **2017**, *104*, 210–220. [CrossRef]
55. Aspé, E.; Fernández, K. The effect of different extraction techniques on extraction yield, total phenolic, and anti-radical capacity of extracts from *Pinus radiata* Bark. *Ind. Crop. Prod.* **2011**, *34*, 838–844. [CrossRef]
56. Lamounier, K.C.; Cunha, L.C.S.; de Morais, S.A.L.; de Aquino, F.J.T.; Chang, R.; do Nascimento, E.A.; de Souza, M.G.M.; Martins, C.H.G.; Cunha, W.R. Chemical analysis and study of phenolics, antioxidant activity, and antibacterial effect of the wood and bark of *Maclura tinctoria* (L.) D. Don ex Steud. *Altern. Med.* **2012**, *2012*, 1–7.
57. Zhu, H.B.; Wang, Y.Z.; Liu, Y.X.; Xia, Y.L.; Tang, T. Analysis of flavonoids in *Portulaca oleracea* L. by UV–vis spectrophotometry with comparative study on different extraction technologies. *Food Anal. Methods* **2010**, *3*, 90–97. [CrossRef]
58. Li, H.; Deng, Z.; Wu, T.; Liu, R.; Loewen, S.; Tsao, R. Microwave-assisted extraction of phenolics with maximal antioxidant activities in tomatoes. *Food Chem.* **2012**, *130*, 928–936. [CrossRef]
59. Cardoso-Ugarte, G.A.; Juárez-Becerra, G.P.; Sosa-Morales, M.E.; López-Malo, A. Microwave-assisted Extraction of Essential Oils from Herbs. *JMPEE* **2013**, *47*, 63–72. [CrossRef]
60. Casazza, A.A.; Aliakbarian, B.; Mantegna, S.; Cravotto, G.; Perego, P. Extraction of phenolics from *Vitis vinífera* wastes using non-conventional techniques. *J. Food Eng.* **2010**, *100*, 50–55. [CrossRef]
61. Pan, Y.M.; He, C.H.; Wang, H.S.; Ji, X.W.; Wang, K.; Liu, P.Z. Antioxidant activity of microwave-assisted extract of *Buddleia officinalis* and its major active component. *Food Chem.* **2010**, *121*, 497–502. [CrossRef]

62. Feng, R.Z.; Wang, Q.; Tong, W.Z.; Xiong, J.; Wei, Q.; Zhou, W.H.; Yin, Z.Q.; Yin, X.Y.; Wang, L.Y.; Chen, Y.Q.; et al. Extraction and antioxidant activity of flavonoids of *Morus nigra*. *Int. J. Clin. Exp. Med.* **2015**, *8*, 22328–22336.
63. Alara, O.R.; Abdurahman, N.H.; Olalere, O.A. Optimization of microwave-assisted extraction of flavonoids antioxidants from *Vernonia amygdalina* leaf using response surface methodology. *Food Bioprod. Process.* **2018**, *107*, 36–48. [CrossRef]
64. Bimakr, M.; Rahman, R.A.; Taip, F.S.; Ganjloo, A.; Salleh, L.M.; Selamat, J.; Hamid, A.; Zaidul, I.S.M. Comparison of different extraction methods for the extraction of major bioactive flavonoid compounds from spearmint (*Mentha spicata* L.) leaves. *Food Bioprod. Process.* **2011**, *89*, 67–72. [CrossRef]
65. Hartonen, K.; Parshintsev, J.; Sandberg, K.; Bergelin, E.; Nisula, L.; Riekkola, M.L. Isolation of flavonoids from aspen knotwood by pressurized hot water extraction and comparison with other extraction techniques. *Talanta* **2007**, *74*, 32–38. [CrossRef] [PubMed]
66. Jha, P.; Das, A.J.; Deka, S.C. Optimization of ultrasound and microwave assisted extractions of polyphenols from black rice (*Oryza sativa* cv. Poireton) husk. *J. Food Sci. Technol.* **2017**, *54*, 3847–3858. [CrossRef] [PubMed]
67. Rodríguez-Pérez, C.; Gilbert-López, B.; Mendiola, J.A.; Quirantes-Piné, R.; Segura-Carretero, A.; Ibáñez, E. Optimization of microwave-assisted extraction and pressurized liquid extraction of phenolic compounds from *Moringa oleifera* leaves by multi-response surface methodology. *Electrophoresis* **2016**, *37*, 1938–1946. [CrossRef]
68. Zekovic, Z.; Vladic, J.; Vidovic, S.; Adamovic, D.; Pavlic, B. Optimization of microwave-assisted extraction (MAE) of coriander phenolic antioxidants—Response surface methodology approach. *J. Sci. Food Agric.* **2016**, *96*, 4613–4622. [CrossRef] [PubMed]
69. Bouras, M.; Chadni, M.; Barba, F.J.; Grimi, N.; Bals, O.; Vorobiev, E. Optimization of microwave-assisted extraction of polyphenols from Quercus bark. *Ind. Crop. Prod.* **2015**, *77*, 590–601. [CrossRef]
70. The, S.S.; Niven, B.E.; Bekit, A.E.A.; Carne, A.; Birch, E.J. Microwave and pulsed electric field extraction of polyphenols from defatted canola seeds cake. *Int. J. Food Sci. Technol.* **2015**, *50*, 1109–1115.
71. Liazid, A.; Guerrero, R.F.; Cantos, E.; Palma, M.; Barroso, C.G. Microwave assisted extraction of anthocyanins from grape skins. *Food Chem.* **2011**, *124*, 1238–1243. [CrossRef]
72. Tan, S.N.; Yong, J.W.H.; Teo, C.C.; Ge, L.; Chan, Y.W.; Hew, C.S. Determination of metabolites in Uncaria sinensis by HPLC and GC-MS after green solvent microwave-assisted extraction. *Talanta* **2011**, *83*, 891–898. [CrossRef]
73. Inoue, T.; Tsubaki, S.; Ogawa, K.; Onishi, K.; Azuma, J.I. Isolation of hesperidin from peels of thinned Citrus unshiu fruits by microwave-assisted extraction. *Food Chem.* **2010**, *123*, 542–547. [CrossRef]
74. Li, J.; Zu, Y.G.; Fu, Y.J.; Yang, Y.C.; Li, S.M.; Li, Z.N.; Wink, M. Optimization of microwave-assisted extraction of triterpene saponins from defatted residue of yellow horn (*Xanthoceras sorbifolia* Bunge.) kernel and evaluation of its antioxidant activity. *Innov. Food Sci. Emerg. Technol.* **2010**, *11*, 637–643. [CrossRef]
75. Ballard, T.S.; Mallikarjunan, P.; Zhou, K.; O'Keefe, S. Microwave-assisted extraction of phenolic antioxidant compounds from peanut skins. *Food Chem.* **2010**, *120*, 1185–1192. [CrossRef]
76. Kong, Y.; Zu, Y.-G.; Fu, Y.-J.; Liu, W.; Chang, F.-R.; Li, J.; Chen, Y.-H.; Zhang, S.; Gu, C.-B. Optimization of microwave-assisted extraction of cajaninstilbene acid and pinostrobin from pigeonpea leaves followed by RP-HPLC-DAD determination. *J. Food Compos. Anal.* **2010**, *23*, 382–388. [CrossRef]
77. Yang, Z.; Zhai, W. Optimization of microwave-assisted extraction of anthocyanins from purple corn (*Zea mays* L.) cob and identification with HPLC–MS. *Innov. Food Sci. Emerg. Technol.* **2010**, *11*, 470–476. [CrossRef]
78. Wang, Y.L.; Xi, G.S.; Zheng, Y.C.; Miao, F.S. Microwave-assisted extraction of flavonoids from Chinese herb *Radix puerariae* (Ge Gen). *J. Med. Plants Res.* **2010**, *4*, 304–308.
79. Périno-Issartier, S.; Zille, H.; Abert-Vian, M.; Chemat, F. Solvent free microwave-assisted extraction of antioxidants from sea buckthorn (*Hippophae rhamnoides*) food by-products. *Food Bioprocess. Technol.* **2010**, *4*, 1020–1028. [CrossRef]
80. Tsubaki, S.; Sakamoto, M.; Azuma, J. Microwave-assisted extraction of phenolic compounds from tea residues under autohydrolytic conditions. *Food Chem.* **2010**, *123*, 1255–1258. [CrossRef]
81. Victório, C.P.; Lage, C.L.S.; Kuster, R.M. Flavonoid extraction from *Alpinia zerumbet* (Pers.) Burtt et Smith leaves using different techniques and solvents. *Eclet. Quim.* **2009**, *34*, 19–24.

82. Yang, L.; Jiang, J.-G.; Li, W.-F.; Chen, J.; Wang, D.-Y.; Zhu, L. Optimum extraction Process of polyphenols from the bark of Phyllanthus emblica L. based on the response surface methodology. *J. Sep. Sci.* **2009**, *32*, 1437–1444. [CrossRef]
83. Hayat, K.; Hussain, S.; Abbas, S.; Farooq, U.; Ding, B.; Xia, S.; Jia, C.; Zhang, X.; Xia, W. Optimized microwave-assisted extraction of phenolic acids from citrus mandarin peels and evaluation of antioxidant activity *in vitro*. *Sep. Purif. Technol.* **2009**, *70*, 63–70. [CrossRef]
84. Zheng, X.; Wang, X.; Lan, Y.; Shi, J.; Xue, S.J.; Liua, C. Application of response surface methodology to optimize microwave-assisted extraction of silymarin from milk thistle seeds. *Sep. Purif. Technol.* **2009**, *70*, 34–40. [CrossRef]
85. Li, W.; Li, T.; Tang, K. Flavonoids from mulberry leaves by microwave-assisted extract and anti-fatigue activity. *Afr. J. Agric. Res.* **2009**, *4*, 898–902.
86. Vian, M.A.; Maingonnat, J.F.; Chemat, F. Clean recovery of antioxidant flavonoids from onions: Optimising solvent free microwave extraction method. *J. Chroma A* **2009**, *1216*, 7700–7707.
87. Chen, L.; Jin, H.; Ding, L.; Zhang, H.; Li, J.; Qu, C. Dynamic microwave-assisted extraction of flavonoids from *Herba epimedii*. *Sep. Purif. Technol.* **2008**, *59*, 50–57. [CrossRef]
88. Wang, J.X.; Xiao, X.H.; Li, G.K. Study of vacuum microwave-assisted extraction of polyphenolic compounds and pigment from Chinese herbs. *J. Chroma A* **2008**, *1198–1199*, 45–53. [CrossRef] [PubMed]
89. Xiao, W.; Han, L.; Shi, B. Microwave-assisted extraction of flavonoids from Radix astragali. *Sep. Purif. Technol.* **2008**, *62*, 614–618. [CrossRef]
90. Chen, L.G.; Ding, L.; Yu, A.M.; Yang, R.L.; Wang, X.P.; Li, J.T.; Jin, H.Y.; Zhang, H.Q. Continuous determination of total flavonoids in *Platycladus orientalis* (L.) Franco by dynamic microwave-assisted extraction coupled with on-line derivatization and ultraviolet-visible detection. *Anal. Chim. Acta* **2007**, *596*, 164–170. [CrossRef]
91. Liu, Z.; Ding, L.; Zhang, H.; Hu, X.; Bu, F. Comparison of the different extraction methods of flavonoids in Epimedium koreamum Nakai by HPLC-DAD-ESI-MSn. *J. Liq. Chromatogr. Relat. Tech.* **2006**, *29*, 719–731. [CrossRef]
92. Japón-Luján, R.; Luque-Rodríguez, J.M.; Luque de Castro, M.D. Multivariate optimisation of the microwave-assisted extraction of oleuropein and related biophenols from olive leaves. *Anal. Bioanal. Chem.* **2006**, *385*, 753–759.
93. Liu, Z.; Yan, G.; Bu, F.; Sun, J.; Hu, X.; Zhang, H. Analysis of chemical composition of *Acanthopanax senticosusleaves* applying high-pressure microwave-assisted extraction. *Chem. Anal.* **2005**, *50*, 851–861.
94. Li, H.; Chen, B.; Zhang, Z.; Yao, S. Focused microwave-assisted solvent extraction and HPLC determination of effective constituents in Eucommia ulmodies Oliv. (*E. ulmodies*). *Talanta* **2004**, *63*, 659–665. [CrossRef]
95. Williams, G.J.; Zhang, C.; Thorson, J.S. Expanding the promiscuity of a natural-product glycosyltransferase by directed evolution. *Nat. Chem. Biol.* **2007**, *3*, 657–662. [CrossRef] [PubMed]
96. Ferreira, T.M.S.; dos Santos, J.A.; Modesto, L.A.; Souza, L.S.; dos Santos, M.P.; Bezerra, D.G.; de Paula, J.A.M. An eco-friendly method for extraction and quantification of flavonoids in *Dysphania ambrosioides*. *Braz. J. Pharmacogn.* **2019**, *29*, 266–270. [CrossRef]
97. Um, M.; Han, T.H.; Lee, J.W. Ultrasound-assisted extraction and antioxidant activity of phenolic and flavonoid compounds and ascorbic acid from rugosa rose (*Rosa rugosa* Thunb.) fruit. *Food Sci. Biotech.* **2018**, *27*, 375–382. [CrossRef]
98. Maran, J.P.; Manikandan, S.; Nivetha, C.V.; Dinesh, R. Ultrasound assisted extraction of bioactive compounds from *Nephelium lappaceum* L. fruit peel using central composite face centered response surface design. *Arab. J. Chem.* **2017**, *10*, 1145–1157. [CrossRef]
99. Ghasemzadeh, A.; Jaafar, H.; Karimi, E.; Rahmat, A. Optimization of ultrasound-assisted extraction of flavonoid compounds and their pharmaceutical activity from curry leaf (*Murraya koenigii* L.) using response surface methodology. *BMC Complement. Altern. Med.* **2014**, *14*, 318. [CrossRef] [PubMed]
100. Wang, C.; Li, Y.; Yao, L.; Wu, G.; Chang, J.; Shu, C.; Chen, M. Optimization of ultrasonic-assisted extraction of flavonoid from *Portulaca oleracea* L. by response surface methodology and chemical composition analysis. *J. Korean Soc. Appl. Biol. Chem.* **2014**, *57*, 647–653. [CrossRef]
101. Memon, A.A.; Memon, N.; Luthria, D.L.; Bhanger, M.I.; Pitafi, A.A. Phenolic Acids Profiling and Antioxidant Potential of Mulberry (*Morus laevigata* W., *Morus nigra* L., *Morus alba* L.) Leaves and Fruits Grown in Pakistan. *Pol. J. Food Nutr. Sci.* **2010**, *60*, 25–32.

102. Babova, O.; Occhipintia, A.; Capuzzo, A.; Maffei, M.E. Extraction of bilberry (Vaccinium myrtillus) antioxidants using supercritical/subcritical CO_2 and ethanol as co-solvent. *J. Supercrit. Fluids* **2016**, *107*, 358–363. [CrossRef]
103. Wang, L.; Yang, B.; Du, X.; Yi, C. Optimisation of supercritical extraction of flavonoids from Pueraria lobata. *Food Chem.* **2008**, *108*, 737–741. [CrossRef]
104. Chen, Y.; Xie, M.-Y.; Gong, X.F. Microwave-assisted extraction used for the isolation of total triterpenoid saponins from *Ganoderma atrum*. *J. Food Eng.* **2007**, *81*, 162–170. [CrossRef]
105. Flórez, N.; Conde, E.; Domínguez, H. Microwave assisted water extraction of plant compounds. *J. Chem. Technol. Biotech.* **2015**, *90*, 590–607. [CrossRef]
106. Krishnan, R.Y.; Chandran, M.N.; Vadivel, V.; Rajan, K.S. Insights on the influence of microwave irradiation on the extraction of flavonoids from *Terminalia chebula*. *Sep. Purif. Technol.* **2016**, *170*, 224–233. [CrossRef]
107. Cassol, L.; Rodrigues, E.; Noreña, C.P.Z. Extracting phenolic compounds from *Hibiscus sabdariffa* L. calyx using microwave assisted extraction. *Ind. Crop. Prod.* **2019**, *133*, 168–177. [CrossRef]
108. Akbari, S.; Abdurahman, N.H.; Yunus, R.M.; Fayaz, F. Microwave-assisted extraction of saponin, phenolic and flavonoid compounds from *Trigonella foenum-graecum* seed based on two level factorial design. *J. Appl. Res. Med. Aromat. Plants* **2019**, *14*, 100212. [CrossRef]
109. Ling, Y.Y.M.; Fun, P.S.; Yeop, A.; Yusoff, M.M.; Gimbun, J. Assessment of maceration, ultrasonic and microwave assisted extraction for total phenolic content, total flavonoid content and Kaempferol yield form *Cassia alata* via Microstructures Analysis. *Mater. Today Proc.* **2019**, *19*, 1273–1279. [CrossRef]
110. Tomaz, I.; Maslov, L.; Stupic, D.; Prenier, D.; Asperger, D.; Karoglan Kontić, J. Multi-response optimization of ultrasound-assisted extraction for recovery of flavonoids from red grape skins using response surface methodology. *Phytochem. Anal.* **2015**, *27*, 13–22. [CrossRef]
111. Castro-López, C.; Rojas, R.; Sánchez-Alejo, E.J.; Niño-Medina, G.; Martínez-Ávila, G.C.G. *Phenolic Compounds Recovery from Grapefruit and By- Products: An Overview of Extraction Methods, Grape and Wine Biotechnology, Antonio Morata and Iris Loira*; IntechOpen: London, UK, 2016. [CrossRef]
112. Chludil, H.D.; Corbino, G.B.; Leicach, S.R. Soil Quality Effects on Chenopodium album Flavonoid Content and Antioxidant Potential. *J. Agric. Food Chem.* **2008**, *56*, 5050–5056. [CrossRef]
113. Wang, X.H.; Wang, J.P. Effective extraction with deep eutectic solvents and enrichment by microporous adsorption resin of flavonoids from *Carthamus tinctorius* L. *J. Pharm. Biomed.* **2019**, *176*, 112804. [CrossRef]
114. Chen, M.C.A.J.; Zhang, H.; Li, Z.; Zhao, L.; Qiu, H. Effective extraction of flavonoids from Lycium barbarum L. fruits by deep eutectic solvents-based ultrasound-assisted extraction. *Talanta* **2019**, *203*, 16–22.
115. Singanusong, R.; Nipornram, S.; Tochampa, W.; Rattanatraiwong, P. Low Power Ultrasound-Assisted Extraction of Phenolic Compounds from Mandarin (*Citrus reticulata* Blanco cv. Sainampueng) and Lime (*Citrus aurantifolia*) Peels and the Antioxidant. *Food Anal. Methods* **2015**, *8*, 1112–1123. [CrossRef]
116. Piana, F.; Ciulu, M.; Quirantes-Piné, R.; Sanna, G.; Segura-Carretero, A.; Spano, N.; Mariani, A. Simple and rapid procedures for the extraction of bioactive compounds from Guayule leaves). *Ind. Crop. Prod.* **2018**, *116*, 162–169. [CrossRef]
117. Nagendra-Prasad, K.; Yang, B.; Zhao, M.; Ruenroengklin, N.; Jiang, Y. Application of ultrasonication or high-pressure extraction of flavonoids from litchi fruit pericarp. *J. Food Process. Eng.* **2009**, *32*, 828–843. [CrossRef]
118. Zhang, O.A.; Fan, X.H.; Li, T.; Zhang, Z.Q.; Liu, Y.K.; Li, X.P. Optimization of ultrasound extraction for flavonoids from semen astragali complanati and its identification by HPLC-DAD-MS/MS. *Int. J. Food Sci. Technol.* **2013**, *48*, 1970–1976. [CrossRef]
119. Xie, Z.; Sun, Y.; Lam, S.; Zhao, M.; Liang, Z.; Yu, X.; Yang, D.; Xu, X. Extraction and isolation of flavonoid glycosides from Flos Sophorae Immaturus using ultrasonic-assisted extraction followed by high-speed countercurrent chromatography. *J. Sep. Sci.* **2014**, *37*, 957–965. [CrossRef] [PubMed]
120. Dassoff, E.S.; Li, Y.O. Mechanisms and effects of ultrasound-assisted supercritical CO_2 extraction. *Trends Food Sci. Tech.* **2019**, *86*, 492–501. [CrossRef]
121. Román Páez, M.; Rivera Narváez, C.; Cardona Bermúdez, L.; Muñoz, L.; Gómez, D.; Passaro Carvalho, C.; Quiceno Rico, J. *Guía de Extracción por Fluidos Supercríticos: Fundamentos y Aplicaciones*; Servicio Nacional de Aprendizaje—SENA: Rionegro, Colombia, 2016.

122. Verma, D.K.; Dhakane, J.P.; Mahato, D.K.; Billoria, S.; Bhattacharjee, P.; Srivastav, P.P. Supercritical Fluid Extraction (SCFE) for Rice Aroma Chemicals: Recent and Advance Extraction Method. In *Science and Technology of Aroma, Flavour and Fragrance in Rice*; Verma, D.K., Srivastav, P.P., Eds.; Apple Academic Press: Waretown, NJ, USA, 2018; pp. 179–198.
123. Belbaki, A.; Louaer, W.; Menial, A.H. Supercritical CO_2 extraction of oil from Crushed Algerian olives. *J. Supercrit. Fluids* **2017**, *130*, 165–171. [CrossRef]
124. Kavoura, D.; Kyriakopoulou, K.; Papaefstahiou, G.; Spanidi, E.; Gardikis, K.; Louli, V.; Aligiannis, N.; Krokida, M.; Magoulas, K. Supercritical CO_2 extraction of Salvia fruticosa. *J. Supercrit. Fluids* **2019**, *146*, 159–164. [CrossRef]
125. Song, L.; Liu, P.; Yan, Y.; Huang, Y.; Bai, B.; Hou, X.; Zhang, L. Supercritical CO_2 fluid extraction of flavonoid compounds from Xinjiang jujube (Ziziphus jujube Mill.) leaves and associated biological activities and flavonoid compositions. *Ind. Crop. Prod.* **2019**, *139*, 111508. [CrossRef]
126. Panja, P. Green extraction methods of food polyphenols from vegetable materials. *Curr. Opin. Food Sci.* **2018**, *23*, 173–182. [CrossRef]
127. Alvarez, M.; Cabred, S.; Ramírez, C.; Fanovich, M. Valorization of an agroindustrial soybean residue by supercritical flfluid extraction of phytochemical compounds. *J. Supercrit. Fluids* **2019**, *143*, 90–96. [CrossRef]
128. Ouédraogo, J.C.; Dicko, C.; Kini, F.; Bonzi-Coulibaly, Y.; Dey, E. Enhanced extraction of flflavonoids from Odontonema strictum leaves with antioxidant activity using supercritical carbon dioxide flfluid combined with ethanol. *J. Supercrit. Fluids* **2018**, *131*, 66–71. [CrossRef]
129. Krakowska, A.; Rafinska, K.; Walczak, J.; Buszewski, B. Enzyme-assisted optimized supercritical flfluid extraction to improve Medicago sativa polyphenolics isolation. *Ind. Crop. Prod.* **2018**, *124*, 931–940. [CrossRef]
130. Kala, H.K.; Mehta, R.; Sen, K.K.; Tandey, R.; Mandal, V. Critical analysis of research trends and issues in microwave assisted extraction of phenolics: Have we really done enough. *Trends Anal. Chem.* **2016**, *85*, 140–152. [CrossRef]
131. Ilina, A.D. The use of enzymes and microorganisms for solving fundamental and applied problems. Herald of the Russian Academy of Sciences. *Rep. Bashortostan* **2013**, *18*, 40–43.
132. Zha, J.; Wu, X.; Gong, G.; Koffas, M.A.G. Pathway enzyme engineering for flavonoid production in recombinant microbes. *Metab. Eng. Commun.* **2019**, *9*, e00104. [CrossRef]
133. Castro-Vazquez, L.; Alañón, M.E.; Rodríguez-Robledo, V.; Pérez-Coello, M.S.; Hermosín-Gutierrez, I.; Díaz-Maroto, M.C.; Jordán, J.; Galindo, M.F.; Arroyo-Jimenez, M.D.M. Bioactive flavonoids, antioxidant behaviour, and cytoprotective effects of dried grapefruit peels (*Citrus paradisi* macf.). *Oxid. Med. Cell. Longev.* **2016**. [CrossRef]
134. Lagaert, S.; Belien, T.; Volckaert, G. Plant cell walls: Protecting the barrier form degradation by microbial enzymes. *Semin. Cell Dev. Biol.* **2009**, *20*, 1064–1073. [CrossRef]
135. Landbo, A.K.; Meyer, A.S. Enzyme-assisted extraction of antioxidative phenols from black currant juice press residues (*Ribes nigrum*). *J. Agric. Food Chem.* **2001**, *49*, 3169–3177. [CrossRef]
136. Kammerer, D.; Claus, A.; Schieber, A.; Carle, R. A novel process for the recovery of polyphenols from grape (*Vitis vinifera* L.) pomace. *J. Food Sci.* **2005**, *70*, C157–C163. [CrossRef]
137. Maier, T.; Göppert, A.; Kammerer, D.R.; Schieber, A.; Carle, R. Optimization of a process for enzyme-assisted pigment extraction from grape (*Vitis vinifera* L.) pomace. *EFRT* **2008**, *227*, 267–275. [CrossRef]
138. Fu, Y.J.; Liu, W.; Zu, Y.G.; Tong, M.H.; Li, S.M.; Yan, M.M.; Efferth, T.; Luo, H. Enzyme assisted extraction of luteolin and apigenin from pigeonpea [*Cajanus cajan* (L.) Millsp.] leaves. *Food Chem.* **2008**, *111*, 508–512. [CrossRef]
139. Zhang, Q.; Zhou, M.M.; Chen, P.L.; Cao, Y.Y.; Tan, X.L. Optimization of ultrasonic-assisted enzymatic hydrolysis for the extraction of luteolin and apigenin from celery. *J. Food Sci.* **2011**, *76*, C680–C685. [CrossRef] [PubMed]
140. Pan, M.; Wang, S.K.; Yuan, X.L.; Xie, R.Y.; Hong, Y.C.; Liu, H.J. Process study on the ultrasonic assisted enzymatic extraction of flavonoids from shepherd's purse. *Adv. Mater. Res.* **2013**, *634*, 1281–1286. [CrossRef]
141. Tchabo, W.; Ma, Y.; Engmann, F.N.; Zhang, H. Ultrasound-assisted enzymatic extraction (UAEE) of phytochemical compounds from mulberry (*Morus nigra*) must and optimization study using response surface methodology. *Ind. Crop. Prod.* **2015**, *63*, 214–225. [CrossRef]

142. Wu, D.; Gao, T.; Yang, H.; Du, Y.; Li, C.; Wei, L.; Zhou, T.; Lu, J.; Bi, H. Simultaneous microwave/ultrasonic-assisted enzymatic extraction of antioxidant ingredients from *Nitraria tangutorun* Bobr. juice by-products. *Ind. Crop. Prod.* **2015**, *66*, 229–238. [CrossRef]
143. Tomaz, I.; Maslov, L.; Stupić, D.; Preiner, D.; Ašperger, D.; Kontić, J.K. Recovery of flavonoids from grape skins by enzyme-assisted extraction. *Sep. Sci. Technol.* **2016**, *51*, 255–268. [CrossRef]
144. Chávez-Santoscoy, R.A.; Lazo-Vélez, M.A.; Serna-Sáldivar, S.O.; Gutiérrez-Uribe, J.A. Delivery of flavonoids and saponins from black bean (*Phaseolus vulgaris*) seed coats incorporated into whole wheat bread. *Int. J. Mol. Sci.* **2016**, *17*, 222. [CrossRef] [PubMed]
145. Xu, S.L.; Zhu, K.Y.; Bi, C.W.; Yan, L.; Men, S.W.; Dong, T.T.; Tsim, K.W. Flavonoids, derived from traditional chinese medicines, show roles in the differentiation of neurons: Possible targets in developing health food products. *Birth Defects Res. Part C Embryo Today* **2013**, *99*, 292–299. [CrossRef]
146. Chen, S.; Xing, X.H.; Huang, J.J.; Xu, M.S. Enzyme-assisted extraction of flavonoids from *Ginkgo biloba* leaves: Improvement effect of flavonol transglycosylation catalyzed by *Penicillium decumbens* cellulase. *Enzym. Microb. Tech.* **2011**, *48*, 100–105. [CrossRef]
147. Huynh, N.T.; Van Camp, J.; Smagghe, G.; Raes, K. Improved release and metabolism of flavonoids by steered fermentation processes: A review. *Int. J. Mol. Sci.* **2014**, *15*, 19369–19388. [CrossRef]
148. Cao, H.; Chen, X.; Jassbim, A.R.; Xiao, J. Microbial biotransformation of bioactive flavonoids. *Biotech. Adv.* **2015**, *33*, 214–223. [CrossRef] [PubMed]
149. Frauzino-Araújo, K.C.; de, M.B.; Costa, E.M.; Pazini, F.; Valadares, M.C.; de Oliveira, V. Bioconversion of quercetin and rutin and the cytotoxicity activities of the transformed products. *Food Chem. Toxicol.* **2013**, *51*, 93–96. [CrossRef] [PubMed]
150. Lee, J.H.; Oh, E.T.; Chun, S.C.; Keum, Y.S. Biotransformation of isoflavones by Aspergillus niger and Cuuninghamella elegans. *J. Korean Soc. Appl. Biol. Chem.* **2014**, *57*, 523–527. [CrossRef]
151. Xin, X.; Fan, G.J.; Sun, Z.; Li, Y.; Lan, R.; Chen, L.; Dong, P. Biotransformation of major flavonoid glycosides in herb epimedii by fungus *Cunninghamella blakesleana*. *J. Mol. Catal. B Enzym.* **2015**, *122*, 141–146. [CrossRef]
152. Jin, S.; Wang, W.; Luo, M.; Mu, F.S.; Li, C.Y.; Fu, Y.J.; Zu, Y.G.; Feng, C. Enhanced extraction genistein from pigeon pea [*Cajanus cajan* (L.) Millsp.] roots with the biotransformation of immobilized edible *Aspergillus oryzae* and *Monacus anka* and antioxidant activity evaluation. *Process Biochem.* **2013**, *48*, 1285–1292. [CrossRef]
153. Huynh, T.N.; Smagghe, G.; Gonzales, G.B.; Camp, J.V.; Raes, K. Extraction and bioconversion of kaempferol metabolites from cauliflower outer leaves through fungal fermentation. *Biochem. Eng. J.* **2016**, *116*, 27–33. [CrossRef]
154. Madeira, J.V., Jr.; Mayumi-Nakajima, V.; Alves-Macedo, J.; Alves-Macedo, G. Rich bioactive phenolic extract production by microbial transformation of Brazilian Citrus residues. *Chem. Eng. Res. Des.* **2014**, *92*, 1802–1810. [CrossRef]
155. Stahlhut, S.G.; Siedler, S.; Malla, S.; Harrison, S.J.; Maury, J.; Neves, A.R.; Forster, J. Assembly of a novel biosynthetic pathway for production of the plant flavonoid fisetin in *Escherichia coli*. *Metab. Eng.* **2015**, *31*, 84–93. [CrossRef]
156. Chiang, C.M.; Ding, H.Y.; Lu, J.Y.; Chang, T.S. Biotransformation of isoflavones daidzein and genistein by recombinant *Pichia pastoris* expressing membrane-anchoring and reductase fusion chimeric CYP105D7. *J. Taiwan Inst. Chem. Eng.* **2016**, *60*, 26–31. [CrossRef]
157. Yu, L.; Gao, F.; Yang, L.; Xu, L.; Wang, Z.; Ye, H. Biotransformation of puerarin into puerarin-6′′-O-phosphate by *Bacillus cereus*. *J. Ind. Microbiol. Biotech.* **2012**, *39*, 299–305. [CrossRef]
158. Sordon, A.; Popłonski, J.; Tronina, T.; Huszcza, E. Regioselective O-glycosylation of flavonoids by fungi Beauveraia bassiana, Absidia coerulea and Absidia glauca. *Bioorg. Chem.* **2019**, *93*, 102750. [CrossRef] [PubMed]
159. Bok, S.H.; Jeong, T.S.; Lee, S.K.; Kim, J.R.; Moon, S.S.; Choi, M.S.; Hyun, B.H.; Lee, C.H.; Choi, Y.K. Flavanone Derivatives and Composition for Preventing or Treating Blood Lipid Level-Related Diseases Comprising Same. U.S. Patent 6455577, 24 September 2002.
160. Hidalgo, A.; Bornscheuer, U.T. Directed evolution of lipases and esterases for organic synthesis. In *Biocatalysis in the Pharmaceutical and Biotechnology Industries*; Patel, R.M., Ed.; CRC Press: Boca Raton, FL, USA; Taylor and Francis: New York, NY, USA, 2006; pp. 159–175.
161. Tian, L.; Dixon, R.A. Engineering isoflavone metabolism with an artificial bifunctional enzyme. *Planta* **2006**, *224*, 496–507. [CrossRef] [PubMed]

162. Kurisawa, M.; Chung, J.E.; Uyama, H.; Kobayashi, S. Enzymatic synthesis and antioxidant properties of poly(rutin). *Biomacromolecules* **2003**, *4*, 1394–1399. [CrossRef] [PubMed]
163. Mandalari, G.; Bennett, R.N.; Kirby, A.R.; Lo Curto, R.B.; Bisignano, G.; Waldron, K.W.; Faulds, C.B. Enzymatic hydrolysis of flavonoids and pectic oligosaccharides from bergamot (*Citrus bergamia* Risso) peel. *J. Agric. Food Chem.* **2006**, *54*, 8307–8313. [CrossRef] [PubMed]
164. Jiao, J.; Gai, Q.Y.; Wang, W.; Zang, Y.P.; Niu, L.L.; Fu, Y.J.; Wang, X. Remarjable enhancement of flavonoid production in a co-cultivation system of *Isatis tinctorial* L. hairy root cultures and immobilized *Aspergillus niger*. *Ind. Crop. Prod.* **2018**, *112*, 252–261. [CrossRef]
165. Ralston, L.; Subramanian, S.; Matsuno, M.; Yu, O. Partial reconstruction of flavonoid and isoflavonoid biosynthesis in yeast using soybean type I and type II chalcone isomerases. *Plant Physiol.* **2005**, *137*, 1375–1388. [CrossRef]
166. Lindahl, S.; Ekman, A.; Khan, S.; Wennerberg, C.; Börjesson, P.; Sjöberg, P.J.; Karlsson, E.N.; Turner, C. Exploring the possibility of using a thermostable mutant of b-glucosidase for rapid hydrolysis of quercetin glucosides in hot water. *Green Chem.* **2010**, *12*, 159–168. [CrossRef]
167. Ihara, N.; Kurisawa, M.; Chung, J.E.; Uyama, H.; Kobayashi, S. Enzymatic synthesis of a catechin conjugate of polyhedral oligomeric silsesquioxane and evaluation of its antioxidant activity. *Appl. Microbiol. Biotech.* **2005**, *66*, 430–433. [CrossRef]
168. Yaipakdee, P.; Robertson, L.W. Enzymatic halogenation of flavanones and flavones. *Phytochemistry* **2001**, *57*, 341–347. [CrossRef]
169. Danieli, B.; Luisetti, M.; Riva, S.; Bertinotti, A.; Ragg, E.; Scaglioni, L.; Bombardelli, E. Regioselective enzyme-mediated acylation of polyhydroxy natural compounds. A remarkable, highly efficient preparation of 6′-acetyl and 6′-O-carboxyacetyl ginsenoside Rg1. *J. Org. Chem.* **1995**, *60*, 3637–3642. [CrossRef]
170. Chung, J.E.; Kurisawa, M.; Uyama, H.; Kobayashi, S. Enzymatic synthesis and antioxidant property of gelatin-catechin conjugates. *Biotechnol. Lett.* **2003**, *25*, 1993–1997. [CrossRef] [PubMed]
171. Xiao, Y.M.; Wu, Q.; Wu, W.B.; Zhang, Q.Y.; Lin, X.F. Controllable regioselective acylation of rutin catalyzed by enzymes in non-aqueous solvents. *Biotechnol. Lett.* **2005**, *27*, 1591–1595. [CrossRef] [PubMed]
172. Vitali, A.; Giardina, B.; Delle Monache, G.; Rocca, F.; Silvestrini, A.; Tafi, A.; Botta, B. Chalcone dimethylallyltransferase from *Morus nigra* cell cultures. Substrate specificity studies. *FEBS Lett.* **2004**, *557*, 33–38. [CrossRef]
173. Moon, Y.H.; Lee, J.H.; Ahn, J.S.; Nam, S.H.; Oh, D.K.; Park, D.H.; Chung, H.J.; Kang, S.; Day, D.F.; Kim, D. Synthesis, structure analyses, and characterization of novel epigallocatechin gallate (EGCG) glycosides using the glucansucrase from *Leuconostoc mesenteroides* B-1299CB. *J. Agric. Food Chem.* **2006**, *54*, 1230–1237. [CrossRef] [PubMed]
174. Nielsen, I.L.F.; Chee, W.S.S.; Poulsen, L.; Offord-Cavin, E.; Rasmussen, S.E.; Frederiksen, H.; Enslen, M.; Barron, D.; Horcajada, M.N.; Williamson, G. Bioavailability is improved by enzymatic modification of the citrus flavonoid hesperidin in humans: A randomized, double-blind, crossover trial. *J. Nutr.* **2006**, *136*, 404–408. [CrossRef] [PubMed]
175. Ozaki, T.; Mishima, S.; Nishiyama, M.; Kuzuyama, T. NovQ is a prenyltransferase capable of catalyzing the addition of a dimethylallyl group to both phenylpropanoids and flavonoids. *J. Antibiot.* **2009**, *62*, 385–392. [CrossRef]
176. Kobayashi, R.; Itou, T.; Hanaya, K.; Shoji, M.; Hada, N.; Sugai, T. Chemo-enzymatic transformation of naturally abundant naringin to luteolin, a flavonoid with various biological effects. *J. Mol. Catal. B Enzym.* **2013**, *92*, 14–18. [CrossRef]
177. Adamczak, M.; Krishna, S.H. Strategies for improving enzymes for efficient biocatalysis. *Food Technol. Biotechnol.* **2004**, *42*, 251–264.
178. Enaud, E.; Humeau, C.; Piffaut, B.; Girardin, M. Enzymatic synthesis of new aromatic esters of phloridzin. *J. Mol. Catal. B Enzym.* **2004**, *27*, 1–6. [CrossRef]
179. Chebil, L.; Humeau, C.; Falcimaigne, A.; Engasser, J.M.; Ghoul, M. Enzymatic acylation of flavonoids. *Process Biochem.* **2006**, *41*, 2237–2251. [CrossRef]
180. Das, S.; Rosazza, J.P.N. Microbial and enzymatic transformations of flavonoids. *J. Nat. Prod.* **2006**, *69*, 499–508. [CrossRef] [PubMed]
181. Viskupicova, J.; Ondrejovic, M.; Maliar, T. Enzyme-mediated preparation of flavonoid esters and their applications. *Biochemistry* **2012**, *10*, 263–286.

182. Peterson, J.J.; Dwyer, J.T.; Jacques, P.F.; McCullough, M.L. Associations between flavonoids and cardiovascular disease incidence or mortality in European and US populations. *Nutr. Rev.* **2012**, *70*, 491–508. [CrossRef] [PubMed]
183. Koirala, N.; Thuan, N.H.; Ghimire, G.P.; Thang, D.V.; Sohng, J.K. Methylation of flavonoids: Chemical structures, bioactivities, progress and perspectives for biotechnological production. *Enzym. Microb. Technol.* **2016**, *86*, 103–116. [CrossRef] [PubMed]
184. Chen, G.L.; Fan, M.X.; Wu, J.L.; Li, N.; Guo, M.Q. Antioxidant and anti-inflammatory properties of flavonoids from lotus plumule. *Food Chem.* **2019**, *277*, 706–712. [CrossRef] [PubMed]
185. Treml, J.; Smejkal, K. Flavonoids as potent scavengers of hydroxyl radicals. *Compr. Rev. Food Sci. Food Saf.* **2016**, *15*, 720–738. [CrossRef]
186. Agati, G.; Tattini, M. Multiple functional roles of flavonoids in photoprotection. *New Phytol.* **2010**, *186*, 786–793. [CrossRef]

© 2020 by the authors. Licensee MDPI, Basel, Switzerland. This article is an open access article distributed under the terms and conditions of the Creative Commons Attribution (CC BY) license (http://creativecommons.org/licenses/by/4.0/).

MDPI
St. Alban-Anlage 66
4052 Basel
Switzerland
Tel. +41 61 683 77 34
Fax +41 61 302 89 18
www.mdpi.com

Processes Editorial Office
E-mail: processes@mdpi.com
www.mdpi.com/journal/processes

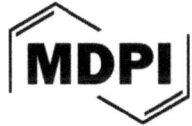